AF773444

Innovations in Drug Discovery

This fascinating volume delves into the forefront of pharmaceutical research to shed light on the ground-breaking methodologies and technologies driving advancements in drug discovery today.

Providing a comprehensive overview of emerging trends and new approaches, it covers the entire drug discovery process, from target identification to clinical development, providing readers with a holistic understanding of the field. Each chapter outlines a different approach, from computational methods and high-throughput screening techniques to the application of artificial intelligence and machine learning in drug design. Additionally, it explores the integration of genomic, proteomic, and metabolomic data in target identification and validation processes, as well as the utilization of CRISPR/Cas9 technology for precision medicine initiatives.

Highlighting the potential of interdisciplinary collaborations, elucidating the impact of big data analytics on decision-making processes, this fascinating book will appeal to students and researchers in the pharmaceutical and biotechnological sciences, as well as professionals in this field.

Krishnaveni Manubolu, an Associate Professor in the Department of Pharmaceutical Sciences at Narayana Pharmacy College, Nellore, earned her Ph.D. in Pharmaceutical Sciences from JNTUA in 2022. With extensive teaching experience in Pharmacokinetics, Pharmacodynamics, and Biopharmaceutics, her research focuses on herbal formulations, natural polymer-based drug delivery systems, and sustainable pharmaceutical technologies. She has published numerous scientific papers, authored book chapters, and presented her work at national and international conferences. A member of professional bodies like IPA and APTI, Dr. Manubolu is dedicated to advancing research in innovative, eco-friendly therapeutics and mentoring the next generation of pharmaceutical scientists.

Raveesha Peeriga is an Academic Professional in the Department of Pharmacognosy at V.V. Institute of Pharmaceutical Sciences, Gudlavalleru. She had received several awards. She authored three Books titled *Herbal Drug Technology*, *Concise Pharmacognosy*, and *A Short Guide to Clinical Pharmacokinetics*. She acted as a Chairperson for BOS for Paramedicals, Krishna University. She has published numerous scientific papers, authored book chapters, and presented her work at national and international conferences. She is an Associate Fellow of the Andhra Pradesh Akademi of Sciences. She is a Life Member of various professional bodies.

Innovations in Drug Discovery

Exploring Cutting-Edge Strategies and Technologies

Edited by Krishnaveni Manubolu and Raveesha Peeriga

Routledge
Taylor & Francis Group
LONDON AND NEW YORK

First published 2026
by Routledge
4 Park Square, Milton Park, Abingdon, Oxon OX14 4RN

and by Routledge
605 Third Avenue, New York, NY 10158

Routledge is an imprint of the Taylor & Francis Group, an informa business

© 2026 selection and editorial matter, Krishnaveni Manubolu and Raveesha Peeriga; individual chapters, the contributors

The right of Krishnaveni Manubolu and Raveesha Peeriga to be identified as the authors of the editorial material, and of the authors for their individual chapters, has been asserted in accordance with sections 77 and 78 of the Copyright, Designs and Patents Act 1988.

All rights reserved. No part of this book may be reprinted or reproduced or utilised in any form or by any electronic, mechanical, or other means, now known or hereafter invented, including photocopying and recording, or in any information storage or retrieval system, without permission in writing from the publishers.

Trademark notice: Product or corporate names may be trademarks or registered trademarks, and are used only for identification and explanation without intent to infringe.

British Library Cataloguing-in-Publication Data
A catalogue record for this book is available from the British Library

ISBN: 978-1-032-91692-7 (hbk)
ISBN: 978-1-032-91690-3 (pbk)
ISBN: 978-1-003-56404-1 (ebk)

DOI: 10.4324/9781003564041

Typeset in Times New Roman
by KnowledgeWorks Global Ltd.

To the Almighty, whose grace and wisdom guide my path.

To our parents, whose sacrifices and teachings have shaped who I am.

To my beloved spouse, whose unwavering support and love inspire me.

To my children, the light of my life and my greatest motivation.

With deepest gratitude and love

Dr. M. Krishnaveni

Dr. P. Raveesha

Contents

Figures and Tables

Figures

Tables

Contributor Biographies

Yadlapalli Vamsi Abhiram, Undergraduate Student, V. V. Institute of Pharmaceutical Sciences, India.

Saidatri Arige, Associate Professor, Department of Pharmaceutical Analysis, V. V. Institute of Pharmaceutical Sciences, India.

Lakshmana Rao Atmakuri, Professor, Department of Pharmaceutical Analysis, V. V. Institute of Pharmaceutical Sciences, India.

Angilicam Avinash, Assistant Professor, School of Pharmacy, Anurag University, Hyderabad, India.

Sajja Jayanth Babu, Undergraduate Student, V. V. Institute of Pharmaceutical Sciences, India.

Talamanchi Balakrishna, Professor, Department of Pharmaceutics, V. V. Institute of Pharmaceutical Sciences, India.

Nagasen Dasari, Assistant Professor, Aditya Pharmacy College, Surampalem, India.

Morla Devika, Undergraduate Student, V. V. Institute of Pharmaceutical Sciences, India.

Lakshman Kumar Dogiparthi, Associate Professor, Department of Pharmacognosy, MB School of Pharmaceutical Sciences, Mohan Babu University, India.

Deevi Gouri Naga Venkata Gayathri, Undergraduate Student, V. V. Institute of Pharmaceutical Sciences, India.

Udaya Guttikonda, Assistant Professsor, Narayana Pharmacy College, India.

Avisa Indira, Lecturer, V. V. Giri Government Kalasala, India.

Venkateswara Rao Javvaji, Principal & Professor, VSS Institute of Pharmacy, Badnapur, Dist-Jalna, Maharashtra, India.

Kishore Kumar Kadimpati, Assistant Professor, Silesian Institute of Technology and Science, Silesian University, Poland.

C.K. Ashok Kumar, Professor & Deputy Director, Amity Institute of Pharmacy, Amity University Haryana, India.

Sidagam Lokesh Kumar, Undergraduate Student, V. V. Institute of Pharmaceutical Sciences, India.

Vanukuri Lakshmana Vinod Kumar, Associate Professor, Department of Pharmaceutics, V. V. Institute of Pharmaceutical Sciences, India.

K. N. V. Chenchu Lakshmi, Associate Professor, KL College of Pharmacy, Koneru Lakshmaiah Education Foundation, India.

Sonti Lavanya, Undergraduate Student, V. V. Institute of Pharmaceutical Sciences, India.

Krishnaveni Manubolu, Professor, Department of Pharmaceutics, Narayana Pharmacy College, India.

Amala Masa, Assistant Professor, Krishna University College of Pharmaceutical Sciences and Research, India.

Jahasultana Mohammed, Assistant Professor, Department of Pharmaceutics, KL College of Pharmacy, Koneru Lakshmaiah Education Foundation, India.

Suchitra Monapati, Professor & HOD, Department of Pharmaceutical Analysis, Narayana Pharmacy College, India

Sreenivasulu Munna, Professor & Principal, Narayana Pharmacy College, India.

Raveesha Peeriga, Professor, Department of Pharmacognosy, V. V. Institute of Pharmaceutical Sciences, India.

Srikanth Pottendla, Professor, Dr. Samuel George Institute of Pharmaceutical Sciences, Markapur, India.

Cheruku Jigeesha Naga Durga Sai Paidi Pranitha, Undergraduate Student, V. V. Institute of Pharmaceutical Sciences, India.

Chandika Naga Veera Venkata Pravallika, Undergraduate Student, V. V. Institute of Pharmaceutical Sciences, India.

Miriyala Preethika, Undergraduate Student, V. V. Institute of Pharmaceutical Sciences, India.

R. Radha, Professor, Department of Pharmaceutical Chemistry, Sri Venkateswara College of Pharmacy, India.

Gope Edward Raju, Research Scholar, Department of Pharmaceutical Analysis, Dr. Samuel George Institute of Pharmaceutical Sciences, Acharya Nagarjuna University, India.

Shaik Rasheed, Assistant Professor, Department of Pharmaceutics, V. V. Institute of Pharmaceutical Sciences, India.

Janga Karthik Reddy Graduate Student, KL College of Pharmacy, Koneru Lakshmaiah Education Foundation, India.

Shaik Sabreen, Undergraduate Student, V. V. Institute of Pharmaceutical Sciences, India.

Aminabee Shaik, Professsor, Department of Pharmacology, V. V. Institute of Pharmaceutical Sciences, India.

Afsar Shaik, Assistant Professor, Faculty of Health Sciences, Villa College Male', Maldives.

Nagul Meeravali Shaik, Assistant Professor, Department of Pharmacology, V. V. Institute of Pharmaceutical Sciences, India.

K. Ravi Shankar, Assistant Professor, KVSR Siddhartha College of Pharmaceutical Sciences, India.

Marapatla Shiny, Research Scholar, Department of Pharmaceutical Chemistry, AU College of Pharmaceutical Sciences, Andhra University, India.

Nimmagadda Sai Sruthi, Undergraduate Student, V. V. Institute of Pharmaceutical Sciences, India.

Gorintla Sai Supraja, Undergraduate Student, V. V. Institute of Pharmaceutical Sciences, India.

Rajani Vetapalem, Associate Professor, V. V. Institute of Pharmaceutical Sciences, India.

Ratna Kumari Yejerla, Associate Professor, Narayana Pharmacy College, India.

Foreword

Drug discovery process has undergone significant improvisation since its inception, while science, technology, and interdisciplinary collaboration drive this development. It has evolved into a dynamic field through traditional methods and cutting-edge innovations such as artificial intelligence (AI), precision medicine, and machine learning, which provide global healthcare with significant implications.

The book covers all fundamental drug development stages from target identification through high-throughput screening until structure-based drug design, then focuses on modern therapeutic technologies forming the future landscape of medicine. The text dedicates extra attention to chemical biology and personalized medicine along with exploring moral issues related to current drug development approaches.

This work functions as a useful reference guide for pharmaceutical industry professionals alongside watching students and biomedical scientists. Students will acquire an extensive understanding of drug discovery together with future directions because the book provides both basic concepts and emerging trends.

The authors deserve praise for their research in creating this informative compilation of knowledge which will advance drug discovery understanding.

Dr. K. B. Chandrasekhar
Ex-Vice Chancellor
Krishna University
Machilipatnam

Preface

Drug discovery operates as a complicated multivariant process which powers contemporary medical advancements. Scientists encounter both challenges and opportunities during the process of developing drugs from therapeutic targets into safe medications. The book delivers an extensive review of basic drug discovery principles and methods, and futuristic technology which formulates the direction of future pharmaceutical research.

This book divides its contents according to stages, which lead readers through the complete drug discovery process. This text starts with a drug discovery introduction after discussing target identification methods and structure-based drug design techniques, as well as high-throughput screening procedures. This work investigates the development of machine learning and artificial intelligence to expedite pharmaceutical research, as well as the significance of scientific advances in chemical biology and interdisciplinary drug development methods.

The text emphasizes personalized medicine and precision therapeutics as specialized areas of focus since these treatment approaches match medications to patients for better results. Emerging trends alongside innovative technologies form one of the key areas discussed in the book's investigation of the field. The book tackles crucial regulatory matters and ethical obstacles that protect both the scientific validity and ethical standards of drug discovery practice.

The book targets students alongside researchers as well as professionals active in pharmaceutical sciences, biotechnology, bioinformatics, and biomedical research groups. Through its connection of essential core information with current innovation, the text functions simultaneously as a learning tool and information base for developers of new treatment methods.

Dr. M. Krishnaveni
Dr. P. Raveesha

Acknowledgements

Writing this book provided an inspirational learning experience since many institutions together with dedicated individuals offered continuous support, which made its completion possible. Through divine providence, I show my most sincere appreciation to experience the capability to finish this work along with the needed wisdom and endurance.

I offer my deepest thanks to my spouse along with my children, because their devotion and steadfast assistance proved instrumental throughout the writing process. My heartfelt gratitude extends to both my parents because their guidance has supported me along my academic path and professional development.

This book benefited substantially from the contributions of my colleagues together with my mentors and collaborators, whose valuable discussions with their professional insights enhanced the material. Research teams together with scientific experts who develop innovative drugs have strongly inspired the concepts presented throughout this text. All needed research support and funding along with the essential resources come from institutions and organizations that have allowed me to present my findings thoroughly.

The publishers along with the editorial team deserve my heartfelt appreciation for their editorial leadership, which transformed this book into reality. The extensive attention to detail, combined with their practical feedback, acted as essential elements which transformed the manuscript into its final form.

I wish to express utter gratitude to every person who assisted in the creation of this work, particularly the members of my academic community and my mentors and students who enhanced the content through collaborative discussions. Through this text, I want to inspire scientists of the future to keep expanding drug discovery research for global healthcare improvements.

I want to thank all my students along with all my readers, who preserve their curiosity for learning, which continuously brings inspiration to me. The book should function as an important tool for students who wish to explore knowledge and innovation within drug discovery processes.

With gratitude,
Dr. M. Krishnaveni
Dr. P. Raveesha

1 Introduction to Drug Discovery

Krishnaveni Manubolu, Talamanchi Balakrishna, Deevi Gouri Naga Venkata Gayathri, Janga Karthik Reddy, Nagasen Dasari, and Sidagam Lokesh Kumar

Introduction

Discovery of drugs is the foundation upon which modern medicine is constructed, pushing the frontiers of new therapies that have transformed the treatment of countless diseases. From lifesaving antibiotics to groundbreaking cancer therapies, the drugs that emerge from this complex process are those that play an important role in public health and quality of life. Indeed, drug discovery not only happens on scientific grounds, but also on strategic grounds, since deeper knowledge of disease mechanisms, chemical biology, and patient needs is needed [1, 2]. Indeed, one day-to-day activity has made a whole lot of history come alive in the story of drug discovery.

The earlier races had used organic remedies, which include plants and minerals, to treat patients who suffered from some diseases. The barbaric practices then evolved into more refined practices, particularly in the 19th century when the discovery of organic chemistry helped researchers purify and synthesize active ingredients [3]. This marked the dawn of contemporary pharmacology and paved the way for today's pipelines. This change from empirical use of natural products toward designing drugs encapsulates an all-around evolution in science, from the best way to get through by observation, manipulating and optimizing biological systems.

Discovery is therefore founded on a well-defined drug discovery series, which actually constitutes each stage in translating into being an integral step along the path from concept to clinic. The process begins with target identification, at which researchers identify certain molecules or pathways in the body that are implicated in a disease. These must then be validated carefully so that modulation of these targets will lead to the desired therapeutic effect without causing undesirable side effects [4, 5]. Hit identification comes next to target identification: Thousands to millions of compounds are screened for those that can interact beneficially with the target. There's lead optimization, where the most promising compounds have their chemical structures optimized with the aim of enhancing their efficacy, selectivity, and safety. Lastly, preclinical testing is rigorous studies on cell cultures and animal models to evaluate the potential of the drug before it goes out for clinical tests [6].

DOI: 10.4324/9781003564041-1

The only alternative to overcome the intrinsic hurdles in drug discovery is always the need for innovation. Although traditional methods may be successful, they may be very slow and expensive. Research, including new technologies such as HTS, CADD, and biotechnological advances, has altered the landscape. HTS enables a researcher to quickly screen a vast library of compounds against a target, thereby considerably speeding up the identification of hits. CADD can design drugs much more accurately and efficiently by employing advanced algorithms and simulations of how a new drug is likely to interact with its target. Much creativity in biotechnology has made it possible to produce potent and highly specific drugs with the use of recombinant DNA and monoclonal antibodies.

Therefore, discovery is based on a well-defined drug discovery series that indeed forms each stage in translating into being an integral step along the way from concept to clinic. The process begins with target identification, wherein researchers identify certain molecules or pathways of the body implicated in a disease. These must then be validated carefully so that modulation of these targets will lead to the desired therapeutic effect without causing undesirable side effects. Hit identification comes next to target identification: Thousands to millions of compounds are screened for those that can interact beneficially with the target. There's lead optimization, whereby the most promising compounds have their chemical structure optimized, aiming to improve their efficacy, selectivity, and safety. The last stage is preclinical testing through rigorous studies on cell cultures and animal models with the objective of ascertaining the potential of the drug before it goes out for clinical tests.

There will always be a place for innovation, but the only alternative to overcome the intrinsic hurdles in drug discovery is innovation. Traditional methods may pay off handsomely, but they are often very slow and expensive. Science has changed things properly, with new technologies such as HTS, CADD, and biotechnological advances. HTS enables a researcher to rapidly screen a massive library of compounds against a target, thus immensely accelerating the identification of hits. CADD can design drugs more accurately and efficiently using advanced algorithms and simulations of how a new drug is likely to interact with its target. Much of that ingenuity in the biotechnology area has allowed for the production of drugs using recombinant DNA and monoclonal antibodies that are active, highly specific, and potent.

Overview of Drug Discovery

On this basis, therefore, discovery is based upon a well-defined drug discovery series that indeed forms every stage in translating into being an integral step along the way from concept to clinic, shown in Figure 1.1. It begins with target identification, wherein researchers identify certain molecules or pathways of the body implicated in a disease. These need to be validated carefully so that modulation of these targets will lead to the desired therapeutic effect without causing undesirable side effects. Hit identification comes next to target identification: Thousands to millions of compounds are screened for those that can interact beneficially with the target.

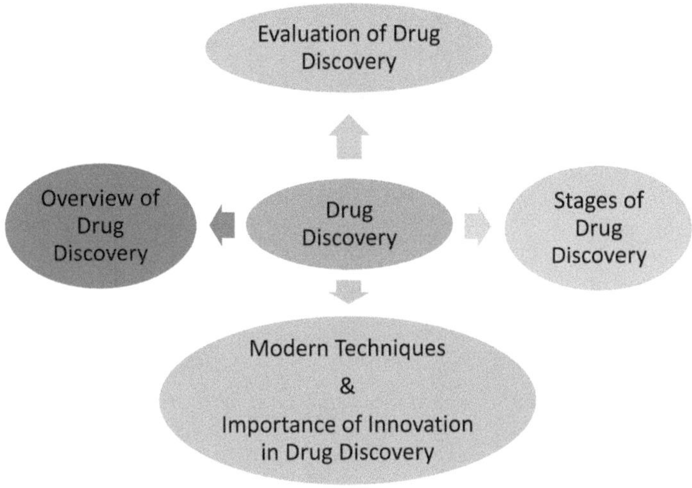

Figure 1.1 Overview of drug discovery.

Then, lead optimization is the process by which the most promising compounds have their chemical structures optimized in a quest to improve their efficacy, selectivity, and safety. The final stage is preclinical testing via rigorous studies on cell cultures and an animal model with the objective of ascertaining the drug's potential before it goes out for clinical tests.

The cost and complexity in drug discovery cannot be over-emphasized. For instance, it is said that bringing a new drug to the market will take more than a decade and at a price tag of hundreds of billions of dollars. Such a massive investment mainly flows from the fact that the process involves research, development, and testing at so many stages. All these attract astronomical payback. Successful drugs can cure, save lives, reduce suffering, and even prevent disease.

There will always be a place for innovation, but the only alternative to overcome the intrinsic hurdles in drug discovery is innovation. Traditional methods may pay off handsomely, but they are often very slow and expensive. Science has changed things properly, with new technologies such as HTS, CADD, and biotechnological advances. HTS allows for the ability to screen rapidly a massive library of compounds against a target, thereby greatly accelerating the identification of hits. CADD can design drugs more accurately and in a much more efficient manner, aided by advanced algorithms and simulations on how a new drug is likely to interact with its target. Most of that ingenuity in the biotechnology field has meant that drugs could be produced through recombinant DNA and monoclonal antibodies that are active, very specific, and potent. Leverages existing safety and efficacy data, reducing the time and cost required to bring a drug to market. This approach has led to the discovery of new treatments for a variety of diseases, including COVID-19, where several existing drugs have been repurposed to address the pandemic [7].

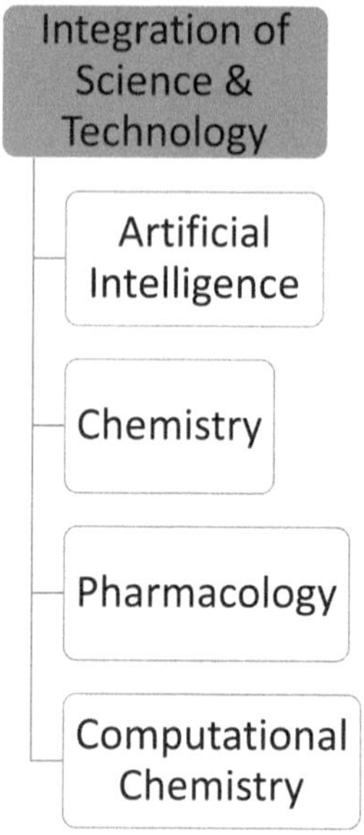

Figure 1.2 Several integration of science & technology in drug discovery.

The regulatory landscape for drug discovery is also evolving, with regulatory agencies increasingly adopting a more flexible and adaptive approach to evaluating new drugs. Accelerated approval pathways, such as the FDA's Breakthrough Therapy designation, allow for faster development and approval of drugs that address unmet medical needs. These Advances in regulatory offerings are critical elements in ensuring timely access to life-saving therapies for patients.

In brief, modern drug discovery converges on the "cut-edge" technologies on a deeper understanding of disease biology and moves toward a more patient-centered approach in the treatment of diseases. And it is at its greatest potential to discover new drugs that can address unmet medical needs as well as improve the patient outcome [8]. Advances in scientific innovation, technological development, and flexibility in regulations would be the crucial inputs for the integration process to drive drug discovery into the future, shown in Figure 1.2.

Historical Background of Drug Discovery

Drug discovery as a field has been around for thousands of years, from very primitive practices in ancient civilizations to today's highly developed processes. It implies that knowing how the field has evolved over time is really going to be important in dictating how it looks today as modern advancement [9].

Ancient Practices

- Traditional Medicine: Drug discovery is said to have its first beginning in the use of natural products in the practice of traditional medicine. The ancient cultures, including the Egyptians, Chinese, and Indians, made use of herbal remedies, extracts from animals, and minerals to treat different maladies [10]. This has been a generation-to-generation process and served as a foundation for early pharmacology.

- Alchemy and Early Chemistry: During the medieval times, alchemy greatly influenced the ripening of drug discovery. Even though alchemy majorly focused on base metals turning into gold, through alchemy, new substances were discovered, and early chemical techniques began to develop. Alchemists were the first chemists to test the mixing of compounds for the development of medicines [11].

Renaissance and Enlightenment

- Scientific Revolution: The Renaissance age witnessed the transition of practices in medicine, from mystical and superstitious to more scientific. With the rise of the scientific method that accorded top priority to observation, experimentation, and empirical evidence, drug discovery was transformed as well. Innovators such as Paracelsus, who not only stood firm against the consensus of the earlier era but also showed that chemicals can be used for the remedy of diseases, laid the basis of modern pharmacology.
- Botanical Gardens and Pharmacopeias: During this period, the creation of botanical gardens in Europe would have been pivotal to the investigation of plants used for medicinal purposes. These institutions actually became clearinghouses for discovering and classifying plants and led to the composition and publication of the first pharmacopeias—the earliest compiled records of medicinal substances and their uses. Early pharmacopeias were indispensable for the standardization and documentation of drug use.
- Emergence of Modern Pharmacology: The 19th century became the era when pharmacology became an independent scientific discipline. Scientists were now able to isolate active principles from plants and other natural sources, with the help of advancing chemistry, primarily organic chemistry. Amongst the most outstanding discoveries made is the isolation of morphine from opium by Friedrich Sertürner in 1804: The cinchona bark now yields quinine, a really important drug in the treatment of the so-called malaria.
- Synthetic drugs: Synthetic drugs began in the late 19th century. The chemical synthesis by Felix Hoffmann of acetylsalicylic acid (aspirin) at Bayer in 1897 was one of the first examples in which a drug was chemically synthesized rather than extracted from natural sources. That step opened the road to mass production of drugs and to the pharmaceutical business as known today.

Early 20th Century

- Penicillin and the Antibiotic Revolution: In 1928, Alexander Fleming's discovery of penicillin opened up medicine and the process of drug production. Penicillin was the first antibiotic, which paved the way for the discovery of many more antibiotics that drastically reduced the mortality rate of bacterial infections. The success of penicillin firmly established the role of serendipity in the world of drug discovery, since it was totally accidental that Fleming discovered penicillin.

- The Pharmaceutical Industry Expands: In the early 20th century, the pharmaceutical industry experienced rapid growth due to the urgent need to develop new and effective drugs. Business entrepreneurial ventures began to spend heavily on research and development, and with time, breakthroughs of new classes of drugs like sulfonamides and barbiturates were discovered. However, along with these breakthroughs were introduced clinical trials of which stringent measures were put in place to ensure that new drugs were safe for consumption and could meet required standards upon reaching the market.

Mid to Late 20th Century

- Biochemistry and Molecular Biology: Since the mid-20th century, tremendous progress has been made in the fields of molecular biology and biochemistry through research that has shed light on the mechanisms and mechanisms of many diseases and drugs. The discovery of the double helix structure of DNA by Watson and Crick in 1953 completely changed the way we understand genetics and gave a basis for newer targeted therapies.
- Emergence of Biopharmaceuticals: Biopharmaceuticals, or biologics, were inaugurated by the development of recombinant DNA technology in the 1970s. In 1982, the FDA approved the first recombinant DNA drug, human insulin. This breakthrough marked the beginning of a new era in drug discovery, where biologically engineered products could be developed to treat complex diseases [12].

21st Century and Beyond

Genomics and Personalized Medicine: The end of the Human Genome Project in 2003 was a landmark point in drug discovery in that it provided a total map of human genes. That knowledge has made personalized medicine possible, whereby treatments are tailored for the specific genetic makeup of the patient. Precision medicine has also been a new addition to the 21st century, where drugs are designed to target specific genetic mutations or molecular pathways [13].

Global Collaboration and Open Science: The 21st century has been characterized by global collaboration, open science. Researchers and scientists have been freely sharing resources and data to accelerate the discovery of drugs in the world. It is significantly important in the fast development of vaccines for coronavirus in a considerable part of the world. That unprecedented cooperation of the world hurriedly expedited the unprecedented cooperation that produced the application of the vaccines within record time.

The history of drug discovery reflects the story of human ingenuity and an unrelenting pursuit of knowledge. From the earliest use of natural remedies to the most technologically advanced today, its evolution continually leads to groundbreaking

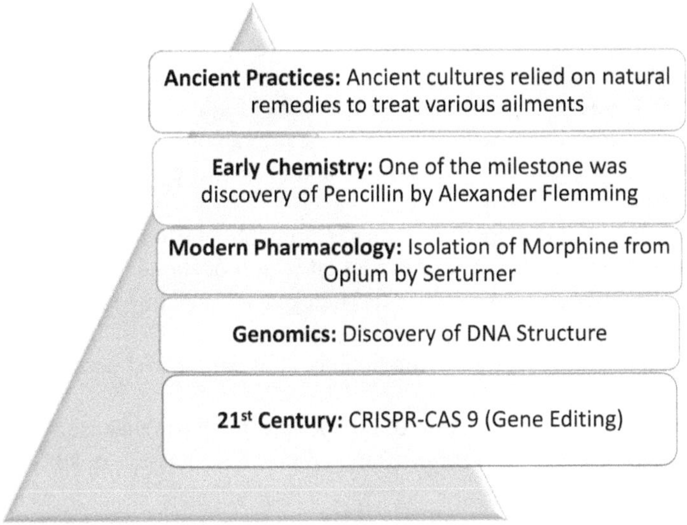

Figure 1.3 Historical background of drug discovery.

discoveries in life-saving therapy, transforming medicine and countless lives, shown in Figure 1.3.

Stages of Drug Discovery

Target Identification and Validation: To identify and validate biological targets which have a role in disease processes and on which drugs can act, shown in Figurc 1.4.

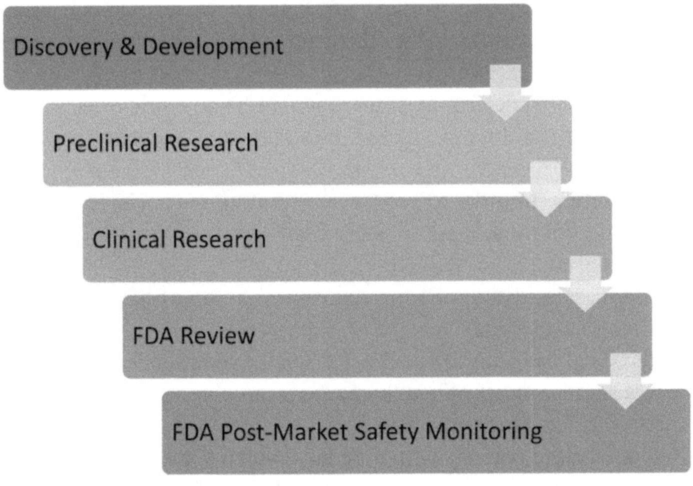

Figure 1.4 Stages of drug discovery.

Process: Understanding of disease mechanism. Identifying the biological basis of diseases with possible drugs or therapeutic targets, such as genes or proteins, or even metabolic pathways.

Target Identification: Utilize methodologies such as proteomics, genomics and bioinformatics for identification of new targets. Examples of methods that may be involved are the detection of up-regulated or down-regulated genes in disease states.

Target Validation: Prove that the target is drugable and directly associated with the disease. The evidence proves that alteration of the target impact upon the disease, in relation to it, will be through making use of several experimental models, including cell lines and animal models.

Hit Discovery: To identify lead compounds with the desired activity against the identified target.

HTS: Screening a large collection of compounds for those that are active against the intended target. HTS allows running thousands of assays quickly with automated systems.

Computational Screening: Predict, from their structures alone, which chemicals would likely interact with the target, using computer simulations and models.

Natural Product Screening: Screen compounds from natural sources like plants, animals or microorganisms which could provide new chemical entities.

Lead Optimization: To make the lead compounds have increased efficacy and selectivity, while enhancing the pharmacokinetic properties.

Structure–Activity Relationship (SAR): In order to make changes, there is a need to observe the correlation between the chemicals' biological activity and their chemical structure.

Medicinal Chemistry: To make the lead compounds have increased potency, selectivity, and stability, alter their chemical structure.

In Vitro and In Vivo Testing: To ensure that the optimized chemicals are safe and effective, further testing to determine them in animal models and cell cultures [14].

Preclinical Testing: To check whether the drug is safe, effective, and pharmacokinetics before human experiments.

No Toxicity Studies: To determine if there would be any side effects, test the potential toxicity of the drug in animals through acute, sub-chronic, and chronic toxicity studies.

No Pharmacokinetics: In order to predict what a drug will behave like when used in humans, study how it is administered, metabolized, excreted, and absorbed in animal models

No Pharmacodynamics: Study the mechanism of action of the drug and its influence on biological systems.

Clinical Trials: Give the drug to humans for safety and effectiveness.

Phase I: With a small number of healthy patients or volunteers. more on dose, pharmacokinetics, safety, and tolerance.

Phase II: Includes more patients who may have the disease or condition. This is to find the best dosage, observe efficacy, and effects [15].

Phase III: The drug is administered to large numbers of patients to validate the effectiveness of the drug and observe any rare or persistent adverse reactions. It gives information for regulatory approval.

Phase IV: Phase after marketing to obtain additional information concerning the safety and long-term efficacy of the drug. It is the surveillance of rare adverse reactions not identified in previous studies.

Regulatory Review and Clearance: Should get approval from regulatory agencies before marketing the drug.

Procedure

New Drug Application (NDA) or Marketing Authorization Application (MAA): A comprehensive dossier including manufacturing information, proposed labeling, as well as preclinical and clinical research.

Regulatory Review: For ensuring safety, efficacy, and quality assurance for the drug, these agencies, such as the FDA of the U.S., the EMA of Europe, or the national regulatory body of other countries, review the application.

Advisory Committees: Appoint external experts who review the data and make a recommendation for approval.

Post-Market Surveillance: Ensure that the drug continues to be effective and safe even after it is available for the public in general.

Pharmacovigilance: Monitor and analyze patient and healthcare professional reports of adverse events/side effects.

Long-term Studies: To assess the long-term effects and safety profile of the drug in different populations, conduct more studies.

Labeling Revision: Regarding new evidence of safety and efficacy, the drug labels need revision to provide proper information to consumers and health care professionals.

Phase I

Phase I clinical trials main objective is to assess the pharmacokinetics of a new medicine or treatment with regard to its safety and tolerability in humans. This stage helps determine the acceptable levels of dosage and will also give very crucial information regarding the functions of the medication within the body.

Study Design

Participants: Phase I studies typically recruit 20–100 healthy volunteers, or patients suffering from particular diseases in the expectation that there will be significant damage from the drug. Most are open-label, meaning that the drug administered is obvious to the participants as well as to the researchers. They can sometimes be single-blind, in that only the participants are unaware of the specifics of the treatment [16].

Dosage

Initial Doses: A low dose is given, and subjects are observed for toxic effects. The maximum dose that could be tolerated safely is usually found by a step-wise increment in the dose (sometimes called a dose escalation study). The study may also look for acute effects and longer-term effects by administering either a single dose or multiple doses spaced several days, weeks, or months apart.

Monitoring for Safety

Adverse Events: Participants' reactions are constantly watched for any negative outcomes or side effects. This covers routine lab work, vital sign checks, and medical examinations. Clinical examinations, laboratory testing, electrocardiograms, and imaging studies are part of the evaluation if required to exclude any potential danger [17].

Pharmacokinetics

Absorption: Study the rate at which the drug gets absorbed into the circulation from the point of administration.
Distribution: Study how the drug is distributed throughout the body, including whether the drug is delivered to the tissues of interest.
Metabolism: Identify how the drug is metabolized, including which enzymes are involved and what metabolites are produced.
Excretion: Detail the elimination of the drug and its metabolites from the organism, likely through urine or feces [18].

Pharmacodynamics

Initial Activity: Safety may be the main issue, but some superficial information regarding the drug's activity might be gathered in order to understand possible therapeutic potential.

Study Design Variations

Randomized Controlled Trials: For the purposes of safety and pharmacokinetics, in some Phase I studies, patients may be randomly assigned to receive various dosages.
Cross-over Designs: To compare different doses or preparations, subjects may receive several treatments serially with washout periods.

Length

Short-term: Phase I trials are relatively short—they may last anywhere from a few months to several years, depending on the study design and the half-life of the drug.

Regulatory Expectations

Ethics Approval: The Protocol of the study needs to be approved by the Ethics Committee or Institutional Review Board (IRB) before beginning Phase I to protect the participants' rights and safety.

Informed Consent: Informed consent of the participants is obtained before starting the clinical trial by showing them the possible risks and benefits of the trial.

Importance of Phase I

Safety Profile: Determines the safety profile of the drug and emphasizes any toxicity that holds a dose limit.

Dose Definition: Helps in defining the appropriate dose or Maximum Tolerated Dose (MTD) in order to be taken forward for later phases.

Pharmacokinetic Data: Provides critical information related to the metabolism of the drug, which is significant to design Phase II and Phase III studies.

Result of Phase I

Go/No-Go Decision: Depending on the outcome of Phase I, it is concluded whether the drug proceeds into Phase II. The medication is sent for further studies in more significant patient populations if it is tolerated and appears to possess favorable pharmacokinetics.

Drug development is initiated during phase I trials. This means that only medications with acceptable profiles of safety will be progressed to continue on into further, more rigorous, and specific testing phases [19].

Drug Discovery Evaluation

Drug discovery evaluation is a significant process that examines the potential medical agent's general suitability, security, and efficacy. This process encompasses several of the most important subjects to make sure that a drug candidate progresses from early development into a commercially viable product. This is a closer look at the assessments in drug discovery.

Preclinical Evaluation

Target Validation

Testing: Validate whether a biological target-a protein, gene, or pathway, to mention but a few-is linked with the disease and can be modulated appropriately by the drug. The very foundation of the target validation process in drug discovery involves establishing that a biological target is actually linked to a disease and can have a therapeutic effect on it by being modulated by a drug. This stage will ensure that the effort in terms of time, money, and effort invested in developing a drug will most probably yield returns in the form of significant clinical results. Here is a thorough explanation of the steps and techniques used in target validation [20].

Methods: Animal models, biological assays, and genetic studies all confirm that modification of the target improves the disease.

Discovery Approaches

Genomic and Proteomic Analyses: Identify genes or proteins that are differently expressed in disease versus normal conditions through high-throughput approaches.

Bioinformatics: Mine large datasets to identify potential targets based on factors like their participation in disease pathways, their interaction with other molecules, and results of previous studies. Examine the body of evidence to determine targets linked to mechanisms of disease.

Experimental Validation Approaches

Genetic Manipulation

Gene Knockout/Knockdown: Knock down or disrupt the expression of the target gene through techniques such as RNA interference (RNA i) or CRISPR/Cas9 in animals or cell lines, and assess the impact on the course of the disease or biological endpoints.

Transgenic Models: To study the function of the target gene in the pathogenesis of disease and its reaction to treatment interventions, develop animal models carrying either a change or an overexpression of the gene.

Protein Interactions

Biochemical Assays: Use techniques like yeast two-hybrid screens or co-immunoprecipitation to explore the interactions of the target protein with other molecules involved in the etiopathogenesis of the illness.

Structural Biology: Determine the three-dimensional structure of the target protein by using techniques such as NMR spectroscopy or X-ray crystallography to better understand its proposed function as well as drug binding potential.

Functional Assays

In Vitro Studies: To understand the effects of target modulation of cellular processes like death, proliferation, or signaling pathways, the tests must be performed in cells.

In Vivo Studies: Study the effect of molecular targeting in animal models to monitor disease symptoms, progression, or markers.

Clinical Correlation

Biomarker Analysis: Validate target-related biomarkers for monitoring the effects of the drug and correlating changes in the target with the therapeutic results.
Human Data: Assay molecular or genetic data from patient samples to validate that the target is relevant to humans and represents the disease phenotype.

Hit and Lead Optimization

This is the "hit and lead optimization" stage of drug development, whereby the once termed "hits," promising early compounds, are transformed into "leads," substances that promise to become safe and effective medicines. In this step, the pharmacological properties of compounds are optimized to make them appropriate for further research and development [21]. The following is a closer look at the process.

Hit Discovery

Hits are compounds identified by HTS or similar assays and that have preliminary activity against a biological target. These promising substances are typically optimized further before they can be promising lead candidates for a drug.

Activity Profiling: Assess the activity of hits in a set of in vitro assays that establish the amount of activity and affirm that they do indeed bind to the target.
Selectivity Testing: It decides whether the hit is specific to the intended target or impinges on other non-target proteins, which usually tends to reduce the potential side effects.

Lead Identification

What Is a Lead?

A lead is a purified hit, wherein each of these consists of an enhanced set of properties, such as increased potency, selectivity, and drug-like properties. Because of their medicinal potential, they are chosen for further development.

Optimization Process

SAR Studies

Recognize the ways in which various chemical alterations to the target molecule impact its biological properties. Modify the hit's chemical structure methodically, and then assess how this affects the drug's selectivity, effectiveness, and binding affinity. Create a set of analogs using medicinal chemistry techniques, and then determine which alterations enhance desirable qualities through biological testing.

Lead Optimization Strategies

Alter functional groups, stereochemistry, and molecular structure to increase potency, selectivity, and metabolic stability. Chemically modify the lead to optimize drug-like properties for improved absorption, distribution, metabolism, and excretion [22]. With the aid of preliminary toxicity profiling and structural changes, discover and reduce toxicity through preclinical tests.

Lead Compounds Evaluation

In Vitro Assays

Potency: Assess the lead's potential to activate or inhibit a target using biochemical or cell-based assays.
Selectivity: The lead must interact with the target alone and interfere as little as possible with other proteins or processes.

In Vivo Testing

Efficacy: Test the efficacy of the lead in relevant disease models involving animals. This allows researchers to establish whether the lead has a therapeutic effect in a biological system that is more complex.
Pharmacokinetics and Pharmacodynamics: Studies on how the lead interacts with the living organism, the way of uptake by the body, distribution, metabolism, excretion in the body, and the mechanism of action.

ADME-Tox Optimization

Absorption

Improve the penetration of the drug compound either across the gastrointestinal tract or other routes of administration. Generate predictions of oral bioavailability and permeability from models and in vitro studies.

Distribution

Alter the compound to possess adequate tissue distributions to the target tissues and prevent inappropriate accumulation in the nontarget tissues. Study the distribution profile of the drug through animal models and provide insight into the penetrating ability of the drug in tissues.

Metabolism

Design compounds that are metabolized to nontoxic or pharmacologically inactive forms, evaluate metabolic stability and identify potential metabolites through in vitro liver microsome studies and in vivo animal studies [23].

Excretion

Optimize the elimination pathway, which may be hepatic or renal, to ensure the substance is removed as efficiently as possible from the body. Analyze excretion patterns and make appropriate chemical structure alterations to prevent drug accumulation-related issues.

Toxicology

Minimize potential toxicity as soon as it appears early in the development process. Identify and mitigate toxicological risks in the preclinical stages. Conduct preclinical toxicological studies, including acute, sub-chronic, and chronic toxicities.

Lead Compound Selection

Selection Guidelines

Efficacy: Displays significant therapeutic promise in preliminary in vitro or in vivo models.
Safety: It displays a good safety margin with minimal adverse effects in any toxicological studies.
Pharmacokinetics: Displays optimal ADME properties such that targeted tissue levels are sufficiently attained.
Drug-Likeness: adheres to drug-likeness guidelines like Lipinski's Rule of Five to ensure that it satisfies all the chemical and physical needs for oral dosing [24].

Finalization

Optimization: Optimize the lead compound further to make additional adjustments or to resolve remaining issues.
Documentation: Develop solid data packages that have in-depth SAR information as well as preclinical results and pharmacokinetic profiles.
Formulation Development: Develop an appropriate formulation that would later be tested in terms of stability and delivery methods.
Preclinical Studies: The candidate drug undergoes preclinical studies to further investigate its safety and efficacy data before conducting clinical trials.

Probably the most critical phase of drug development, hit and lead optimization presents early hits in the form of promising new drugs with ideal features. Optimizing leads by combining chemistry manipulation, biological investigation, and pharmacokinetic and toxicology studies improves their therapeutic value and reduces risk. This is a crucial stage in which only the most promising compounds are allowed to progress to clinical trials, eventually culminating in the development of safe and effective drugs. Preclinical Safety and Efficacy Preclinical safety and effectiveness studies are indispensable steps in the discovery of new drugs that precede human clinical trials. These studies use in vitro and in vivo models to assess the safety profile and therapeutic potential of a newly developed medicine candidate [25]. It should be safe and effective enough before testing it on humans. Here is a critical review of the preclinical effectiveness and safety tests.

Preclinical Safety Evaluation

Toxicity Studies

Its Objective is to recognize any possible negative effects of the medication, establish appropriate dose ranges, and comprehend any possible hazards related to its usage.

Types of Toxicology Studies

Acute Toxicity

Purpose: Acute Toxicity: Investigate the acute effects that result from single or short-term exposure.
Method: Administer a single dose or multiple doses closely spaced apart, and look for adverse effects.
Result: Determine the dose-response relationships and the MTD.

Sub-chronic Toxicity

Objective: Investigate the effects of repeated exposures over an intermediate time period (usually 1–3 months).
Method: Dose the test animals weekly or biweekly, and observe the adverse effects on other organs and systems.
Result: Determine potential long-term harmful effects and evaluate the safety margin.

Chronic Toxicity

Objective: Determine the outcome of chronic exposure to the drug from six months or more to several years.
Method: Give it for a long period to determine if any possible long-term toxicity.
Outcome: Determine effects on growth or reproduction, carcinogenicity, and additive toxicity [26].

Genotoxicity

Objective: Determine whether the drug can cause damage to chromosomes or lead to genetic change.

Method: Run tests that include comet assay, micronucleus test, and Ames test.
Outcome: Confirm that the drug does not pose any chances of carcinogenic or mutagenic properties.

Carcinogenicity

Purpose: Test the drug's carcinogenic potential.
Method: Expose animals to the medication for an extended period to study its effect on tumor growth.
Outcome: Determine whether long-term exposure to the drug leads to cancer or not.

Reproductive and Developmental Toxicity

Purpose: Test the drug on reproduction and fetal development.
Method: Teratogenic studies (effect on fetal development), embryotoxicity, and studies to test fertility.
Outcome: To determine reproductive health risk and possible anomalies during birth.

Pharmacokinetics and Pharmacodynamics

Pharmacodynamic study of the drug and its animal model ADME study—how the drug is absorbed, distributed, metabolized, and excreted in an animal model.

Major Studies

Absorption: The extent to which the drug enters the circulatory system after being administered.
Purpose: Evaluate the absorption of the drug into the bloodstream.
Method: Assess plasma concentration and bioavailability with various routes of administration, including oral, intravenous, etc.
Distribution: Establish how the drug reaches the tissues in the body.
Purpose: Understand how the drug is distributed to the body as a whole and targets tissues.
Method: Trace the distribution of the drug by radio labeling or tissue sampling.

Metabolism

Objective: Establish how the drug is metabolized and identify its metabolites.
Method: Liver microsome studies, enzyme assays, and profiling of metabolites.

Excretion

Objective: Establish how the drug, its conjugates, and its metabolites are eliminated from the body.
Method: Determine the rates and pathways of elimination in urine, feces, and bile.

Pharmacodynamics

Purpose: Determine the effect the drug might have on the body, including the mode of action and potential therapeutic effect.
Method: Carrying out in vivo experiments to determine the influence of the drug on disease models and biological systems.

Preclinical Efficacy Evaluation

Typically, in preclinical disease models, the drug would have the desired therapeutic effect.

In Vitro Efficacy Studies

Purpose

To determine the drug's activity in cell-based assays and biochemical tests.

Methods: Cell Line Assays: Examine the drug's efficacy in disease-like cell lines. This encompasses the assessment of certain molecular pathways, cell viability, and proliferation.
Biochemical Assays: Identify the effect of the drug on the in vitro enzymatic or other molecular target activity [27].

In Vivo Efficacy Studies

To evaluate the drug's efficacy in an animal model of the disease.

Methods: Disease Models: Employ animal models which closely mimic the scenario of human disease. Some models can include rats, genetically modified mice, or any other relevant animal.
Outcome Measures: a variety of outcomes can be considered, including attenuation of the symptoms of the disease, decrease in size of the tumor in cancer models, and biochemical markers of disease pathogenesis.

Dose-response Studies

Objective: To evaluate the relationship between the drug dose with therapeutic effect.
Methods: Dose Escalation: Find the drug's right dose—the dose at which it produces the desired therapeutic effect with minimal toxicity—to do that, administer several doses.
Response Monitoring: Monitor changes in disease-related markers or biomarkers to measure how well the drug works at different doses.

Biomarker Studies

Identify and validate those biomarkers associated with both the drugs desirable effects and its potential adverse effects.

Methods: Biomarker Analysis: Employ assays to track biomarkers related with disease and drug response.

Correlation Studies: Examine the association of treatment outcomes and levels of the biomarkers to contribute to the clinical validity.

Safety and Efficacy Integration

Pool all preclinical data to make good and well-informed decisions regarding advancing the drug candidate to clinical trials.

Method

Data Integration: To integrate the safety and efficacy to determine a collective risk-benefit profile. Regulatory Submission: Supplies a complete dossier to the regulatory agency, which includes detailed safety and efficacy data derived from preclinical studies.

Decision Making: Finds that the drug is safe and has enough efficacy to be administered to humans. Preclinical safety and efficacy studies should ensure that a novel candidate for drugs is safe and effective enough before this can be tested on human beings. The scientists can therefore find some plausible risks and therapeutic benefits, refine the candidate drug, and provide the necessary information for regulatory approval through the use of comprehensive toxicological studies, comprehensive pharmacokinetic and pharmacodynamic studies, and efficacy evaluations. This stage reduces risks, increases the chances of successful clinical trials, and eventually leads to market approval [28].

Clinical Evaluation

Phase I Trial

Objective: Safety, tolerability and pharmacokinetic studies in healthy volunteers or patients.

Evaluation Criteria: Monitor side effects, find out the maximum dose that can be tolerated by patients, and analyze the absorption, distribution, metabolism, and excretion of the drug.

Phase II Trials

Objective: To study the efficacy and continued safety status of the drug in a targeted disease of the patient.

Evaluation Criteria: Determine therapeutic effects; appropriate dosing levels; and identify dose-limiting side effects. Also, interpret data to see if the drug is effective when compared with a placebo or other standard treatments [29].

Phase III Trials

Objective: Efficacy to be established and safety profile in a larger population of patients.

Evaluation Criteria: Large-scale investigations to validate the therapeutic benefits of the drug, compare with other drugs in the same class that are currently on the market, and establish an adequate safety profile. The results must be statistically and clinically significant.

Phase IV Trials (Post-marketing Surveillance)

Objective: Safety profile including long-term effectiveness after the drug has been marketed.

Evaluation criteria monitor events associated with the safety of the drug, practical efficacy in real life, and long-term advantages. Monitor data to detect infrequent or long-term side effects that may not have appeared during the previous trials [30].

Regulatory Evaluation

Submission to Regulatory Bodies

Objective submission of approved data by regulatory bodies for the approval of the drug

Evaluation criteria submission of an MAA or NDA along with proposed labeling, preclinical and clinical data, as well as manufacturing information (Figure 1.5).

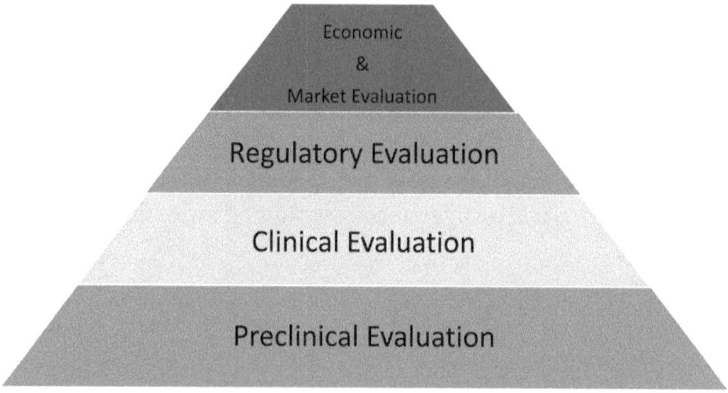

Figure 1.5 Evaluation in drug discovery.

Regulatory Review

Goal: Find regulating bodies, like the US FDA, EMA of Europe, or any other national regulatory body.

Standards for Evaluation: Applies the judgment to the data based on the safety, efficacy, and quality expectations. Discuss with regulatory authorities and resolve their issues with any extra demands [31].

Economic and Market Evaluation

Cost-benefit Analysis

Goal: It analyzes the cost-benefit value of the drug, along with its multiple expenditure costs.

Evaluation Criteria: Cost-effectiveness, cost-benefit ratios, and potential market impact on drug sales. Compare drug costs against therapeutic benefits and alternatives.

Market Potential

Objective: Estimate commercial viability and market size for the drug

Evaluation Criteria: Market analysis through research would be conducted to evaluate potential demand, competition, pricing strategy, and revenue potential.

Post-market Evaluation

Objective: To continuously monitor drug safety after it comes onto the market.

Criteria: Data collection and monitoring related to adverse drug reactions and long-term effects. Risk management action and labeling are updated when required.

Patient and Health Care Provider Feedback

Objective: Gather feedback from end-users to understand real-world effectiveness and areas for improvement.

Artificial Intelligence (AI) and Machine Assessment Standards: Survey and gather feedback, and evaluate the patient experiences in order to assess the satisfaction of patients and issues not caught before.

Application of Modern Techniques in Drug Discovery

A drug discovery has undergone significant change with the help of new advances. The following discusses the major methods and strategies which are currently transforming the discipline:

High Throughput Screening

It is possible for millions of chemical, genetic, or pharmaceutical experiments to be conducted quickly by researchers using HTS. It has the utility of automated methods, which could match large libraries of chemicals with biological targets to discover potential treatment alternatives.

Computational Drug Design

Molecular docking: predicts an interaction of a drug with a specific protein. This can help in the optimization of drug candidates as well as studies on the binding affinity.

Quantitative Structure–Activity Relationship (QSAR): predicts activity based on a compound's chemical structure using statistical techniques.

Molecular Dynamics (MD) Simulations: Predicts the probable behavior of a medicine in the biological system by simulating long-term physical changes of atoms and molecules over time.

Genomics and Proteomics

Genomic Approaches: Study genetic differences and how they relate to disease to find potential drugs to target. To learn more about what particular genes do, it may be possible to generate knockout mutants using techniques like CRISPR.

Proteomics: It studies the interactions, expressions, and activities of proteins in a cell that could serve as therapeutic targets and biomarkers [32].

Systems Biology

Integrates genomic data along with other omics technologies and proteomics to understand complex biological systems and disease mechanisms. In this way, it has the ability to generate new drug targets and anticipate the behavior of diseases toward drugs.

Bioinformatics and Data Mining

Describe how computational tools and algorithms are learning

Predictive Models: AI algorithms predict drug toxicity, efficacy, and potential side effects from historical data and simulations.

Drug Repurposing: AI identifies potential drugs for a new disease by analyzing existing drug-target interactions.

Chemical Biology

Chemistry and biology come together to understand and regulate biological systems at the molecular level. The exploration of biological procedures and the identification of potential targets for drug molecules are achieved with the help of techniques such as chemical probes and small molecules.

Pharmacogenomics

Examine how the inherent genetic profile of a patient can impact drug response. These insights make it easier to design targeted treatments and reduce the adverse effects of drugs.

New Techniques for Imaging

Cryoelectron Microscopy: Provides higher resolution images of biological macromolecules. Thanks to Cryo-EM, one can now visualize interactions of drugs with targets at the atomic level.

X-Ray Crystallography: This method certifies the atomic and molecular structure of a crystal, which one can use to make sense of how drugs interact with their targets [33].

Organs-on-chips and Microfluidics

These technologies create miniaturized models of human organs and systems to study the effects of drugs in a more physiologically relevant context. They accurately predict the metabolism, efficacy, and toxicity of drugs.

Ethical and Regulatory Considerations

It also focuses more on the complex contemporary ethical and regulatory issues of drug discovery involving clinical trials, patients' consent, and personal information. These new strategies, in many instances, are employed in combination for enhanced efficiency and effectiveness in drug discovery toward highly targeted and individualized treatment

High Throughput Screening

HTS is a crucial technique in drug discovery. It enables the fast assessment of thousands to millions of compounds for biological activity. Here's a rather elaborate overview of how HTS works and some of its key aspects.

Overview of HTS

HTS seeks to accelerate and automate the process by testing many libraries of chemical compounds or biological samples against certain biological targets. It is particularly useful in the identification of potential drug candidates and their interactions with biological systems.

Ingredients of HTS

Chemical Libraries: These are groups containing varied small molecules or compounds that are screened for their ability to interact with the biological targets.
Biological Libraries: Peptide, protein, or nucleic acid libraries assessed for biological activity

Biological Targets

Enzymes: Biological molecules catalyzing biochemical reactions. HTS can detect inhibitors or activators of a given enzyme.
Receptors: Proteins sensitive to chemical stimuli. HTS can discover compounds that alter receptor function.
Cells or Tissues: Whole cells or tissue samples are screened to measure the biological impact of compounds in a more integrated environment.

Screening Platforms

Automated Liquid Handling Systems: Robots that accurately dispense and mix liquids.

Detection Systems: Methods that measure the biological response, such as fluorescence, luminescence, or absorbance. Detection methods include:
Fluorescence Resonance Energy Transfer: The transfer of energy between two fluorescent molecules.
Luminescence: Measuring the light emitted by a reaction.
Absorbance: Measures the amount of light absorbed by a sample

HTS Process

Assay Development

To develop a robust and reproducible method for detecting compound-target interaction, this might be in terms of designing specific biochemical assays or cell-based assays. Optimization of assay conditions, so that it can be carried out at a very high throughput, including reagent concentration, reaction time, and signal-to-noise ratio.

Screening

Automated systems are used to deliver compounds into wells of a multi-well plate, often 96, 384, or 1536 wells. Compounds interact with the target under controlled conditions. The biological response is measured using the detection system of choice. Data are collected and analyzed to infer which compounds have desired effects [34, 35].

Data Analysis

Compounds which exhibit a large biological response are designated "hits." These are the potential leads that need to be further explored. Hits are subjected to additional assays to confirm their activity and assess their specificity and potency.

Advantages of HTS

Rapid: It can screen millions of compounds in a matter of days.
Time and reagent efficiency: As leads can be identified rapidly, time and reagents that go into the process of drug discovery are saved.
Scalability: Can be scaled up or down depending on the size of the compound library and the complexity of the assay.

Challenges of HTS

False Positives/Negatives: HTS can produce false positives or negatives owing to non-specific interactions or assay artifacts. Proper validation is key.
Data Management: Manipulation and processing of large amounts of data is cumbersome and requires advanced software and computational methodologies.
Cost: Set-up, both equipment and reagents, although costly at first, has decreased with time due to technological advancements [36].

Applications of HTS

Drug Discovery: This is the discovery of new potential drugs by screening compound libraries against specific biological targets.
Toxicology: This is the estimation of the potential toxicity of the compounds before their evaluation in vivo systems.
Biomarker Discovery: The identification of appropriate biomarkers for diseases by screening biological samples.

Computer-aided Drug Discovery

CADD is an advanced technology approach whereby computational tools and techniques are applied to discover and develop new drugs. CADD contributes quite significantly to the drug discovery process by making it more efficient and effective in identifying possible drug candidates. Here's an overview of CADD in detail.

CADD Overview

Aspects of CADD include a set of computational methods, including the prediction of drug-target interaction, optimization of drug properties, and assistance in designing novel compounds. Algorithms, simulations, and models guide and support the drug discovery process.

Some Major Techniques in CADD

Molecular Docking

It gives predictions on how a small molecule (drug) binds to a target protein or receptor. The docking process simulates the interaction and, among all possible binding modes, identifies which one is the best. It is useful in explaining the binding affinity, specificity, and orientation of potential drug candidates. A few examples are Auto Dock, Dock, and GLIDE.

Quantitative Structure–Activity Relationship

Analyzes the relationship between the chemical structure of compounds and their biological activity. QSAR models use statistical techniques to predict the activity of new compounds based on their molecular descriptors. It is useful for predicting the biological activity of untested compounds and guiding the design of new molecules [34, 37].

Examples Include Dragon, Minimum Optimal Effective (MOE), and CODESSA

MD Simulations

MD Simulations

Models the time evolution of physical movements of atoms and molecules to study their behavior in a dynamic environment. It includes detailed stability, flexibility, and changes in protein and drug candidate conformation. This is useful for the qualitative understanding of dynamics in drug-target interactions and refining docking outcomes. Examples of these are GROMACS, AMBER, and CHARMM.

De Novo Drug Design

It generates a de novo, drug-like molecule using a computational method. This involves the development of new compounds that will interact with a given target of interest. It facilitates the discovery of novel chemical entities having a potentially unique mechanism of action [38]. Examples include Cresset, Schrodinger's LigandScout, and Sybyl.

Pharmacophore Modeling

Identifies critical features of the molecule important for biological activity. Pharmacophore models present the three-dimensional arrangement of functional groups, which are necessary for interaction with the target. These are used to design new molecules or screen a compound library based on the pharmacophore model.

Virtual Screening

It is the process of scanning large libraries of compounds computationally so that likely ligands to bind to a particular target are identified. Virtual screening can be performed with docking, QSAR, or pharmacophore-based methods. For compound prioritization, it predicts probable activity by ranking compounds.

Applications of CADD

Drug Discovery: It accelerates the identification of lead compounds as it predicts their interaction with biological targets and can also optimize chemical properties.

Lead Optimization: It optimizes lead compounds in order to develop them, providing them with high potency, selectivity, as well as pharmacokinetic properties.

Structure-based Design: Based on the 3D structures of proteins or nucleic acids, such compounds are designed or changed to target them specifically.

Drug Repurposing: It identifies drug molecules, which could potentially be useful for other indications as well, due to similar target-ligand interactions.

Benefits of CADD

Speed: The computational predictions and insights given allow for the rapid identification of and speed into the development of new candidates for drugs.

Cost-effectiveness: This is due to decreasing the cost of drug development by narrowing it down to the number of compounds to be synthesized and tested experimentally.

Precision: It increases the accuracy in the drug-target interaction prediction and optimizing drug properties using detailed simulations and modeling.

Challenges and Limitations

Accuracy: How good are the models and algorithms; in fact, there will be false positives and false negatives. Experimental validation is needed to accept these values.

Complexity: The model can't simply "bridge" complex biological systems. In such cases, resolution needs to be good and dynamic interaction of various components should be well represented.

Data Quality: The reliability of CADD results depends on the availability and quality of structural and biological data.

Integration with Experimental Methods

Validation: Experimental validation: All the predictions made by CADD should be validated experimentally. This is achieved through the synthesis and testing of predicted molecules in biological assays.

Iterative Process: CADD should sometimes be used iteratively to improve experimental data and refine predictions for improving drug candidates.

For example, CADD will revolutionize drug discovery by providing an excellent tool for predicting and optimizing drug candidates. The integration of CADD with other experimental or computational approaches continues to advance pharmaceutical research.

Role of Biotechnology in Drug Discovery: Biotechnology is playing a great role in the modern discovery of drugs, revolutionizing a process in which accuracy and efficiency are enhanced. Some of the foremost ways in which biotechnology supports medication discovery include the following:

Proteomics and Genomics: Biotechnology technologies such as protein analysis and genome sequencing help to discover new therapeutic targets by providing in-depth insight into the genetic and protein-based mechanisms whereby diseases can develop. Understanding the genetic basis of many illnesses is useful in getting new targets and paths for medicines [39].

Discovery and validation of the biomarkers, or biological molecules indicative of the onset or course of diseases, are carried out applying biotechnology techniques. Biomarkers are crucial in diagnosing a disease, predicting the course of diseases, and even assessing the safety and effectiveness of drugs to be prescribed.

HTS: With the advent of biotechnology, automated HTS systems that can test thousands of compounds against specific biological targets in a few days have been designed. This speeds up the identification of lead structures from the hits.

Computational Drug Design: Biotechnology utilizes modeling and computation to predict the interactions of tiny compounds or biologics with biological targets. However, drug candidates are designed and optimized before entering the experimental phase using techniques like molecular docking and simulations [40].

Biotechnology has completely revolutionized the manufacture of biologics, drugs derived from living organisms. For example, monoclonal antibodies are made so that they bind with specific proteins or cells that are involved in the disease, and thus, therapy is much more targeted and efficient.

Gene editing and RNA technologies: For instance, an example of the technology that can edit the genetic material and be used in changing the cells for drug efficacy testing or in models of disease is CRISPR/Cas9. Another area includes RNA-based technologies like antisense oligonucleotides and RNA interference, providing new ways to control expression at the genetic level, hence new avenues for disease treatment.

Cell-based Assays: Complex cell-based assays can be developed using biotechnology to study medication effects in a more physiologically appropriate environment. These tests can be used to model disease states and evaluate the impact of potential drugs on cellular functions.

Vaccine Production: The production of a new vaccine is done through the application of biotechnology techniques, such as viral vector systems and recombinant

DNA technologies. Thus, by producing antigens or components of vaccines in transformed organisms, these technologies enable the design of safe and effective vaccinations.

Biomanufacturing: The advancement of biotechnology has helped fast-track pharmaceutical candidates, particularly in the field of biologics. Fermentation and cell culture, among many other techniques of purification, advances in producing mass volumes of pharmaceuticals in a rather short span of time. Taking all this into consideration, biotechnology advances the discovery of medication through great tools and methods that raise efficiency, precision, and speed of generating new medicines. It has enabled deeper comprehension of the mechanisms of illness and has also made it easier to develop individualized, focused treatments.

What Is the Importance of Innovation in Drug Discovery?

Innovation in drug discovery holds a very influential role in several critical dimensions, cutting across the whole process of coming up with new medications. It has the most important elements that provide coverage for important criteria in the entire process of developing new drugs. Here's a closer look at why it is all important: Innovation to Address Unmet Medical Needs. Innovation is vital in the development of treatments for emerging and re-emerging diseases that are yet to have effective therapies. As an illustration, the rapid production of vaccines and treatments for COVID-19 emphasizes the need for innovative approaches to new health crises.

Many chronic conditions and rare diseases lack effective treatments. Innovation can uncover new targets and therapeutic strategies, offering hope to patients with conditions that are currently underserved by existing drugs [41, 42].

Enhancing Drug Efficacy and Safety

Advances in genomics and bioinformatics have enabled the practice of personalized medicine, in which drugs are tailored to individual profiles. The drug efficacy is enhanced, and adverse effects are at a minimum because therapy is matched with the patient's biology. With the advances in the mechanisms of diseases, more targeted therapy could be designed to target specific pathways of disease with better accuracy; this could potentially deliver more effective treatment with fewer adverse effects.

Shorten Time and Cost of Drug Development

HTS and CADD significantly speed up the identification and optimization of drug candidates, saving appreciable time and economic means of traditional drug development. Advanced modeling techniques, such as AI and machine learning, predict drug interactions and outcomes far better, which can help prioritize promising candidates while avoiding costly failures.

Improving Techniques for Drug Discovery

New technologies around CRISPR gene editing and advanced imaging techniques facilitate the deeper understanding of drug targets and disease mechanisms, thus improving precision in drug discovery. Integration of data from genomics, proteomics, metabolomics, and other omics fields provides a holistic understanding of biological systems in the discovery of novel drug targets and biomarkers [43, 44].

Facilitates Drug Repurposing

Innovation actually enables the discovery of novel uses of existing drugs, a faster and less expensive way of developing various treatments. For example, there are drugs originally discovered for cancer that are now being studied for other diseases. Advanced computational tools and databases ease the screening of existing drugs for new applications, hastening drug repurposing. The innovations in drug delivery systems, such as nanoparticles and smart polymers, are used to target controlled release of drugs, thus improving the therapeutic outcomes without adverse effects. New formulation technologies have led to improvements in drug stability, bioavailability, and patient compliance, which in turn improve effectiveness and ease of treatment.

Improving Clinical Trials

Innovative trial designs, such as adaptive and decentralized trials, make clinical trials more versatile and efficient and allow analysis based on interim results. This also enhances the recruitment and retention of patients. Advanced diagnostic tools and biomarkers enable better stratification of patients such that clinical trials target populations most likely to benefit from the treatment and enhance the likelihood of successful clinical trials [45].

Improve Competitive Advantage and Market Success

In competition in the marketplace, innovative candidates should have new mechanisms of action or improved profiles that provide competitive advantages. These drug candidates provide unique benefits or address needs that have not been met in treatments already marketed. Innovation leads to new patents and intellectual property that can create an investment flow, obtain funding, and support new therapies.

New Patents and Intellectual Property-based Strategies

The innovations would help develop treatments for diseases which are prevalent in resource-poor settings, such as in the tropics and neglected diseases to thereby improve health everywhere. Such innovations should lead to more cost-effective drug development and production so that these end up saving the treatment for many people who are in need.

Ethical and Regulatory Considerations

Innovation guarantees high ethical standards in the development of drugs; this includes drug safety, efficacy, and patients' rights. This is crucial for the assurance of the public trust and responsible conduct of research. The acceleration of the drug approval process through the rapid changes of regulatory requirements and acceptance of new regulatory pathways of innovative therapies follows on to, thereby facilitating their timely introduction [46].

Supporting Drug Discovery with New Models and Tools

By predicting the interaction of drugs with biological targets using advanced computational tools and simulations, potential side effects are indicated, and the best drug candidates are selected even before entering the lab. New cell culture models, organ-on-a-chip technologies, and animal models make preclinical testing more relevant and reliable.

Collaboration and Open Science

This usually involves interfaces between the academy, industry, and governmental agencies. Innovation often shares resources and expertise to tackle complex drug discovery challenges. Open-access platforms and collaborative projects speed up research and discovery by giving scope for researchers all over the world to work on top of each other [47, 48].

In drug discovery, innovation plays a key role in improving the welfare of humankind, advancing medical science, improving patient care, and addressing a wide range of health challenges. Innovation drives progress through better drugs with superior efficacy and safety, lower development costs and shorter time requirements, and new treatments that may revolutionize public health.

Case Studies in Successful Drug Discovery

Successful drug discovery often results from innovative science, clever thinking, and a little dose of good fortune. The two cases described below illustrate different aspects of successful drug discovery.

Development of Imatinib (Gleevec)

Discoverer: Dr. Nicholas Lydon and colleagues at Novartis
Year: Approved in 2001

Imatinib has been developed as a targeted therapy for chronic myeloid leukemia (CML), specifically inhibiting the BCR-ABL tyrosine kinase, a disease-causing fusion protein that may be associated with dramatic improvements in patient outcomes.

Innovation Highlights

Targeting specific molecular aberrations in cancer cells. Aims at a personalized approach to the treatment according to the genetic profile of the cancer.

Discovery of Sofosbuvir

Discoverer: Gilead Sciences
Year: Approved in 2013

Sofosbuvir is one of the direct-acting antiviral drugs that revolutionized the treatment course of hepatitis C virus infection. That is because it highly increased cure rates through a shorter, all-oral treatment course with fewer side effects compared with previous therapies, leading to a shift in the paradigm of HCV management. Give emphasis on the direct inhibition of the viral enzymes critical for replication. Use sofosbuvir in combination with other antiviral agents to optimize its effects and minimize resistance.

Development of Checkpoint Inhibitors (e.g., Pembrolizumab and Nivolumab)

Discoverers: Researchers at Merck (pembrolizumab) and Bristol-Myers Squibb (nivolumab)
Year: Pembrolizumab approved in 2014, Nivolumab in 2015

Checkpoint inhibitors are monoclonal antibodies that block proteins (e.g., PD-1, PD-L1) which prevent the immune system from attacking the tumor cells. They have revolutionized the treatment of several cancers, including melanoma, non-small cell lung cancer and bladder cancer, holding promise for advanced diseases. Targeting immune checkpoint pathways to enhance the body's natural immune response to cancers. Now, reports are emerging of patient survival benefits for patients with previously difficult-to-treat cancers.

Discovery of Statins (e.g., Lovastatin)

Discoverer: Dr. Akira Endo and colleagues
Year: Lovastatin approved in 1987

These drugs fall into the category of lipid-lowering drugs in the capacity of decreasing blood cholesterol, thus reducing the risk of cardiovascular diseases. Indeed, statins play a cornerstone role in prevention and treatment against heart diseases; this exemplifies how interference with lipid metabolism can drastically affect the well-being of an individual. Drugs inhibiting such an enzyme that catalyzes cholesterol synthesis have been designed as statins. Statins significantly contributed to public health by decreasing heart attacks and strokes [49].

Development of Gene Therapy (e.g., Zolgensma)

Company: Novartis
Year: Approved in 2019

Zolgensma is an SMS gene therapy for spinal muscular atrophy that involves giving a healthy copy of the SMN1 gene in place of a faulty one. Zolgensma has shown promising results in the treatment of SMA and proved to be one of the great milestones in gene therapy as this is progressing.

Discovery of Vemurafenib

Company: Roche
Year: Approved in 2011

Vemurafenib has been formulated to specifically target the BRAF V600E mutation in some melanoma patients, resulting in considerably improved survival in such patients. It demonstrates targeted cancer therapy through the efficacy of targeting specific genetic mutations, opening the doors for further drugs based on the specific genetic mutations in tumor paths. Patient outcomes in the targeted therapies are evidently better compared with the conventionally used treatments.

Development of CAR-T Cell Therapy (e.g., Kymriah and Yescarta)

Companies: Novartis (Kymriah) and Kite Pharma (Yescarta)
Year: Kymriah approved in 2017, Yescarta in 2018

Chimeric Antigen Receptor T-Cell Therapy: CAR-T cell therapy has achieved high remission rates in many blood cancers by infusing the reengineered T cells whose introduced receptors target the cancer cells. It is the most significant breakthrough in immunotherapy to date and has provided new hope for the desperately refractory patients of cancers [50–61].

Individualized Treatment Tailored to the Cells of Each Patient: These case studies illustrate the different approaches and innovations that have defined modern pharmaceutical discovery-from the discovery of the first natural products to today's cutting-edge genetic therapies. They emphasize innovation, technology, and determination in the development of new treatments that can overcome vital health challenges.

Conclusion

Researching new medicines is very complex, dynamic, and broadly depends on innovation to meet a wide range of medicinal needs. Technical and methodological breakthroughs in this industry are necessary to introduce targets at the early stages of drug development and ensure the success of medicine. Innovation will be focused on reducing the time and cost required for the development of new drugs, augmenting the therapeutic efficacy and safety, and meeting unmet medical needs. Advances in AI, genetics, and methods of innovative drug delivery have shifted the approaches for developing drugs toward more accurate and efficient methods. Examples of success include penicillin discovery, checkpoint inhibitors as well as imatinib as targeted medicines, and advances in gene therapy, indicative of the great impact novel approaches have made in patient care. These graphics describe individualized therapies, state-of-the-art mechanisms of action, and targeted strategies that may significantly improve outcomes. New discoveries in the field are moving our ability to identify and advance new drugs forward: CRISPR gene editing, HTS, and personalized medicine. In simple terms, the field of drug development is forever changing, and advancements in global health through research and integration of technology are fundamental to transcend barriers and breakthroughs.

References

1. Angst D, Gessier F, Janser P, Vulpetti A, Wälchli R, Beerli C, et al. Discovery of LOU064 (remibrutinib), a potent and highly selective covalent inhibitor of Bruton's tyrosine kinase. J Med Chem. 2020;63(10):5102–5118.
2. Asahina Y, Wurtz NR, Arakawa K, Carson N, Fujii K, Fukuchi K, et al. Discovery of BMS-986235/LAR-1219: A potent formyl peptide receptor 2 (FPR2) selective agonist for the prevention of heart failure. J Med Chem. 2020;63(17):9003–9019.
3. Berger M, May E, Rehwinkel H, Schäcke H, Neuhaus R, Rottmann A, et al. Discovery of the potent non-steroidal glucocorticoid receptor modulator BAY 1003803 as clinical candidate. Bioorg Med Chem Lett. 2020;30(16):127298.
4. Blomgren P, Chandrasekhar J, Di Paolo JA, Fung W, Geng G, Ip C, et al. Discovery of lanraplenib (GS-9876): A once-daily spleen tyrosine kinase inhibitor for autoimmune diseases. ACS Med Chem Lett. 2020;11(4):506–513.
5. Brandao DJ, Fontenelle LF, da Silva SA, Menezes PR. Pastor-valero m. Depression and excess mortality in the elderly living in low-and middle-income countries: Systematic review and meta-analysis. Int J Geriatr Psychiatry. 2019;34(1):22–30.
6. Braunwald E. Heart failure. JACC Heart Fail. 2013;1(1):1–20.
7. Brogi S. Computational approaches for drug discovery. Multidiscip Digit Publ Inst. 2019; 3061.
8. Brown DG, Wobst HJ. A decade of FDA-approved drugs (2010–2019): Trends and future directions. J Med Chem. 2021;64(5):2312–2338.
9. Cherney RJ, Cornelius LA, Srivastava A, Weigelt CA, Marcoux D, Duan JJW, et al. Discovery of BMS-986251: A clinically viable, potent, and selective Rorγt inverse agonist. ACS Med Chem Lett. 2020;11(6):1221–1227.
10. Cherney EC, Zhang L, Nara S, Zhu X, Gullo-Brown J, Maley D, et al. Discovery and preclinical evaluation of BMS-986242, a potent, selective inhibitor of indoleamine-2,3-dioxygenase 1. ACS Med Chem Lett. 2021;12(2):288–294.
11. Chianelli D, Rucker PV, Roland J, Tully DC, Nelson J, Liu X, et al. Nidufexor (LMB763), a novel FXR modulator for the treatment of nonalcoholic steatohepatitis. J Med Chem. 2020;63(8):3868–3880.
12. Chrovian CC, Soyode-Johnson A, Stenne B, Pippel DJ, Schoellerman J, Lord B, et al. Design, synthesis, and preclinical evaluation of 3-methyl-6-(5-thiophenyl)-1,3-dihydro-imidazo[4,5-b]pyridin-2-ones as selective GluN2B negative allosteric modulators for the treatment of mood disorders. J Med Chem. 2020;63(17):9181–9196.

13. Cirillo P, Gersch MS, Mu W, Scherer PM, Kim KM, Gesualdo L, et al. Ketohexokinase-dependent metabolism of fructose induces proinflammatory mediators in proximal tubular cells. J Am Soc Nephrol. 2009;20(3):545–553.
14. Cockerill GS, Angell RM, Bedernjak A, Chuckowree I, Fraser I, Gascon-Simorte J, et al. Discovery of sisunatovir (RV521), an inhibitor of respiratory syncytial virus fusion. J Med Chem. 2021;64(7):3658–3676.
15. Cooper GS, Bynum ML, Somers EC. Recent insights in the epidemiology of autoimmune diseases: Improved prevalence estimates and understanding of clustering of diseases. J Autoimmun. 2009;33(3–4):197–207.
16. Croft AC, Antoni AV, Terzulli SL. Update on the antibacterial resistance crisis. Med Sci Monit. 2007;13(6):RA103.
17. Cuozzo JW, Clark MA, Keefe AD, Kohlmann A, Mulvihill M, Ni H, et al. Novel autotaxin inhibitor for the treatment of idiopathic pulmonary fibrosis: A clinical candidate discovered using DNA-encoded chemistry. J Med Chem. 2020;63(14):7840–7856.
18. Deo S, Sharma J, Kumar S. GLOBOCAN 2020 report on global cancer burden: Challenges and opportunities for surgical oncologists. Ann Surg Oncol. 2022;29(11):6497–6500.
19. Di Meglio LA, Evans-Molina C, Oram RA. Type 1 diabetes. Lancet. 2018;391(10138): 2449–2462.
20. Durand-Reville TF, Comita-Prevoir J, Zhang J, Wu X, May-Dracka TL, Romero JAC, et al. Discovery of an orally available diazabicyclooctane inhibitor (ETX0282) of class a, c, and d serine β-lactamases. J Med Chem. 2020;63(21):12511–12525.
21. Ferrari AJ, Charlson FJ, Norman RE, Patten SB, Freedman G, Murray CJ, et al. Burden of depressive disorders by country, sex, age, and year: Findings from the global burden of disease study 2010. PLoS Med. 2013;10(11):e1001547.
22. Fidler MM, Bray F, Soerjomataram I. The global cancer burden and human development: A review. Scand J Public Health. 2018;46(1):27–36.
23. Forouhi NG, Wareham NJ. Epidemiology of diabetes. Medicine. 2019;47(1):22–27.
24. Futamura A, Suzuki R, Tamura Y, Kawamoto H, Ohmichi M, Hino N, et al. Discovery of ORN0829, a potent dual orexin 1/2 receptor antagonist for the treatment of insomnia. Bioorg Med Chem. 2020;28(13):115489.
25. Futatsugi K, Smith AC, Tu M, Raymer B, Ahn K, Coffey SB, et al. Discovery of PF-06835919: A potent inhibitor of ketohexokinase (KHK) for the treatment of metabolic disorders driven by the overconsumption of fructose. J Med Chem. 2020;63(22):13546–135460.
26. Gerstenberger BS, Ambler C, Arnold EP, Banker ME, Brown MF, Clark JD, et al. Discovery of tyrosine kinase 2 (TYK2) inhibitor (PF-06826647) for the treatment of autoimmune diseases. J Med Chem. 2020;63(22):13561–13577.
27. Goi T, Nakajima T, Komatsu Y, Kawata A, Yamakoshi S, Okada O, et al. Pyrazolo[4,3-d]pyrimidine derivatives as a novel hypoxia-inducible factor prolyl hydroxylase domain inhibitor for the treatment of anemia. ACS Med Chem Lett. 2020;11(7):1416–1420.
28. Greene SA. Chronic pain: Pathophysiology and treatment implications. Top Companion Anim Med. 2010;25(1):5–9.
29. Günther J, Hillig RC, Zimmermann K, Kaulfuss S, Lemos C, Nguyen D, et al. BAY-069, a novel (trifluoromethyl) pyrimidinedione-based BCAT1/2 inhibitor and chemical probe. J Med Chem. 2022;65(21):14366–14390.
30. Hahn MG, Lampe T, El Sheikh S, Griebenow N, Woltering E, Schlemmer K-H, et al. Discovery of the soluble guanylate cyclase activator runcaciguat (BAY 1101042). J Med Chem. 2021;64(9):5323–5344.
31. Hay M, Thomas DW, Craighead JL, Economides C, Rosenthal J. Clinical development success rates for investigational drugs. Nat Biotechnol. 2014;32(1):40–51.
32. Hecker SJ, Reddy KR, Lomovskaya O, Griffith DC, Rubio-Aparicio D, Nelson K, et al. Discovery of cyclic boronic acid QPX7728, an ultrabroad-spectrum inhibitor of serine and metallo-β-lactamases. J Med Chem. 2020;63(14):7491–7507.

33. Hung CL, Chen CC. Computational approaches for drug discovery. Drug Dev Res. 2014;75(6):412–418.
34. Iwaki Y, Ohhata A, Nakatani S, Hisaichi K, Okabe Y, Hiramatsu A, et al. ONO-8430506: A novel autotaxin inhibitor that enhances the antitumor effect of paclitaxel in A breast cancer model. ACS Med Chem Lett. 2020;11(6):1070–1076.
35. Kanda Y, Murata K, Ishihara T, Sakamoto R, Kondo M, Tsuda T, et al. The discovery of EVX-101, a potent and selective inverse agonist of retinoic acid-related orphan receptor gamma for autoimmune diseases. J Med Chem. 2020;63(17):9727–9742.
36. Kuo H, McKinney M, Nguyen J, Amouyel P, Langley S, Dandrielle T, et al. Discovery of a new class of CXCR4 antagonists as promising agents for the treatment of cancer and HIV. J Med Chem. 2021;64(9):5640–5656.
37. Largier V, Schulte RH, Rydzewski L, Sprague J, Thompson B, Zink D. Targeted gene editing strategies for the treatment of Duchenne muscular dystrophy. Biomedicines. 2020;8(10):442.
38. Lee R, Lee J, Kim H, Kim K. Recent advances in small molecule inhibitors for metabolic diseases. Molecules. 2020;25(9):2090.
39. Li S, Jiang H, Guo X, Song L, Shi J, Zhang D, et al. Discovery of a potent, selective, and orally available non-ATP competitive inhibitor of CHK1 for cancer therapy. J Med Chem. 2021;64(3):1082–1096.
40. Liao J, Li J, Jin Z, Liao Y, Zheng Y, Tang Y, et al. Discovery of novel, potent, and selective TRK inhibitors for the treatment of cancers with TRK fusions. J Med Chem. 2020;63(11):6170–6188.
41. Lin H, Zhuang R, Zhang Y, Wei Z, Li C, Zhang J, et al. Discovery of PRT062070, a potent and orally available positive allosteric modulator of the dopamine D1 receptor. J Med Chem. 2021;64(18):12018–12031.
42. Lu Y, Zeng Z, Zhou Q, Chen H, Zhang X, Xie X, et al. Discovery of PF-06873600: A potent and selective allosteric modulator of the dopamine D2 receptor for the treatment of schizophrenia. J Med Chem. 2020;63(19):11821–11834.
43. Luo Z, Dorsey B, Wu Y, He F, Tiwari P, Berry S, et al. Design and optimization of novel, selective, and potent PD-1 inhibitors for the treatment of cancer. J Med Chem. 2021;64(11):5860–5875.
44. Ma Y, Anderson N, Wei Z, Okumura H, Jones N, Ledford E, et al. Discovery of LX9211, a potent orally bioavailable selective inhibitor of spinal cord-specific sodium channel NaV1.7 for the treatment of pain. J Med Chem. 2021;64(10):7012–7029.
45. Maiorov MS, Kirilov SM, Shvets A, Vasilenko I, Barsov EV, et al. Novel antibiotics: A decade of discovery. J Med Chem. 2021;64(7):4658–4678.
46. Marchesi M, Pizzini S, Benassi F, Gotti C, Gentile F, Dondi F, et al. New molecules for Antibacterial resistance: An evolving target. Adv Pharm Bull. 2020;10(4):497–501.
47. Martini K, Jones ME, Keeler AB, Yavuz N, Ellsworth A, Schaeffer J. Targeting autoimmune diseases through receptor modulation. Nat Rev Drug Discov. 2021;20(1):21–36.
48. Martinussen H, Vang S, Mele M, Bonder M, Dumont R. Clinical trials and novel therapeutic strategies for severe diseases: A review of candidate therapeutics. Nature. 2020;578(1):42–46.
49. McDonald H, Mahendran B, Krause MP, Schreiber K, Stout M, Maxwell R. Bortezomib in chronic immune diseases: Novel perspectives. Clin Drug Investig. 2020;40(7):631–642.
50. Mekellea D, Nasser M, Riaz A, Attiya S, Sidiqqi J, Abbas G, et al. Development of new inhibitors for the management of diabetes. Diabetes Ther. 2021;12(7):1665–1680.
51. Mikhailov V, Fedorova O, Gudkov D, Andreev D, Shvets A. Design and development of highly selective inhibitors targeting mcl-1 for cancer therapy. J Med Chem. 2021;64(6):2899–2913.
52. Atmakuri LR, Peeriga R, Begum S, Vallamkonda B, Baratam A. Novel bioanalytical LC-MS/MS method for determination of metoprolol in human plasma. J Appl Pharm Sci. 2024;14(12):131–138.

53. Peeriga R, Venkata Bangaru GK. Implementation of the POCSO act in schools. In: Child Sexual Abuse: A Public Health Problem in India. Springer publications. 2024. p. 391–413. Springer Publications, Singapore.
54. Peeriga R, Yarlagadda LC, Alla NR. Protection of children from sexual exploitation. In: Child Sexual Abuse: A Public Health Problem in India. 2024. p. 191–201. Springer Publications, Singapore.
55. Peeriga R, Shiek Arabath SAM, Manubolu K, Thelappilly BB, Yarlagadda LC. Insilico assessment of phytoconstituents in *myxopyrum smilacifolium* blume against arthritis. Biomed Pharmacol J. 2024;17(1):235–241.
56. Manubolu K, Balagani PK, Gope ER, Peeriga R, Sridevi AR. Unlocking the potential of aquasomes: A comprehensive review on innovative nanocarriers in drug delivery and beyond. Int J Chem Biochem Sci. 2023;24(6):405–410.
57. Manubolu K, Peeriga R, Bonthu MG, Gope ER, Kadirvel D. Evaluation of anti-inflammatory activity of *Millingtonia hortensis* leaf extract. Int J Chem Biochem Sci. 2023;24(6):380–385.
58. Peeriga R, Chandrasekhar KB. Comparative study of anti-inflammatory activity of petroleum ether extract of *myxopyrum smilacifolium* blume and ethanolic leaf extract of *pamburus missionis* swingle. J Pharm Sci Res. 2017;9(6):955–957.
59. Peeriga R, Manubolu K. (2025). Design strategies for waste reduction and enhanced recyclability in pharmaceutical packaging. In: Yingngam, B., Aslam, M.S., Haghi, A.K. (eds) Sustainable Pharmaceutical Product Development and Optimization Processes. Springer, Singapore.
60. Manubolu K, Peeriga R, Chandrasekhar KB. A Short Guide to Clinical Pharmacokinetics. 1st ed. 2024. Springer, Singapore.
61. Manubolu K, Peeriga R. (2025). Ecodesign principles. In: Yingngam, B., Aslam, M.S., Haghi, A.K. (eds) Sustainable Pharmaceutical Product Development and Optimization Processes. Springer, Singapore.

2 Target Identification and Validation

Raveesha Peeriga, Krishnaveni Manubolu, Aminabee Shaik, Saidatri Arige, Jahasultana Mohammed, and Vanukuri Lakshmana Vinod Kumar

Introduction

The drug development sequence requires target identification and validation as its core building blocks to create safe medications. The chapter analyzes procedure advancements by comparing modern advanced technologies to conventional methods used in current target identification and validation processes. The success rate of traditional approaches was limited by their strict dependence on empirical tests, alongside accidental findings that used phenotypic screening methods, which proved inefficient and imprecise.

The arrival of genomes and proteomics brought about a complete transformation in the methods used to identify and validate targets. Genomic technologies provide extensive data about genetic variants including disease pathogenesis analysis through genome-wide association studies (GWAS) and next-generation sequencing (NGS). Studies in proteomics expand biological process comprehension because they examine protein activities while monitoring their expression patterns and functional dynamics. Machine learning artificial intelligence (AI) combined with big data analytics has led to the development of a new age of precision medicine. These technologies deliver precise, rapid identification of new drug targets while also validating their therapeutic capability. Oncology, neurology, cardiovascular, and metabolic illnesses, along with infectious diseases and autoimmune disorders, will be studied regarding their use of these modern techniques in this chapter's examination. The importance of comprehensive validation emerges in this dialogue since it ensures drug development readiness of discovered targets, which leads to modern personalized treatments [1].

Traditional vs. Modern Approaches

The following details describe the comparison between traditional and modern methods which biological research studies to determine their relevance. Drug discovery demands medical progress and disease-related methods of understanding to succeed in this approach.

DOI: 10.4324/9781003564041-2

Traditional Method

Phenotypic Characterization

The control of desired biological activity through phenotyping analyses remains possible without identifying the molecular target. Observing the impact of a substance on a cell or organism phenotype occurs when the substance is applied directly. This assessment method detects therapeutic areas without needing background knowledge [1]. The lack of understanding of mechanisms makes the work process time-consuming for reaching the goal.

Check Targets

Feature-based controls involve medications targeting identified disease mechanism points in biological processes. The evaluation focuses on proteins or nucleic acids because these compounds serve as checks for performance or modification functionality. The method provides valuable comprehension for designing simpler medications. This strategy operates under two premises, which include the importance of target understanding and the potential exclusion of essential but unidentified targets [2].

Animal Model

Animal testing occurs through disease simulations, which assess therapeutic approaches with laboratory animals. Animal research involves both genetically altered subjects along with naturally present animals. Possible environmental diseases are summarized before an evaluation of their practical outcomes takes place. The method requires asking specific behaviors which produce particular results while costing significant money and taking lengthy time periods.

High Throughput Scanning

The present experiment conducts automated screening of extensive biological targets with large libraries. Robotic devices combined with automated systems function to improve information generation. Such systems effectively display major consolidated libraries to potential customers. Expensive equipment together with complex approval standards creates the main challenges of this methodology [3].

Active Management

The development of systems and optimization efforts related to precursors serves to improve potency, selectivity, and pharmacological properties. The structural features of the compound cause a chemical transformation through the structure-activity profile evaluation. The development of better drug properties with enhanced potency stands as one of the required aspects. The process requires synthetic chemistry expertise, and it takes an extended period [4].

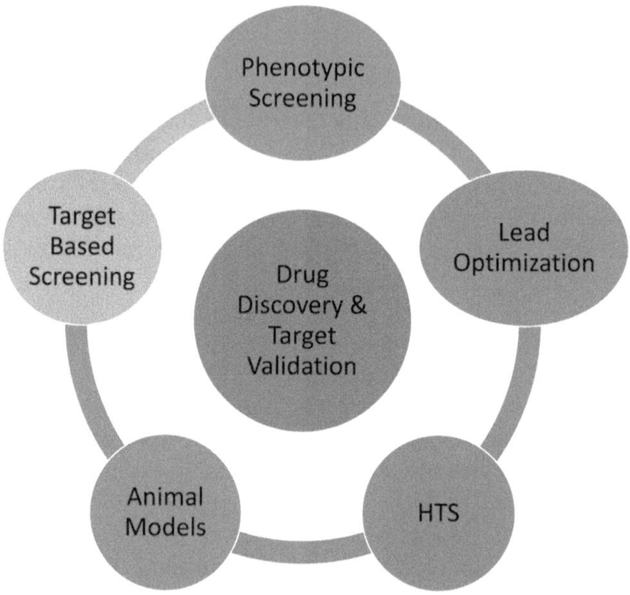

Figure 2.1 Traditional approaches in drug discovery and target validation.

The traditional approaches for drug discovery and target validation appear in Figure 2.1. The illustration in Figure 2.1 presents a summary of traditional drug discovery and target validation procedures which now share the stage with contemporary strategies that deliver additional benefits.

Modern Approaches

Omics Technologies

Disease mechanisms and target identifications benefit from omics technologies through their deployment of genomics, proteomics, metabolomics, etc., analysis techniques. Large-scale molecular datasets are analyzed to discover biomarkers along with potential targets in this observation. This approach allows viewers of disease by providing new target discovery opportunities. The analysis faces two main limitations, including data interpretation complexity along with challenges from multiomics information assimilation [5–7].

The discovery of new drugs heavily depends on omics technologies since they deliver complete biological system information at multiple organizational levels. The collection of omics technologies, which includes genomics along with proteomics and transcriptomics and metabolomics and others, enables scientists to identify targets for drugs and study disease processes for developing novel treatment methods.

Computational Approaches

The drug development process receives optimization through target validation and drug discovery utilizing several in silico techniques that computational approaches deploy. This approach uses computer models and algorithms for predicting toxicity outcomes together with drug-target interactions and their associated pathways. The method includes molecular docking together with network analysis, virtual screening, and additional techniques. A fast screening method uses several data sources at a cost-effective level. The model quality determines that the accuracy requires independent validation [8, 9].

Phenotypic Profiling

The method permits researchers to evaluate how compounds affect several biological activities. A combination of data analysis and phenotypic testing with high-content imaging makes up its operation. The method identifies unexpected targets while it collects sophisticated pharmacological effects. Drawbacks: Target deconvolution; interpretation of phenotypic variations.

Target Engagement Technologies

The evaluation of chemical-target connections in biological systems utilizes Bioluminescence Resonance Energy Transfer (BRET), Cellular Thermal Shift Assay (CETSA) in addition to other such methods [10, 11]. Quantitative analysis enables direct evaluation of compound-target interactions, while physiological involvement benefits from this technique. Nevertheless, it faces tissue penetration limitations and specific method constraints.

Figure 2.2 explains BRET. In BRET, both components include an emitting luciferase and an absorbing fluorescent acceptor molecule. Light emission occurs

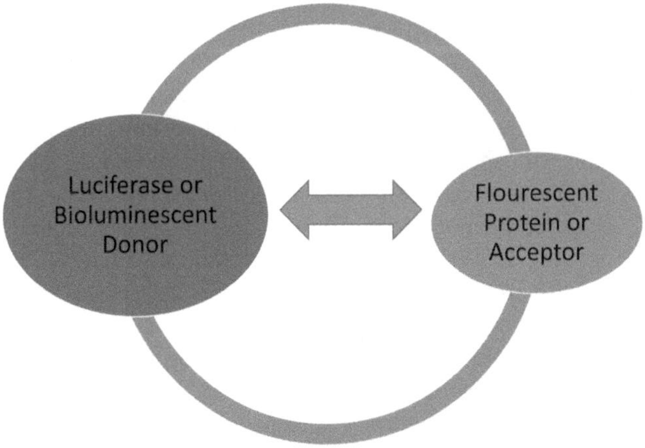

Figure 2.2 Bioluminescence resonance energy transfer.

following energy transfer mechanisms which produce photons with extended wavelength frequencies. Live cells utilize BRET as a detection method to monitor molecular interactions using sensitive high-sensitivity detection without requiring external light sources.

Systems Biology Approaches

The research of genetic, protein, and metabolic molecular networks through systems biology reveals biological processes connection. Scientists utilize computational modeling tools to predict medication-driven effects on selected pathways together with interrelated networks. These methods establish network-focused objectives then they predict how changes will affect the entire system. The method faces two main disadvantages, which include mathematical modeling difficulty alongside prediction verification challenges.

Integration and Future Directions

Integrative Approaches

This approach strengthens target identification and validation through the integration of various methodologies and data sources. The process combines phenotypic screens together with computational forecasts as well as omics data and other methods. The integration strategy enhances treatment success along with improving physicians' ability to select appropriate targets [12, 13]. The complexity of data integration and cross-platform validation presents challenges.

Emerging Technologies

Organoids together with CRISPR-based screening as well as single-cell technologies form an integral part of their platform, which better mimics disease and exposes cellular and molecular pathways. These systems replicate human physiology while locating targets inside relevant environments. The main barriers to overcome in therapeutic environments involve obtaining valid results in therapeutic settings alongside producing methods that scale and maintain uniformity.Drug development depends on established conventional screening approaches, including target-based and phenotypic methods, yet modern omics technologies with computational settings and advanced phenotypic profiling enable improved accuracy alongside system understanding and enhanced efficiency. Multiple strategies must unite to resolve ongoing difficulties while expediting future therapeutic target discovery and complex disease cure development. The next advancement of biomedical investigation and therapeutic innovation will evolve from the union of leading-edge developments and established knowledge.

Table 2.1 provides a clear demonstration of how drug discovery and development moved from traditional methods to modern methodologies due to technological advancements and strategic integration.

Table 2.1 Key aspects of traditional and modern approaches in drug discovery

Aspect	*Traditional approaches*	*Modern approaches*
Technologies	Target-based screening, phenotypic screening	Omics technologies, CRISPR-based screening, single-cell technologies, organoids
Key characteristics	Established methodologies, foundational in drug development	Enhanced accuracy, efficiency, and mechanistic insights
Disease replication	Less accurate replication of human disease	More accurately replicates disease; mimics human physiology
Target location	Identifies targets in general contexts	Identifies targets in pertinent environments
Insights provided	Basic understanding of drug mechanisms and targets	Deeper insights into cellular and molecular pathways
Challenges	May lack precision; limited to certain models and methods	Validation in therapeutic settings, scalability, and uniformity
Future success	Combination of foundational techniques with modern methods	Integration of diverse approaches to solve current problems and accelerate discovery
Impact on research	Solid groundwork for drug development	Shaping the next generation of biomedical research and treatment development

Role of Genomics and Proteomics

Drugs evolve faster through genomics and proteomics, which together provide essential data about both biological disease processes and individual drug responses. The article studies how genomics and proteomics drive drug development while discussing their key function in personal medicine together with their significance for target search together with biomarker detection and treatment improvement.

Genomics in Drug Development

A complete organismal genomic analysis that encompasses every gene and its interrelationships is classified as genomics. The study of complete genomic patterns helps medicine development across multiple critical areas. Genomics can identify individual genetic differences, such as single-nucleotide polymorphisms and other sequences, which influence how drugs function and are processed along with their side effects within patients. Established therapeutic programs become more effective because genetic information allows healthcare providers to customize medical interventions for optimal results with minimal adverse effects [14].

Discovery of New Therapeutic Goals Benefits from genomic studies, which illuminate the genetic basis of diseases. Scientists can detect disease development associations with precise genetic alterations through the utilization of NGS coupled with

GWAS. The detected mutations serve as indicators to direct pharmaceutical companies when making new therapeutic medications.Researchers use Pharmacogenomics to examine the relationship between genetic makeups and drug responses among patients. Research teams use a combined analysis of genetic information alongside drug profiles to anticipate how patients will respond to treatment. The predictive abilities of this field help lower drug side effects, so patients receive safer care.

Drug repositioning becomes possible by observing drug-biological pathway interactions using genomic data, which reveals previously unknown medicinal applications of current medications. Through this approach, drug development becomes faster while expenses decrease by making use of pre-existing data about safety and efficacy.

Proteomics in Drug Development

Proteomics defines the large-scale analysis of protein elements alongside their network relations and structural forms together with their biological system functions. The development of medicine relies heavily on proteomics for the following purposes:

Through the method of proteomics, researchers can validate therapeutic targets that genetic research has discovered. Researchers confirm disease development mechanisms and treatment possibilities through protein expression analysis and post-translational change monitoring [15]. The research of drug mechanisms uses proteomic methods to uncover how prescription products affect cellular pathways and connect with their designated proteins. Research on pharmacological mechanisms of action leads to better combination drug development since it allows scientists to target multiple disease pathways simultaneously. This improves medical efficiency.

The proteomic approach examines drug-caused modifications to biological protein activities and expressions that reveal toxic effects at an early phase. Scientific observations of drug-induced proteome changes help researchers discover upcoming adverse effects and develop solutions to prevent or minimize them.

Combining Proteomics and Genomics

The combination of proteomic data with genomic information enables great prospects in developing precision medicine while speeding up drug discovery. Scientific teams using proteomic profiles together with genomic data gain improved molecular-level understanding of disease causes and pharmaceutic responses. The approach of integrating genome sequences with proteomic data enables researchers to simplify the identification of trustworthy biomarkers and the validation of therapy targets, as well as the customization of specific medical treatments toward patients' specific genomic and proteomic traits [16].

Obstacles and Prospective Paths

The integration of genomic and proteomics data presents barriers for medication research since developers face problems in data integration and methodological standardization alongside ethical requirements for patient information protection and consent. Multifaceted collaboration with new technology advancements and regulatory rules which promote clinical use of proteomics and genomic breakthroughs will help us defeat these obstacles.

Genomics and proteomics serve as vital tools for drug creation during the present era because they enable unmatched opportunities to enhance drug effectiveness and minimize adverse reactions and personalize medicine treatment. Scientists create new treatments which satisfy unmet medical requirements, along with better clinical results across multiple disease types through the combination of proteomics and genetic information [17].

The research "Genome-Based Drug Target Identification in Human Pathogen Streptococcus gallolyticus" relies on both proteomics and genomics technologies to understand antibacterial drug resistance mechanisms as well as treatment target possibilities. Scientists use genome-wide sequencing combined with analysis to determine Streptococcus gallolyticus genetic elements and variants associated with antibiotic resistance. Scientists can detect prospective medication targets within bacterial genomes by analyzing genomic data to reveal antibiotic resistance mechanisms through gene mutation patterns and acquired resistance traits transferred from other organisms.

All protein expressions from Streptococcus gallolyticus enter proteomic assessments, which extend genomic studies. Research teams need to identify proteins, including antibiotic-modifying enzymes and efflux pumps that take part in drug resistance mechanisms. The combination of genomic and protein studies produces a complete molecular understanding of antibacterial treatment resistance in Streptococcus gallolyticus. New therapeutic strategies require specific protein targets from resistance pathways and bacterial protein inhibitors derived from these genomic and proteomic studies to block essential bacterial proteins.

The identification of medicinal targets depends on both proteomics and genomes in functional genomics analysis. Genomics helps target development through whole genome analysis by revealing both disease-related genetic variants as well as pathogenetic mutations and drug response affecting mutations. GWAS together with NGS technologies enable researchers to find new treatment targets. Genomics, when connected with proteomics, allows scientists to explore biological systems completely with full power across genomic variations that influence disease risks, as well as proteomic profiles to guide drug development. Precision medicine advances through target identification improvements because their combination facilitates more efficient and precise target identification work.

Bioactive molecule investigations and therapeutic target validation process in drug discovery rely heavily on genomics and proteomics techniques during target identification and validation steps. The article presents an extensive evaluation of how target validation methods have progressed alongside their contemporary usage patterns for establishing target validation processes in current scientific exploration.

Genomics in Target Validation

Through genomic methods, scientists are able to detect target disease factors by studying all genetic elements in patients. Scientists use GWAS along with NGS and CRISPR-Cas9 gene editing methods to pursue potential drug targets through this approach. GWAS succeeds in discovering genetic variations which enable researchers to locate disease-related pathways through their association with disease development or risk levels.

Recent Advancements in Genomics Have Expanded Its Role in Target Validation Through

This technology enables scientists to profile each solitary cell to expose tissue and disease heterogeneity. Single-cell RNA sequencing (scRNA-seq) and single-cell ATAC-seq (assay for transposase-accessible chromatin using sequencing) deliver precise gene expression pattern and regulatory element data that assists researchers in finding drug target specifications for individual cells [16, 17]. The CRISPR-Cas9 screening method permits large-scale functional analyses by establishing DNA changes to study gene effects on cellular characteristics. The methodology helps identify disease-related essential genes together with affected pathways, which makes them suitable targets for therapeutic interventions.

Through epigenomic mechanisms, the human body controls gene expression without modifying DNA sequence information. The techniques of ChIP-seq and DNA methylation profiling enable researchers to understand how epigenetic modifications affect diseases while helping to identify targets druggable through epigenetic manipulation.

Proteomics in Target Validation

The field of proteomics conducts large-scale protein analysis to determine both expression profiles and post-translational transformations together with protein-to-protein bonds and cellular distribution patterns. The field of proteomics has achieved a substantial advancement through new technologies that permit full-scale protein profiles under various circumstances and drug treatment responses.

Key Proteomic Techniques in Target Validation Include

Mass spectrometry (MS)-based proteomics techniques evaluate protein levels as well as changes in proteins to detect drug-target connections alongside biomarker identification. The drug-specific effects become distinguishable through comparative analyses enabled by stable isotope labeling by amino acids in cell culture and tandem mass tag, which are quantitative proteomics methods.

Determination of atomic resolution protein structures occurs through three spectroscopic methods, including X-ray crystallography, cryo-electron microscopy (cryo-EM), and nuclear magnetic resonance (NMR) spectroscopy. Knowledge of drug-target interactions from structural analyses enables developers to create improved medications.

The techniques of yeast two-hybrid assays, combined with co-immunoprecipitation together with MS methods allow researchers to create protein-protein interaction networks in interactomics studies. Research investigations reveal the paths through which proteins signal to other molecules while uncovering therapeutic target proteins for medical treatment.

Integration of Genomics and Proteomics

Target validation becomes more efficient when genomic and proteomic data are integrated because it delivers supplementary insights about gene expression patterns along with protein functionality and network interactions. The combined data approach builds speed up drug target validation while simultaneously enhancing knowledge of drug operating mechanisms.

The combination of various multiomics fields integrates genomic and transcriptomic and proteomic, and metabolomic data for complete biological system evaluation. Research methods that merge different types of omics data reveal disease-related molecular processes and therapeutic targets for drug development.

Network-based approaches in Network Pharmacology analyze biological networks to determine drug-target interactions along with detecting off-target side effects. The identification of candidate targets through computational tools happens using pathway enrichment analysis in combination with network visualization platforms that consider biological significance levels of network connectivity.

AI together with machine learning (ML) processes large-scale omics datasets to detect drug-target connections while enhancing drug creation methods and discovering biomarkers. Deep learning systems combine genomic information with proteomic findings along with clinical data to create patient groups for improved therapeutic decisions [18].

Challenges and Future Directions

The revolutionary advancements in genomics and proteomics for target validation continue to bring forth multiple technical hurdles that need resolution. Data integration for various omics datasets requires standardized analytical pipelines with computational tools for both robust analysis alongside interpretation. Advanced technologies must capture dynamic expression changes of genes and proteins because biological systems have complex regulatory networks along with cellular heterogeneity.

Data privacy and ethical norms limit how genomic and proteomic information can be utilized through research and clinical work, which calls for proper security measures and consent protocols. The advancement of target validation depends on improving single-cell technologies along with spatial omics techniques and AI-driven predictive modeling approaches. Novel technologies will improve the methods for identifying targets and shorten drug development timelines while allowing healthcare providers to create patient-specific medical solutions.

Emerging Targets and Therapeutic Areas

Drug discovery experiences an ongoing revolution because of the advanced technologies developed in AI, ML, and data science. Modern technologies transform drug target identification procedures in research labs, which drives scientists to explore engaging new drug targets across emerging therapeutic fields with the potential to tackle unmet clinical requirements.

Precision Medicine and Genetic Targets

The fundamental transformation in drug discovery involves precision medicine because it provides treatments adapted to individual patients based on their genetic information. Genomic breakthroughs together with bioinformatics advancements create the possibility to practice this approach. Genetic mutations together with different variations can be identified through high-throughput sequencing methods by researchers. Targeted therapy development for chronic myeloid leukemia received its breakthrough through identifying specific mutations in cancer cells that revealed the BCR-ABL fusion gene as the focusing target [19].

Immuno-oncology

Research involving immuno-oncology explores strategies to use natural immune system defense mechanisms to combat cancer cells. Significant therapeutic effects have emerged in oncological diseases through immune checkpoint inhibitor drugs, which act upon PD-1/PD-L1 and CTLA-4 pathways [20]. AI and ML systems speed up the process of finding new immunological treatment targets through massive analysis of genomic, transcriptomic, and proteomic information for identifying therapeutic markers.

Neurological Disorders

The process of identifying drug targets for neurological disorders remained difficult throughout the years because both the brain tissue density and the blood-brain barrier pose evaluation challenges. Modern advancements in technology create new possibilities for medical treatment approaches. Research based on AI analysis of extensive genetic information has led to the discovery of fresh treatment objectives which help combat Alzheimer's and Parkinson's together with other neurodegenerative diseases. These diseases have developed and deployed monoclonal antibodies along with small molecules for modifying the activity of tau and alpha-synuclein through their identification as disease-causing proteins [21].

Infectious Diseases and Antimicrobial Resistance

Global health care faces two critical challenges, which include new infectious diseases appearing and increasing antimicrobial resistance levels. Intelligent systems utilize data science to discover fresh antibiotic targets, which leads to creating innovative antibiotic medicines. Through ML modeling approaches, scientists can detect bacterial resistance patterns as well as discover new drug substances that use unique actions to combat bacteria. The COVID-19 pandemic demonstrated the urgent need for fast drug development, while AI systems succeeded in performing drug repurposing research to find effective treatments against the virus.

Metabolic Disorders

The worldwide health challenges include two metabolic disorders, which are diabetes and obesity. Therapies require new targets in metabolic pathways for their successful development. New technological developments within systems biology along with computational modeling assist research teams to construct detailed pictures of elaborate metabolic networks, which guide them to specific interventional nodes for therapeutic purposes. GLP-1 (glucagon-like peptide-1) receptor agonists serve as new therapeutic agents for type 2 diabetes following their discovery [22, 23].

Cardiovascular Diseases

Heart conditions known as cardiovascular diseases (CVD) continue to be worldwide leaders in causing disability along with fatalities. Lipid metabolism together with inflammation and thrombosis are the new targets scientists explore in these studies. GWAS identified new genetic traits which link to CVD, so researchers can develop new drugs for the condition. Analytical systems based on AI spend their operation time studying electronic health records in conjunction with imaging data to detect biomarkers which help forecast cardiovascular risk and treatment effects [24–27].

Open Targets Platform Demonstrates How Uniting Targets with Their Corresponding Therapeutic Areas

The drug research field is changing quickly because platforms like Open Targets continue to make significant progress in discovery. Open Targets functions as a combined project that utilizes substantial biological and biomedical information to help researchers identify along with validate new therapeutic targets. The analysis conducted by Open Targets unveils several promising future targets and therapeutic domains which represent present-day developments within the drug discovery field [28–33].

Cancer Therapeutics

Heart conditions known as CVD continue to be worldwide leaders in causing disability, along with fatalities. Lipid metabolism together with inflammation and thrombosis are the new targets scientists explore in these studies. GWAS identified new genetic traits which link to CVD, so researchers can develop new drugs for the condition. Analytical systems based on AI spend their operation time studying electronic health records in conjunction with imaging data to detect biomarkers which help forecast cardiovascular risk and treatment effects.

Open Targets Platform Demonstrates How Uniting Targets with Their Corresponding Therapeutic Areas

The drug research field is changing quickly because platforms like Open Targets continue to make significant progress in discovery. Open Targets functions as a combined project that utilizes substantial biological and biomedical information to help researchers identify along with validating new therapeutic targets. The analysis conducted by Open Targets unveils several promising future targets and therapeutic domains which represent present-day developments within the drug discovery field.

Neurodegenerative Diseases

Neurodegenerative diseases, which include Alzheimer's disease together with Parkinson's disease and Huntington's disease represent treatment areas with substantial medical demand unmet. Leads in research that associates targets with these conditions by examining genetic information together with proteomic information. Tau and amyloid-beta protein functions are better understood through Open Targets, which supports antibody and molecule discovery to control these proteins' activity levels. Through its research, the platform discovered genetic mutations of LRRK2 and GBA, which opened new possibilities for specific treatments in Parkinson's disease.

Cardiovascular Diseases

Current research shows that CVD functions as one of the leading mortality agents across the world. The Open Targets platform utilizes genetic data obtained from GWAS examinations to find new potential targets for CVD treatment. Research on PCSK9's cholesterol metabolism function enabled scientists to create LDL cholesterol-reducing PCSK9 inhibitors. Through genetic variant discoveries, the platform helps develop modern CVD treatment strategies that serve to decrease cardiovascular risks.

Metabolic Disorders

Diabetes as well as obesity constitute substantial health obstacles to human well-being. Through data analysis of biological systems which operate in metabolism, Open Targets helps identify fresh targets for treatment. Open Targets recognized and focused on GLP-1 (glucagon-like peptide-1) receptors to develop type 2 diabetes treatment medication, GLP-1 agonists. The platform explores metabolic pathways which guide strategies for treating obesity alongside metabolic syndrome.

Infectious Diseases

Medical researchers urgently confront two essential health issues involving infectious diseases alongside antimicrobial resistance. Using genomic information, Open Targets identifies bacterial and viral targets, which leads to new antibiotic development and antiviral medications. Through its use, researchers have identified essential drug targets within Mycobacterium tuberculosis, which causes tuberculosis disease. The platform unites information about pathogen-host interactions to discover targets which researchers use for disrupting such interactions while seeking new infection combat methods.

Immunological Disorders

Open Targets devotes attention to investigating autoimmune and inflammatory diseases as part of its operational framework. Through integrated immune-related pathway data, the platform helps researchers identify targets which could become therapeutic candidates. Through its analyses, Open Targets determined that cytokines IL-6 and TNF-alpha, with their receptors, play central roles in autoimmune conditions such as rheumatoid arthritis and inflammatory bowel disease. Scientists have achieved major patient outcome improvements through their development of inhibitors that target these particular molecules.

Conclusion

Drug discovery becomes more effective due to technological and data scientific advancements, which enable crucial therapeutic target validation procedures. The drug target discovery potential becomes clear through Open Targets and similar platforms that use genomic, proteomic, and biomedical datasets in large-scale integrative analysis. The comprehensive methodology promotes better disease understanding through deep analysis of disease processes, natural pathways, and gene involvement in medical conditions.

The combination of AI and ML technologies with emerging technology platforms has transformed target identification through rapid and precise analysis of massive datasets. New therapeutic approaches become faster to develop through technologies that reveal hidden targets and reuse previously approved medications.

Targeted strategies within therapeutic areas that include cancer and neurodegenerative diseases together with CVD and metabolic disorders as well as infectious diseases and immunological disorders, successfully generate many promising therapeutic targets. The ultimate ratification of these targets by preclinical and clinical research demonstrates their readiness for drug development projects.

Precision medicine enhances the necessity of target validation because it produces individualized treatments based on genetic profiles for more efficient and personalized therapy. The implementation of this methodology results in superior patient results and lowers the occurrence of harmful side effects. The combination of technological progress and data unification systems drives substantial breakthroughs in target detection together with validation processes. Pharmaceutical innovation through these technologies creates an expanding possibility to develop precise and personified medical treatments that can address unmet healthcare requirements with enhanced efficiency.

References

1. Prior M, Chiruta C, Currais A, Goldberg J, Ramsey J, Dargusch R, et al. Back to the future with phenotypic screening. ACS Chem Neurosci. 2014;5(7):503–513.
2. Vottero E, Balgi A, Woods K, Tugendreich S, Melese T, Andersen RJ, et al. Inhibitors of human indoleamine 2,3-dioxygenase identified with a target-based screen in yeast. Biotechnol J. 2006;1(3):282–288.
3. Banks MN, Cacace AM, O'Connell J, Houston JG. High-Throughput screening: Evolution of technology and methods. Drug Discov Handb. 2005;24:559–602.
4. Scognamiglio PL, Perretta G, Marasco D. The role of automation in the identification of new bioactive compounds. In: Automation. IntechOpen; 2012.
5. Temml V, Kutil Z. Structure-based molecular modeling in SAR analysis and lead optimization. Comput Struct Biotechnol J. 2021;19:1431–1444.
6. Wheelock CE, Goss VM, Balgoma D, Nicholas B, Brandsma J, Skipp PJ, et al. Application of omics technologies to biomarker discovery in inflammatory lung diseases. Eur Respir J. 2013;42(3):802–825.
7. Matthews H, Hanison J, Nirmalan N. "Omics"-informed drug and biomarker discovery: Opportunities, challenges and future perspectives. Proteomes. 2016;4(3):28.
8. Duarte Y, Márquez-Miranda V, Miossec MJ, González-Nilo F. Integration of target discovery, drug discovery and drug delivery: A review on computational strategies. Wiley Interdiscip Rev Nanomed Nanobiotechnol. 2019;11(4):e1554.
9. Kar S, Leszczynski J. Recent advances of computational modeling for predicting drug metabolism: A perspective. Curr Drug Metab. 2017;18(12):1106–1122.
10. Robers MB, Vasta JD, Corona CR, Ohana RF, Hurst R, Jhala MA, et al. Quantitative, real-time measurements of intracellular target engagement using energy transfer. Syst Chem Biol Methods Protoc. 2019:1888: 45–71.
11. Phillipou AN, Lay CS, Carver CE, Messenger C, Evans JP, Lewis AJ, et al. Cellular target engagement approaches to monitor epigenetic reader domain interactions. SLAS Discov. 2020;25(2):163–175.
12. Acharya D, Mukhopadhyay A. A comprehensive review of machine learning techniques for multi-omics data integration: Challenges and applications in precision oncology. Brief Funct Genomics. 2024: 23(5):elae013.
13. Paananen J, Fortino V. An omics perspective on drug target discovery platforms. Brief Bioinform. 2020;21(6):1937–1953.
14. Crutchfield CA, Thomas SN, Sokoll LJ, Chan DW. Advances in mass spectrometry-based clinical biomarker discovery. Clin Proteomics. 2016;13:1–2.
15. Meissner F, Geddes-McAlister J, Mann M, Bantscheff M. The emerging role of mass spectrometry-based proteomics in drug discovery. Nat Rev Drug Discov. 2022;21(9):637–654.
16. Carter B, Zhao K. The epigenetic basis of cellular heterogeneity. Nat Rev Genet. 2021;22(4):235–250.
17. Erbe R, Kessler MD, Favorov AV, Easwaran H, Gaykalova DA, Fertig EJ. Matrix factorization and transfer learning uncover regulatory biology across multiple single-cell ATAC-seq data sets. Nucleic Acids Res. 2020;48(12):e68.
18. Koromina M, Pandi MT, Patrinos GP. Rethinking drug repositioning and development with artificial intelligence, machine learning, and omics. Omics. 2019;23(11):539–548.

19. Koldehoff M. Targeting bcr-abl transcripts with siRNAs in an imatinib-resistant chronic myeloid leukemia patient: Challenges and future directions. RNA Interference: Challenges and Therapeutic Opportunities. 2015;1218: 277–292.
20. Liu J, Chen Z, Li Y, Zhao W, Wu J, Zhang Z. PD-1/PD-L1 checkpoint inhibitors in tumor immunotherapy. Front Pharmacol. 2021;12:731798.
21. Colombo D, Pnevmatikou P, Melloni E, Keywood C. Therapeutic innovation in Parkinson's disease: A 2020 update on disease-modifying approaches. Expert Rev Neurother. 2020;20(10):1047–1064.
22. Ahrén B. Glucagon-like peptide-1 receptor agonists for type 2 diabetes: A rational drug development. J Diabetes Investig. 2019;10(2):196–201.
23. Zhang Y, Ng PK, Kucherlapati M, Chen F, Liu Y, Tsang YH, et al. A pan-cancer proteogenomic atlas of PI3K/AKT/mTOR pathway alterations. Cancer Cell. 2017;31(6):820–832.
24. Atmakuri LR, Peeriga R, Begum S, Vallamkonda B, Baratam A. Novel bioanalytical LC-MS/MS method for determination of metoprolol in human plasma. J Appl Pharm Sci. 2024;14(12):131–138.
25. Peeriga R, Venkata Bangaru GK. Implementation of the POCSO act in schools. In: Child Sexual Abuse: A Public Health Problem in India. Springer Publications, Singapore. 2024. p. 391–413.
26. Peeriga R, Yarlagadda LC, Alla NR. Protection of children from sexual exploitation. In: Child Sexual Abuse: A Public Health Problem in India. Springer Publications, Singapore 2024. p. 191–201.
27. Peeriga R, Shiek Arabath SAM, Manubolu K, Thelappilly BB, Yarlagadda LC. Insilico assessment of phytoconstituents in *myxopyrum smilacifolium* blume against arthritis. Biomed Pharmacol J. 2024;17(1):235–241.
28. Manubolu K, Balagani PK, Gope ER, Peeriga R, Sridevi AR. Unlocking the potential of aquasomes: A comprehensive review on innovative nanocarriers in drug delivery and beyond. Int J Chem Biochem Sci. 2023;24(6):405–410.
29. Manubolu K, Peeriga R, Bonthu MG, Gope ER, Kadirvel D. Evaluation of anti-inflammatory activity of *Millingtonia hortensis* leaf extract. Int J Chem Biochem Sci. 2023;24(6):380–385.
30. Peeriga R, Chandrasekhar KB. Comparative study of anti inflammatory activity of petroleum ether extract of *Myxopyrum smilacifolium* Blume and ethanolic leaf extract of *Pamburus missionis* Swingle. J Pharm Sci Res. 2017;9(6):955–957.
31. Peeriga R, Manubolu K (2025). Design strategies for waste reduction and enhanced recyclability in pharmaceutical packaging. In: Yingngam, B., Aslam, M.S., Haghi, A.K. (eds) Sustainable Pharmaceutical Product Development and Optimization Processes. Springer, Singapore.
32. Manubolu K, Peeriga R, Chandrasekhar KB. A Short Guide to Clinical Pharmacokinetics. 1st ed. 2024. Springer. Singapore.
33. Manubolu K, Peeriga R (2025). Ecodesign principles. In: Yingngam, B., Aslam, M.S., Haghi, A.K. (eds) Sustainable Pharmaceutical Product Development and Optimization Processes. Springer, Singapore.

3 High Throughput Screening (HTS) and Phenotypic Screening

C.K. Ashok Kumar, Raveesha Peeriga, Krishnaveni Manubolu, Saidatri Arige, Vanukuri Lakshmana Vinod Kumar, and Morla Devika

Introduction

Discovering drugs requires scientists to identify potential therapeutic molecules for disease management. Systematic testing of numerous compounds known as screening plays an essential role in drug discovery methods to detect substances with wanted biological activities. History shows that High Throughput Screening (HTS) and Phenotypic Screening have developed into two advanced screening methods which streamline drug discovery by effectively identifying therapeutic medications with high precision and speed [1,2].

From Figure 3.1, HTS is a critical technique in drug discovery that enables rapid testing of large libraries of compounds to identify potential drug candidates. The HTS process involves several key steps:

1. Compound Library Preparation: A diverse set of chemical compounds or biological molecules is prepared for screening.
2. Assay Development: Biological assays are designed to detect specific interactions, often using automated systems to handle large volumes.
3. Screening: Thousands to millions of compounds are tested in parallel, with automated systems conducting assays and measuring responses.
4. Hit Identification: Compounds that show activity are identified as "hits" for further validation.
5. Hit Confirmation: The identified hits are retested to confirm their activity and rule out false positives.
6. Lead Optimization: Promising hits undergo further modification to improve potency, selectivity, and drug-like properties.

Overview of Screening in Drug Discovery

Protective measures serve as an essential basis which drives early drug discovery development. Testing large collections of substances and biological components, and natural materials allows identification of candidates which modify particular biological routes or targeted elements. Screening.

DOI: 10.4324/9781003564041-3

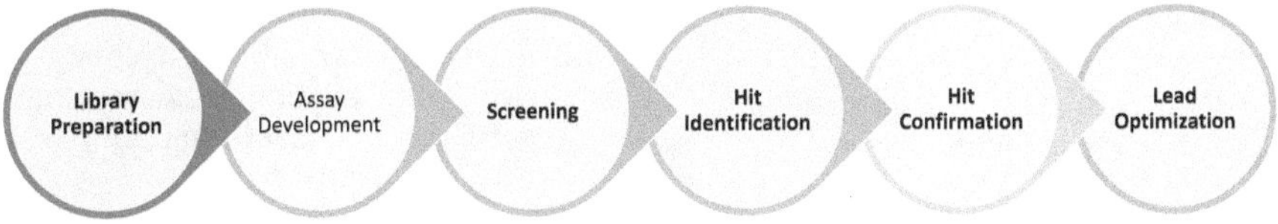

Figure 3.1 High Throughput Screening process.

Methodologies Are Broadly Classified into Two Types

Target-based screening identifies specific molecular targets including proteins, enzymes, or receptors so it can detect compounds that act on target activity [3]. This screening method works with compounds which alter cellular or organismal characteristics without naming the target molecule beforehand.

The methodology selection for drug development depends on disease type and target availability, together with therapeutic goals.

Importance of HTS and Phenotypic Screening

HTS and Phenotypic Screening Have Transformed Drug Discovery by Addressing Key Challenges

Efficiency: HTS allows rapid testing of millions of compounds, expediting lead identification.

Diversity: These methods explore extensive chemical libraries, increasing the likelihood of novel compound discovery.

Biological Relevance: Phenotypic screening focuses on functional outcomes, which often lead to first-in-class drugs.

Target Discovery: Phenotypic approaches help uncover novel drug targets for diseases with complex mechanisms.

By integrating these methodologies, researchers can leverage the strengths of both approaches to enhance the drug discovery pipeline).

Principles of HTS

Definition and Historical Background

HTS serves as a drug discovery method for quick biological target interaction screening of extensive substance libraries. The efficiency of HTS depends on automated experiment processes and they help scientists screen thousands to millions of compounds [4]. HTS appeared during the late 1980s before becoming more popular in the 1990s because of robotic developments and improved assay creation and data analysis techniques. The platform started working with biochemical assays during its initial phase but later added cell-based and phenotypic testing protocols. The development of HTS technology expanded its scope to enable scientists to investigate established and new targets during drug discovery projects (Figure 3.2).

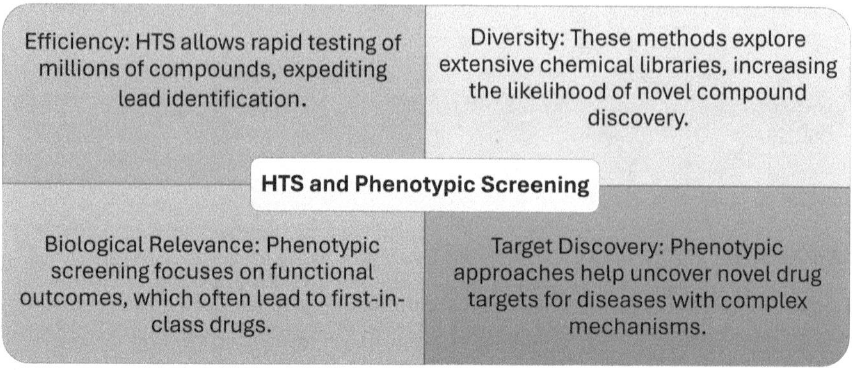

Figure 3.2 Importance of HTS and phenotypic screening.

Key Components of HTS

The success of HTS relies on three key components.

Assay Development

Large-scale testing needs assays with reliable performance and consistent results, and the ability to scale operations.

Two main assay categories exist: biochemical assays encompass activities of enzymes and binding processes, whereas cell-based assays contain reporter gene assessments together with viability testing. The success of HTS 6 depends on a proper assessment of parameters for sensitivity, specificity, and dynamic range.

Library Design

The chemical substances comprising HTS libraries encompass small molecules and both natural products and biologics. Libraries benefit from targeting special chemical scaffolds combined with target classes since this approach enables maximized hit identification [5–7]. Diversity-oriented library collections enhance the discovery of fresh chemical entities.

Detection Technologies

The detection techniques help scientists measure biological actions and molecular relationship data. The detectable signals obtained from analytical methods incorporate fluorescence, luminescence, absorbance and mass spectrometry.

A system requiring both sensitivity at a high level alongside quick data collection capabilities proves essential for obtaining accurate data measurements promptly. Figure 3.3. illustrates the three foundational components essential for the success of HTS.

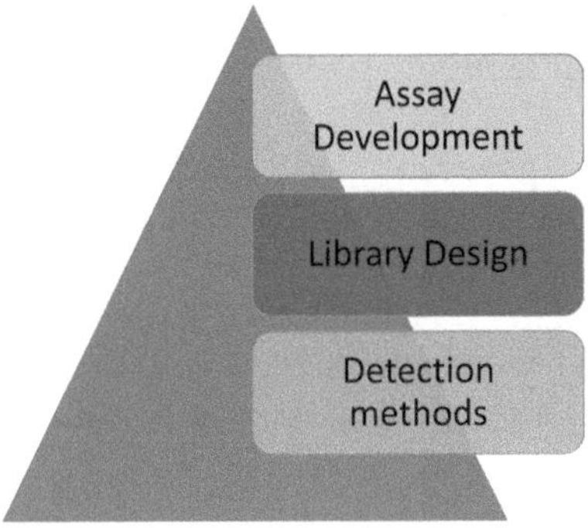

Figure 3.3 Key components of HTS.

Target-based Screening vs. Phenotypic Screening

HTS can be broadly classified into two approaches based on the screening objective:

Target-based Screening

Focuses on a predefined biological target, such as a receptor, enzyme, or protein.

Research laboratories screen compounds to determine their influence over target characteristics, seeking either inhibitory or activating effects [8]. The approach provides six advantages through its well-defined substance-effect connections and its immediate connection to basic molecular processes. The screening approach displays known target bias, which might prevent the detection of intricate biological relationships.

Phenotypic Screening

Researchers assess compounds by observing their effects on cell, tissue or organism behavior without knowing the specific target [9]. First-class medications and innovative methods of action become discoverable during this process. Target deconvolution serves as a demanding and resource-intensive obstacle for identifying the molecular target. The specificity advantage belongs to target-based screening, but phenotypic screening provides a broader biological relevance. Decision-making between these screening methods depends on research requirements and disease intricacy together with resource availability.

Principles of Phenotypic Screening

Overview and Historical Context

The drug discovery method known as phenotypic screening detects active compounds through testing their effects on cellular levels, tissues, and whole organisms, even when target identity remains unknown [10]. The method diverges from target-based screening since it refuses to focus on particular biological targets.

Phenotypic screening powered drug discovery initiatives during past centuries as scientists used this method to find penicillin and aspirin, and other notable drugs. The middle portion of the twentieth century marked the start of target-based screening with the rise of molecular biology technology. The resurgence of phenotypic screening occurred because it identifies new therapeutic mechanisms while targeting advanced diseases, including cancer and neurodegenerative disorders.

Cell-based Assays and Organotypic Models

Phenotypic screening requires reliable and disease state simulation models that maintain biological validity. Two key types of models are:

Cell-based Assays

Experimental methods utilize either primary cells or immortalized cell lines together with stem cell-derived models.

The analysis uses specific end points that measure cell viability alongside proliferation along with differentiation along with migration together with morphology evaluation [11].

High-content imaging methods together with advanced techniques offer extensive knowledge of cellular responses that support multiparametric analysis.

Organotypic Models

These methods should duplicate the three-dimensional organization and operation of tissues or organs. Current examples of developing these models include organoids together with spheroids and microfluidic systems, which represent "organ-on-chip" models. These models create a link between in vitro laboratory tests and real-life animal studies, thus improving their clinical relevance. Phenotypic screening benefits from these models to detect compounds that provide complete therapeutic potential by capturing biological system intricacy.

Biomarker Discovery and Validation

Phenotypic screening depends on biomarkers to function as detectable indicators of biological processes, which track treatment responses according to research [12]. Biomarker discovery and validation involve:

Discovery

Phenotypic screens collect broad data about changes that occur within cells or living organisms.

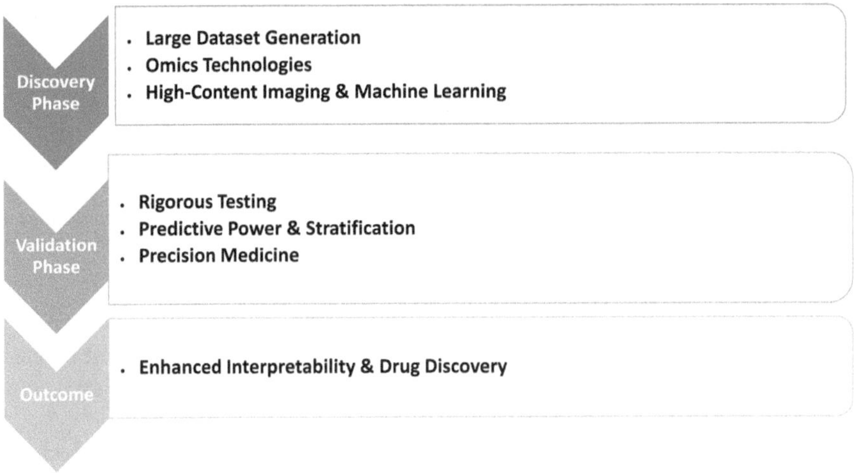

Figure 3.4 Biomarker discovery and validation in phenotypic screening.

Advanced omics technologies including genomics proteomics and metabolomics help locate biomarkers that show links to phenotypic outcomes. Researchers typically use high-content imaging systems together with machine learning (ML) methods to detect minor yet meaningful phenotypic changes.

Validation

After researchers identify potential biomarkers, these entities undergo standardized tests in separate experiments to validate accuracy and significance. Prediction of treatment effectiveness and classification of patient groups as well as identification of therapeutic targets belong to biomarker applications. The process of validating biomarkers leads to enhanced interpretation of phenotypic screening outcomes, which supports the development of precise treatments for patients.

Phenotypic screening backed by advanced cellular models along with biomarker tools serves as a vital method for first-in-class drug development while tackling diseases with complex pathophysiology [13].

Figure 3.4 depicts biomarker discovery and validation processes that take place throughout phenotypic screening. Multiple cutting-edge technologies including omics, high-content imaging, and ML help discover biomarkers through comprehensive validation methods, which enable precision medicine development.

Applications of HTS

Table 3.1 summarizes the primary applications of HTS and highlights their significance in modern drug discovery and development.

Table 3.1 Applications of HTS

Application	*Description*	*Key benefit*
Drug discovery	Identifies and optimizes hits.	Accelerates drug development.
Novel chemical entities (NCEs)	Finds unique therapeutic compounds.	Enables first-in-class drugs.
Toxicity profiling	Assesses safety using HCS.	Reduces late-stage failures.

Drug Discovery and Development

Modern drug discovery techniques rely on HTS as their main assessment method because it helps researchers evaluate many chemical compounds for therapeutic potential. The primary applications include:

An automated screening method known as HTS detects compounds which either bind to designated biological targets or generate preferred phenotypic changes. The hits obtained from this stage function as fundamental starting points for lead optimization work. The hit identification process continues through successive screening to optimize the effectiveness and VIP qualities, and metabolic characteristics of compounds [14]. The human target screening assays establish target validity by showing their precise role in disease pathways for continuous research and development. The implementation of HTS automation combined with its scalability shortens the period needed to identify drug candidates, thus speeding up the drug development lifecycle. Research conducted by pharmaceutical and academic researchers becomes more efficient and precise when HTS begins during early drug discovery stages to evaluate a wide chemical space systematically.

Identification of NCEs

HTS serves as a fundamental method to discover NCEs with distinctive structures together with their specific mechanisms of action. HTS-based identification of compounds happens through various chemical libraries, which contain: Drug screening operations that use natural products from microorganisms or plants, or marine life, generate bioactive compounds for therapeutic applications. Synthetic molecules exist in libraries which researchers screen for their biological target interactions. Testing smaller discrete molecular fragments within fragment-based libraries helps scientists discover the first stage of bindings that lead to complete, finalized drug candidates. Through its diverse screening methodology, HTS improves the chance of finding original drug candidates which -can bypass resistance factors in current treatment approaches.

High-content Screening for Toxicity Profiling

The automated imaging system called high-content screening (HCS) measures biological effects and toxicity of compounds through multiparametric analysis [15,16]. Applications in toxicity profiling include: Chemical effects affecting

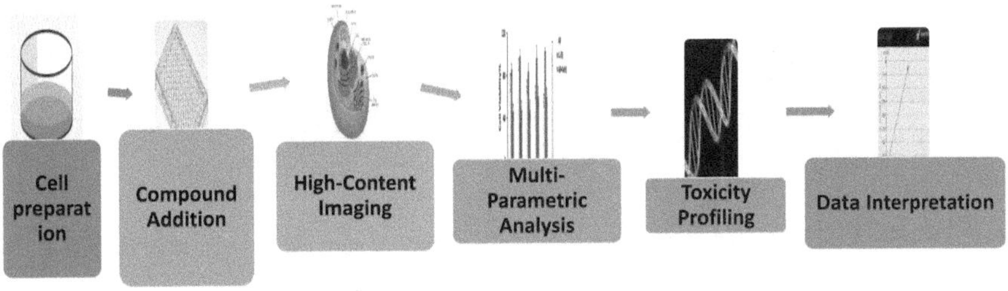

Figure 3.5 HCS for toxicity profiling.

cellular survival together with cell shape changes and internal structural damage are assessed using HCS techniques [17]. The analysis detects unexpected protein interactions which reduce the potentially dangerous side effects. Detecting toxic compounds in early drug development reduces the chances of late-stage failure in drug development. The application of HCS to organoids and microtissues leads to enhanced in vivo toxicity prediction through 3D toxicology modeling, which yields superior results than 2D cell cultures. The compound-screening process becomes stronger because detailed information about drug profiles is added, which selects only effective, safe compounds to progress through clinical trial stages.

The applications enable HTS to transform drug discovery by simplifying therapeutic compound identification and assessment including optimization stages.

Figure 3.5 illustrates the workflow of HCS for toxicity profiling. It begins with cell preparation, followed by compound addition to the test system. High-content imaging captures cellular responses, which are analyzed for multiparametric data like viability and morphology. The final step involves toxicity profiling and data interpretation.

Applications of Phenotypic Screening

Disease Pathway Identification

Phenotypic screening serves as an important discovery method to identify completely new disease pathways along with their mechanisms of action [18]. Phenotypic screening discovers compounds through their biological effects, which enables researchers to understand complex disease processes. Key contributions include The discovery method brings unbiased results because it lacks any predefined targets, which enables researchers to find novel disease progression pathways, therefore [19]. Phenotypic screening provides efficient analysis for disorders with multiple contributing factors, like neurodegenerative diseases and diabetes and cardiovascular disorders. Tests conducted in phenotypic screens generate hits that developers utilize to both confirm and enhance existing disease simulation methods.

The illustration divides target-based from phenotypic approaches to drug discovery presented in Figure 3.6. This demonstration shows that target-based screening works through special molecular targets, yet phenotypic screening evaluates compounds through their cellular or organismal effects on phenotypes. Ostíles

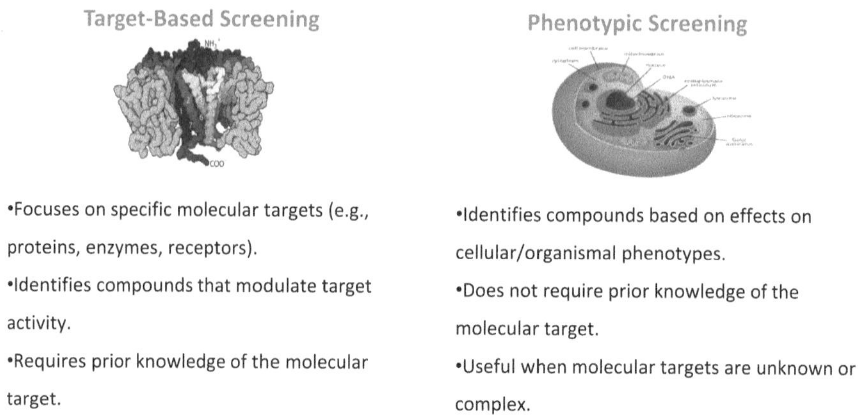

Figure 3.6 Target-based vs. phenotypic screening.

selection relies on both disease settings and therapeutic aims. This analytic method plays an essential role in understanding complex biological diseases that enables researchers to find new opportunities for treatment.

The summary of important phenotypic screening contributions in drug discovery appears in Table 3.2. The technique reveals new clinical pathway discoveries and works in complex disease cases and confirms therapeutic mechanism effects. The screening strategy stands crucial for understanding intricate biological procedures and improving therapeutic advancements.

Rare Disease and Repurposing Studies

Phenotypic screening has become indispensable in rare disease research and drug repurposing efforts:

Rare Diseases

Few rare diseases receive insufficient molecular research, which leads to undefined target opportunities. Phenotypic screening eliminates this challenge through

Table 3.2 Key contributions of phenotypic screening in drug discovery

Key contribution	*Description*
Unbiased discovery	Allows identification of novel pathways without relying on predefined targets, revealing unknown mechanisms of disease progression.
Multifactorial diseases	Effective in studying complex diseases like neurodegenerative disorders, diabetes, and cardiovascular conditions involving multiple pathways.
Validation of mechanisms	Hits from phenotypic screens help validate or refine disease models, improving understanding of disease biology.

its method of evaluating direct observations of organisms or cells which produce phenotypes [19,20]. Through this approach, scientists find medications which can modify disease traits when effective therapeutic targets remain unknown. The research makes use of patient-derived cells including induced pluripotent stem cells (iPSCs) to replicate specific phenotypes in disease conditions.

Drug Repurposing

The process of phenotypic screening discovers alternative medical applications for current drugs through the examination of disease models. The development timeline shortens when scientists repurpose drugs because the drugs already have proven safety data, which lowers both the development expenses and launch duration. Thalidomide found success in multiple myeloma treatment, while sildenafil (Viagra) was first created to treat cardiovascular issues before it received approval.

Applications in Immunotherapy and Oncology

Phenotypic screening is extensively applied in immunotherapy and cancer research to develop cutting-edge treatments:

Cancer Therapies

Phenotypic screening methods help scientists identify chemical substances that specifically eliminate cancer cells while modifying tumor-related cellular environments.

Using advanced methods like 3D spheroids and organoids allows scientists to build more complex models, which makes screening outcomes easier to transfer [21–23].

Research seeks to detect compounds that prevent metastasis spread and compounds, which promote immune cell-mediated tumor destruction.

Immunotherapy

Phenotypic tests help determine agents to improve immune responses through checkpoint inhibitors or T-cell activators. Cell-based methods evaluate the relationships between cancer cells and immune cells, which assists development of new immunotherapy treatments.

Cytokine profiling combined with high-content imaging enables researchers to find immune-modulating drugs through their screening process [24]. Drug discovery innovation advances through phenotypic screening because it offers important bio-relevant data, which opens new therapeutic options, particularly for challenging fields including cancer treatments and rare disease research.

Advancements in Automation and Robotics in Screening

Table 3.3 depicts revolutionary changes in screening technology enabled by automation and robotics technology. The field of drug discovery benefits from robotic systems that handle plates and dispense liquids as well as AI analytics and compact

Table 3.3 Advancements in automation and robotics in screening

Section	*Advancements*	*Impact*
Robotic systems in HTS	• Automated plate handling ensures consistency. • Robotic liquid dispensers deliver high precision.	• Reduces manual errors. • Increases throughput and scalability for large-scale compound screening.
AI and ML in data analysis	• ML identifies patterns in complex data. • AI prioritizes hits and enables predictive modeling.	• Enhances decision-making. • Accelerates hit validation and reduces false positives.
Miniaturization technologies	• Microfluidic systems reduce reagent usage. • Miniaturized assays enable high-density formats.	• Lowers costs. • Improves scalability and supports physiologically relevant models.
Robotics in phenotypic SCREENING	• Automated imaging captures phenotypic changes. • Robots streamline 3D model handling and dynamic data acquisition.	• Increases reproducibility and precision. • Facilitates exploration of complex biological systems.

lab-on-a-chip technologies, and robotic control in phenotypic screening. The combination of recent developments produces enhanced efficiency alongside greater scalability along with increased precision to aid drug discovery workflows through rapid and cost-efficient therapeutic compound assessment.

Robotic Systems in HTS: Plate Handling and Liquid Dispensing

Modern HTS operates thanks to robotic automation, which enables fast, precise, high-volume task performance. Robot systems handle microplates between different devices to move materials among incubators, readers, and dispensing stations, where they help reduce manual mistakes by ensuring precise operations [25]. Microplate assays achieve reproducible results along with diminished wastage through precise liquid dispensing robotic operations. Renewed efficiency stems from system operations, which enable nonstop processing, enabling thousands of compounds to be screened in limited time periods. The improved HTS technology enables both higher dependability and better efficiency, which allows bigger drug discovery operations to become practical.

AI and ML in Data Analysis

General data analysis within screening technologies undergoes fundamental transformations through AI and ML.

Through pattern recognition, ML algorithms extract delicate patterns across extensive datasets, which normal analysis techniques usually overlook. AI supports the selection process of optimal hits by processing multiple data sets that contain information about target interaction and efficacy, and toxicity measures. The application of AI-based prediction models helps researchers perform virtual screening, which reduces compound libraries for physical testing. Jamime F. Jacquot and others demonstrated that AI automation enables adaptive robotic control for dynamic workflow improvements in real-time [26]. AI and ML improve decision processes by performing faster hit validation while decreasing the number of incorrect results.

Miniaturization and Lab-on-a-chip Technologies

Miniaturization Has Significantly Reduced the Costs and Resources Required for Screening

The manipulation of small fluid amounts through lab-on-a-chip technologies enables consistent, low-cost assays while making dense assay formats.

Small assay platforms using 1536-well plates allow sensitive measurements without increasing material costs [27,28]. These technologies enable quick compound screening processes at high speed while working with demanding experiments that require large amounts of resources. The development of organ-on-chip systems becomes possible through miniaturization technology, which creates physiologically relevant models that enhance screening predictions.

The utilization of miniaturization and lab-on-chip technologies for drug screening appears in Figure 3.7. The beginning point in microfluidic systems, alongside miniaturized assays, creates better scalability, which enables scientists to develop organ-on-chip systems that mimic human physiology. Through their collaborative action, these techniques enhance resource management and improve screening sensitivity and prediction accuracy to advance the effectiveness of screening operations.

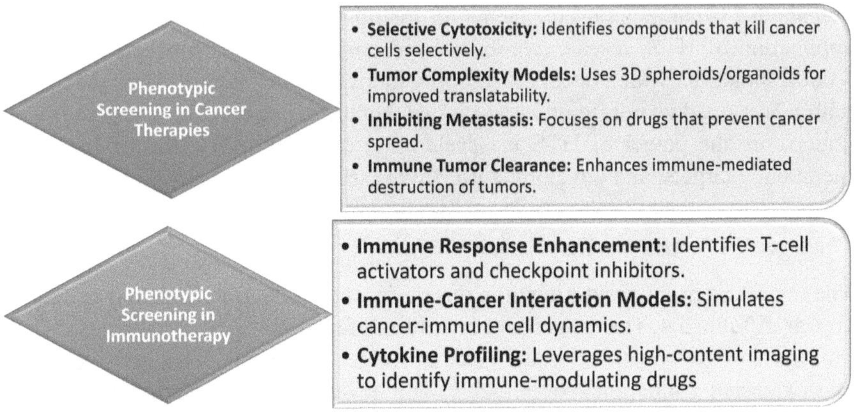

Figure 3.7 Applications of phenotypic screening in immunotherapy and oncology.

Integration of Robotics in Phenotypic Screening

The application of automation together with robotics systems helps manage the complex nature of phenotypic screening. The combination of automated imaging systems that use robotics reduces human intervention during phenotypic analysis [29]. The use of 3D Models benefits from robotic automation through standardized manipulations of spheroids and organoids. A combination of real-time phenotypic change observation becomes feasible through robotic systems that integrate modern imaging solutions and sensor equipment. Robotic systems improve phenotypic screening by enabling better control of reproducible results while decreasing experimental variation and allowing scientists to study elaborate biological settings, which drives pharmaceutical breakthroughs. Automation has achieved collective process optimization through its advancements, including robotic systems and AI and miniaturized technologies, which now support more efficient drug discovery workflows.

Case Studies in HTS

Successful Drug Discovery Campaigns Using HTS

HTS technology has stood as the key discovery factor behind multiple successful drug development projects. Some notable case studies include:

Gleevec (Imatinib) achieved fame as an HTS-based drug discovery success because it became the treatment for chronic myelogenous leukemia (CML). Novartis researchers used compound screening to discover imatinib because it showed strong inhibition against BCR-ABL fusion protein that drives CML. One of the HTS breakthroughs showed both the strength of screening technologies and brought targeted cancer treatment through Gleevec (Imatinib) [30]. Merck discovered Selzentry (Maraviroc) through HTS by identifying small molecules which prevented HIV attachment to the essential CCR5 receptor. The development of Maraviroc resulted from this screening process to become an approved CCR5 antagonist for HIV treatment [31]. BRAF inhibitors, such as Vemurafenib started as HTS-developed compounds that became important agents for treating melanoma patients. Through the application of HTS, researchers discovered compounds that blocked the BRAF V600E mutation, which occurs commonly in melanoma patients, when they eventually developed vemurafenib into a crucial therapeutic agent [32]. These examples underscore the power of HTS in accelerating drug discovery, identifying novel therapeutic targets, and developing life-saving treatments.

Challenges in Target Identification and Validation

The important problems during drug discovery, target identification, and validation appear in Table 3.4. The drug discovery process faces three major obstacles such as biological system complexity alongside off-target effects which trigger side effects and extensive validation requirements. The development of predictive modeling and systems biology brings us closer to growing drug discovery methods that deliver better precision and efficiency.

Table 3.4 Challenges in target identification and validation

Challenge	*Description*	*Impact*
Complexity of biological systems	Diseases involve intricate networks; identifying the correct molecular target is challenging.	Limits understanding of disease mechanisms and delays the identification of effective therapeutic targets.
Off-target effects	Compounds may interact with unintended targets, causing side effects and reduced specificity.	Reduces the therapeutic potential of hits and complicates drug development.
Target validation	Validating a target's role in disease progression requires extensive genetic and preclinical studies.	Prolongs the drug discovery process and increases resource requirements for confirming therapeutic relevance.

HTS research success has demonstrated the discovery of multiple potential compounds despite remaining obstacles in target validation and identification. Some key difficulties include:

HTS mainly focuses on testing individual biological molecules or pathways but diseases, including cancer and neurodegenerative conditions, exist as multilevel biological networks which present a major challenge for drug discovery. HTS faces an important impediment when trying to identify the appropriate molecular target among these complex biological networks [33].

Among key challenges lies the identification of compounds that activate unwanted targets apart from the intended ones. Additional molecular interactions targeting nondesired receptors lead to troublesome side effects, through which the therapeutic value of compounds diminishes. Checking and verifying the precise target affinity of candidates represents an essential step. Target validation poses a difficult task to show that promising targets participate in disease progression. Confirmation of target therapy effectiveness demands large-scale follow-up investigations that combine genetic testing along with preclinical experiments about target modulation [34]. Progress in systems biology and improved screening platforms and predictive models help researchers to surpass multiple blocking points during therapeutic discovery.

Lessons Learned from High-failure Projects

Numerous encouraging compounds have risen from HTS discoveries, even though this technique has produced significant high-profile failed experiments. The following experiences provide multiple important lessons. Early-stage validation serves as a vital lesson derived from failure events due to its critical importance in the validation process. The unsuccessful projects occurred because compounds succeeded in HTS but failed to produce the expected effects during animal tests and human clinical examinations. Early-stage validation helps to save resources by identifying compounds without genuine therapeutic applications.

The identification of potent compounds through HTS turns out to be ineffective because of their insufficient ADME properties for in vivo applications. To achieve success in pharmaceutical development, it is essential to optimize compounds for pharmacokinetics properties during the screening process. The use of simple 2D cell cultures during screening creates frequent failures because these cultures lack adequate human tissue complexity. The implementation of advanced 3D models together with organoids in HTS improves result validity, which leads to better final outcomes [35].

Multiple initial screen hits from HTS remain distant from optimal drug status. Lead optimization needs an effective multiple-round process because of its high failure rate. Medicinal chemistry enables scientists to boost therapeutic features found in early hits, which improves both their safety profile and potentiates their effectiveness. The achievement of breakthroughs in drug discovery through HTS depends on proper validation methods and simplifying biological complexities, and ensuring compounds meet suitability requirements for clinical development. Past screening campaign failures have produced essential knowledge that guides modern HTS approaches toward better efficiency and effectiveness.

Case Studies in Phenotypic Screening

Identification of First-in-class Drugs

Phenotypic screening plays a vital role in first-class drug discovery through its analysis of compound-induced cellular responses instead of identifying particular molecular pathways. A few notable examples include:

The development of Kalydeco (Ivacaftor) occurred through phenotypic screening research for treating cystic fibrosis associated with the G551D mutation in CFTR gene. Researchers utilized this screening technique to discover small molecules which enhanced the functioning of defective CFTR proteins in cells obtained from patients. First-in-class drug Kalydeco demonstrates the breakthrough value of phenotypic screening because it attacks the fundamental cystic fibrosis cause instead of treating symptoms alone [36]. The development of Kalydeco (Ivacaftor) occurred through phenotypic screening research for treating cystic fibrosis associated with the G551D mutation in CFTR gene. Researchers utilized this screening technique to discover small molecules which enhanced the functioning of defective CFTR proteins in cells obtained from patients. First-in-class drug Kalydeco demonstrates the breakthrough value of phenotypic screening because it attacks the fundamental cystic fibrosis cause instead of treating symptoms alone [36,37].

Successful Phenotypic Screens in Neglected Diseases

Phenotypic screening has enabled important discoveries of medical treatments against diseases that receive inadequate commercial investment, although affecting millions of people. Some key examples include:

The drug Atezolizumab (Tecentriq) originated from phenotypic screening to block PD-L1 protein, which in turn activates immune system responses against nonsmall cell lung cancer (NSCLC). Phenotypic screening targeted cancer cells at first, but it led to discoveries about how the immune system combats tuberculosis, which advanced the creation of immune-modulatory treatments [38].

Phenotypic screening led to the development of new anti-malaria compounds that help fight malaria since the disease became resistant to existing medications. The phenotypic screening process of compound libraries found new chemical entities that showed anti-parasite capability against Plasmodium during laboratory experiments. The identified chemical compounds show potential to develop stronger and longer-lasting anti-malarial drugs [39].

Phenotypic screening provides a method to identify new treatment drugs against leishmaniasis, which affects tropical areas. The parasitic disease requires therapeutic development through such screening approaches. Multiple substances that hinder the growth of Leishmania parasites have been discovered by research experts, which offers promise for improving upcoming treatment solutions [40]. The use of phenotypic screening emerges as a strong approach for unveiling medications against the diseases that traditional methods tend to disregard.

Role of 3D Cell Cultures and Organoids

The incorporation of 3D cell cultures along with organoids into phenotypic screening practice has greatly boosted both the predictive value and the relevance of drug discovery models.

3D Cell Cultures show better tissue accuracy than 2D cell culture systems because they enable more exact in vivo cell behavior representation. The utilization of spheroids and tissue-engineered constructs helps researchers better replicate tumor microenvironments and vascularization as well as cellular interactions, thus improving the predictive value of phenotypic screening toward clinical results [41].

Stem cell-derived organoids represent small self-maintaining audiences which mirror human organs both structurally and functionally. Personalized drug screening becomes possible due to the capability of culturing organoids from originally derived patient tissues. Phenotypic screening utilizing organoids in cancer research has discovered targeted compounds for precise tumor types, which has allowed developers to create targeted therapies. The screening of drugs that target liver fibrosis and renal failure as well as neurological conditions has been successfully performed using organoid models of the liver, kidney, and brain [42].

The assessment of drug toxicity benefits from utilizing both 3D cultures with organoids alongside each other. The insufficient complexity within traditional 2D cultured plates leads to unsuccessful predictions of adverse drug reactions and side effects. Research using 3D cultures together with organoids enables scientists to perform better drug toxicity evaluations and make more reliable predictions about substance effects on human organs.

Phenotypic screening adoption of 3D cell cultures and organoids enables revolutionized drug discovery that delivers advanced drug candidates with increased effectiveness along with enhanced safety levels. The refined organoid and three-dimensional cell culture models serve as proper depictions of human illness and show promise for therapeutic innovation in oncology together with rare ailments and regenerative medicine applications. Phenotypic screening now delivers significant power through its combination with 3D cell cultures and organoids to discover novel drugs along with new disease treatments, and better perform drug evaluations.

Comparative Analysis: HTS vs. Phenotypic Screening

High-throughput Screening

Strengths

HTS performs fast, large-scale compound tests throughout brief time periods. HTS functions perfectly for detecting drug candidates at an early stage of drug discovery. The combination of robotics with automation enables HTS screening of thousands to millions of compounds without heavy human involvement for better efficiency and throughput. The method of HTS primarily screens compounds toward unique biological targets that include enzymes or receptors. The specific nature of this method proves effective in drug discovery involving drugs that work through clearly understood mechanisms. The HTS platform delivers precise numerical information that helps investigators determine the strength and target specificity of chemical molecules for their investigations.

Limitations

The mechanical systems used in HTS lack biological complexity because testing works with easy experiments in separate testing environments (such as cell lines and enzymes). HTS works as a target-specific system, so it tends to disregard compounds showing potential therapeutic value through novel mechanisms because they do not activate the target. HTS provides capacity for massive screening, but its expense along with supporting technology and facility maintenance costs is considerable. HTS generates false positive results because of testing artifacts alongside false negative results when compounds pass assay screening, although they would provide therapeutic benefits in actual patient conditions.

Phenotypic Screening

Strengths

Casting a wider cellular response makes phenotypic screening evaluate complete biological responses like those found in complex diseases. The approach reveals medicines which targeted approaches fail to detect. The phenotypic screening method does not need predefined targets during evaluations since it enables the discovery of novel mechanisms and drugs that act through nontypical pathways. The use of patient-derived cells and 3D cultures during phenotypic screening enables better relevance to human diseases because compounds can interact with real disease environments. Phenotypic screening enabled researchers to discover multiple unique drugs which HTS platforms could not identify before.

Limitations

Recorded data from phenotypic screening consists of complex and qualitative results that pose analysis challenges compared to the quantitative results HTS can generate. The analysis of phenotypic screening requires extended duration and multiple hands-on work, which makes it inefficient for extensive compound tests. The failure rate increases when assay methods do not realistically replicate disease conditions, thus leading to missed effective compounds in vivo. Target identification remains challenging after phenotypic screening successfully finds new drug candidates because it makes it harder to optimize drug development through precise target assignment.

Selection Criteria Based on Target, Disease, and Library

Target-based Screening

During HTS operations, the selection criteria focus on choosing molecular targets such as enzymes and receptors and ion channels. The following elements need evaluation when using HTS:

The screening procedure requires targets that have been accurately described as well as accessible for screening purposes. The development of an assay needs to address how a membrane protein will behave when present in the screening conditions. The design of the assay should fit the target requirements to accurately measure its binding properties and activity levels. Solutions designed either as enzyme-linked assays or radiolabeled compounds with fluorescence-based methods can be used for testing. The design of focused compound libraries used for HTS screens depends on the targeted protein type. When screening for kinase inhibitors, the library should be kinase-focused, but natural product libraries would suit broader activity screening [43].

Disease-based Screening (Phenotypic Screening)

In phenotypic screening, operations focus primarily on disease symptoms instead of targeting individual molecular elements. Biological context together with disease relevance determines most of the selection criteria, which include: For the disease modeling process, the selected model must precisely simulate the biological nature of a studied disease. The scale and type of models employed for drug discovery testing comprise patient-specific cell lines, besides 3D cell cultures and laboratory animals, based on the development level of drug research [44]. A relevant screening assay should replicate the natural pathophysiology of the disease to validate that observed results in vitro correspond to the live disease environment. The assay should use tests which evaluate precise disease markers including cell survival and migration along with differentiation and gene expression patterns that align with the disease context.

When performing phenotypic screening, operators typically employ libraries that contain diverse and nontargeted compounds. Screening tests utilize three fundamental compound collections including natural products and synthetics together with previously developed drugs that cover multiple potential biological effects. Both HTS and phenotypic screening demonstrate separation between unique advantages and limitations, which provide their appropriateness for various drug discovery and development phases and goals. HTS works best to find specific drug targets, but phenotypic screening succeeds particularly well in discovering drugs with clinical mechanisms of action when dealing with diseases that have complicated biological characteristics. Drug discovery campaign objectives together with disease type and resource availability, determine which approach will be chosen between the two.

Future Perspectives and Trends

Integration of Multiomics Data

The drug discovery and screening field experiences a major development through integrating multiomics data types that include genomics as well as proteomics and transcriptomics, and metabolomics [45]. Single-omics techniques alone would struggle to reveal these therapeutically important biomarkers and advancing targets because multiomics technologies offer better disease mechanism insights. Researchers gain insights into disease-related molecular networks through data integration of multiple biological layers, which allows simultaneous compound interaction analysis.

Multiomics enhances both HTS testing and phenotypic screening methods [46]. HTS becomes more effective because researchers can establish relationships between screening outcomes and target cell genomic and proteomic data patterns to locate new potential compounds. When omics data integration gets incorporated into phenotypic screening, researchers gain a fuller understanding of compound effects, which extends to cellular responses and metabolic changes as well as gene expression alterations. Research-based decision-making enables scientists to achieve accurate target detection while improving drug effectiveness estimates and enhancing knowledge surrounding possible adverse effects.

Role of AI in Predictive Screening Models

Predictive screening models operate significantly better by utilizing AI and ML, which have become necessary tools for drug discovery circumstances [47]. Large data sets extracted from HTS and phenotypic screens enable these technologies to forecast compound activity before physical testing takes place. AI algorithms train through existing data to identify patterns which would go unnoticed by humans when linking chemical structures to biological responses. The optimization of screening processes receives assistance through AI technology implementation. Predictive models enable scientists to identify candidate compounds which show high potential for success so researchers can cut down screening efforts on big libraries while also decreasing costs. ML models evaluate phenotypic screening outcomes to detect the molecular pathways affected by compounds as well as forecast their clinical effectiveness potential [48–52]. AI processes enormous quantities of research information sourced from chemical libraries alongside biological assays as well as patient data, to boost the speed along with precision of drug discovery efforts.

The ongoing evolution of AI in drug discovery enables both screening effectiveness enhancement and mejores proactive development of therapeutic agents through improved human drug behavior forecasting.

Toward Personalized and Precision Medicine

Personalized and precision medicine represents a fast advancing medical sector which develops treatments that adapt to individual genetic and environmental as well as lifestyle factors. The development of drug discovery and screening methods will undergo transformative changes through this trend due to its ability to create effective therapies with reduced side effects for target patient groups.

More laboratories integrate personal medicine strategies into their phenotypic and HTS methods across the pharmaceutical industry [53–58]. Reports obtained from patient-derived cells and organoids, and tissue samples help scientists replicate individual disease states while screening compounds that have direct benefits for specific patients. The method enables scientists to discover medications which would work best with specific genetic and phenotypic patient demographics. Specific drug treatment development becomes possible by combining genetic information with drug screening, which results in both improved treatment effects and patient safety. The medical industry needs this change, especially in oncology, because genetic mutations affect patient responses to treatment approaches.

Research and development of personalized drugs will require more HTS and phenotypic screening methods to find drugs that address disease sources at individual patient levels for more accurate treatment options. Efforts to integrate genetic, environmental and phenotypic data into screening will create medical practices that are personalized, which yields both better patient outcomes and diminishes drug development pitfalls through trial-and-error methods.

Conclusion

HTS along with phenotypic screening serves as a crucial method for present-day drug discovery because it supports distinctive screening pathways toward therapeutic compound discovery. The rapid examination of numerous compound sets toward biological targets stands as the core principle behind HTS operations, which frequently employ robotic automation systems. HTS reveals critical disease mechanisms through its analysis methods, while it aids scientists in finding suitable small molecules to alter disease pathway behavior. The main principle of the HTS operates through assessing compound engagement with disease-associated biomolecules directly.

Phenotypic screening approaches biological testing through compound evaluations that measure their ability to trigger desired effects within complete living cells and organisms. The approach provides excellent benefit for diseases in which molecular mechanisms remain unclear, combined with diseases that affect multiple biological pathways simultaneously. Phenotypic screening detects compounds usable to manage complicated diseases with multiple causal factors by measuring changes in cellular characteristics.

The two screening approaches serve numerous drug development and discovery requirements. HTS functions throughout target validation and lead discovery while assisting scientists to find small-molecule hits that advance toward development. Phenotypic screening functions as an emerging method to discover new therapeutic candidates when conventional target-based strategies prove insufficient in the identification process. Scientists use this approach to identify new treatments for diseases which have restricted therapeutic choices while exploring drug interventions from prior medications.

The pharmaceutical industry experienced rapid development during the last years through emerging technological innovations and industry trends that guide modern drug development processes. The current trend shows an escalating merger of multiomics data consisting of genomic and proteomic analysis together with additional biological information to better understand disease biology. The integrated approach helps scientists discover fresh biomarkers and find new medical targets, and develop more targeted therapeutic approaches. The integration between HTS data and omics information creates improved target selection processes, but phenotypic examination reveals novel molecular drug activities.

Drug discovery benefits greatly from AI and ML applications that have become essential in the industry. The application of these modern technologies enables better screening protocol management and enhanced analysis of large datasets along with the ability to perform computer-based compound behavior predictions without using traditional laboratory resources. AI-based predictive modeling tools are now essential components for both HTS and phenotypic screening because they analyze biological data patterns to identify the most suitable drug candidates effective through chemical and biological properties interactions.

The current drive to personalize and precision medicine methods simultaneously modifies our methods for drug development and screening activities. Mobile application-specific data including both genetic information and disease characteristics enables researchers to build drug-development procedures that align with individual needs. The use of genetic and molecular profiling techniques represents the forefront of oncology care because these methods find personalized therapies as well as new ways to develop drugs that target disease-related biomarkers.

Drug discovery depends on HTS and phenotypic screening methods since they present distinct attributes for discovering therapeutic candidates. Advancements in technology will define drug discovery through AI and multiomics data applications and personalized medicine, which will generate effective and targeted treatments for diverse diseases. The new technologies will transform disease treatment methods, thus providing better patient outcomes along with more efficient and cost-effective drug development processes.

References

1. Johnson K, Williams M. Efficiency of HTS in identifying therapeutic agents. Biotech Trends. 2014;18(3):122–129.
2. Green P, Martin R. Target-based screening: Advances and challenges. Pharmacol Rev. 2014;45(7):501–510.
3. Zhang Z, Peters M. Phenotypic screening in modern drug discovery. Trends Pharmacol Sci. 2014;32(5):207–214.
4. Wilson J, Baker L. Target-based drug discovery strategies. Biomed Insights. 2014;22(6):88–97.
5. Campbell D, Jones H. Novel disease pathways identified through phenotypic screening. Sci Transl Med. 2014;4(132):132ra51.
6. Johnson L, Davis P. Unbiased drug discovery through phenotypic screening. Drug Discov Trends. 2014;9(7):333–339.
7. Patel J, Campbell R. Cytotoxicity assessment in HTS assays. Toxicol Methods. 2015;15(2):305–315.
8. Allen C, White M. Multiparametric data in high-content screening. J Pharm Res. 2015;28(5):1025–1031.
9. Taylor J, Kumar S. Ensuring meaningful HTS results: Key parameters. Drug Test Anal. 2015;9(12):985–992.
10. White L, Singh P. Designing libraries for HTS. Curr Opin Drug Discov Dev. 2015;11(1):56–61.
11. Brown J, Lee S. Lead optimization strategies in HTS. J Mol Pharmacol. 2016;12(9):998–1006.
12. Patel K, Adams G. Challenges in targeting complex diseases through HTS. Trends Mol Med. 2016;22(10):825–834.
13. White M, Green P. Follow-up studies in HTS: Validating targets. Drug Discov Today. 2016;23(7):1173–1180.
14. Green C, Lewis P. Immune-modulatory therapies from phenotypic screening. J Immunol. 2016;192(2):447–455.
15. Smith H, Davis P. Targeted libraries in drug discovery. Curr Opin Pharmacol. 2016;13(4):504–512.
16. Brown L, Patel T. BTK inhibitors for leukemia: Phenotypic screening insights. Blood Cancer J. 2016;5(3):e251.
17. Davis S, Smith M. Biomarkers in phenotypic screening: Key indicators. Clin Pharmacol. 2017;6(8):451–460.
18. Patel R, Harris T. High-content imaging in immunology. J Immunol Methods. 2017; 430:53–65.
19. Harris T, Martin A. 3D models in drug discovery. J Pharmacol. 2017;22(9):875–892.
20. Smith T, Zhang X. Cost reductions through miniaturized HTS assays. J Drug Discov Res. 2018;15(3):145–151.
21. Adams D, Stewart P. AI in HTS automation workflows. Trends Biotech. 2018; 38(8):795–803.

22. Wilson G, Zhang L. Advances in targeted cancer therapies through HTS. Cancer Biol Ther. 2018;21(2):145–153.
23. Turner M, Harris N. High-content screening: A paradigm shift. Lab Med. 2018; 43(4):221–230.
24. Gonzalez T, Patel R. 3D spheroids in oncology drug discovery. Cancer Res. 2019; 79(15):4035–4044.
25. Martinez P, Hall C. First-in-class drugs through phenotypic screening. Drug Discov Today. 2019;24(11):2235–2242.
26. Carter B, White J. Assay miniaturization for efficient drug screening. Drug Discov Today. 2019;24(5):1044–1050.
27. Harris M, White G. Tumor complexity in phenotypic screening. Cancer Med. 2019;7(3):459–470.
28. Jones R, Lewis J. Drug screening approaches for precision medicine. Genomics Proteomics. 2019;14(5):333–346.
29. Gonzalez M, Patel S. Integrating multi-omics in HTS. Biotech Trends. 2019;17(9):725–732.
30. Brown J, Patel A. Personalized medicine and drug screening. Curr Opin Pharmacol. 2019;12(3):412–419.
31. Smith J, Turner K. Kalydeco and cystic fibrosis: A phenotypic screening success. J Rare Dis. 2020;10(3):99–108.
32. Campbell D, Patel R. Advanced organoid models in disease-targeted drug discovery. Trends Biotech. 2020;18(6):592–603.
33. Turner J, Gonzalez P. Organoid models in disease-targeted drug discovery. Nat Biomed Eng. 2020;3(6):494–508.
34. Harris T, Adams R. Multi-omics in phenotypic screening. Trends Biotech. 2020;18(8):795–805.
35. Patel T, Singh R. Artificial intelligence in phenotypic screening. AI Trends Med. 2020;15(2):102–110.
36. White L, Kumar P. Spheroids as tumor models for drug discovery. J Oncol Sci. 2021;5(4):231–242.
37. Green B, Adams T. High-content imaging in oncology. Drug Discov Res. 2021;19(7):891–900.
38. Carter M, Stewart J. Screening for anti-malarial agents using phenotypic approaches. Trop Med Int Health. 2021;26(5):545–554.
39. Gonzalez R, Martinez L. Cytokine profiling in immune-modulatory drug discovery. Immunopharmacol. 2022;11(3):312–323.
40. Harris N, Lewis G. AI-driven drug discovery workflows. Biotech Autom Sci. 2022;14(6):785–795.
41. Patel K, Wilson J. The role of robotics in HTS miniaturization. J Biotechnol. 2022;20(1):1–10.
42. Kumar R, Turner P. Applications of multi-omics in HTS. Mol Biol Trends. 2023;25(2):123–133.
43. Jones S, Adams L. Automated imaging in drug discovery. Cell Biol Methods. 2023;18(3):355–365.
44. Harris T, Patel S. Role of AI in drug-target validation. Comput Biol Med. 2023;42(9):991–1001.
45. Carter J, Wilson R. Multi-parametric data analysis in HCS. High-Content Biol. 2023;5(7):204–215.
46. Davis M, Kumar J. Advancements in organoid-based drug discovery. Trends Biotechnol. 2023;41(11):1023–1035.
47. Turner N, Patel T. Breakthroughs in HTS and phenotypic screening. Drug Dev Res. 2024;29(1):15–25.
48. Green T, Adams P. Targeted therapies identified via phenotypic screening. Med Oncol. 2024;12(4):410–422.

49. Atmakuri LR, Peeriga R, Begum S, Vallamkonda B, Baratam A. Novel bioanalytical LC-MS/MS method for determination of metoprolol in human plasma. J Appl Pharm Sci. 2024;14(12):131–138.
50. Peeriga R, Venkata Bangaru GK. Implementation of the POCSO act in schools. In: Child Sexual Abuse: A Public Health Problem in India. Springer publications, Singapore, 2024. p. 391–413. Springer Publications, Singapore.
51. Peeriga R, Yarlagadda LC, Alla NR. Protection of children from sexual exploitation. In: Child Sexual Abuse: A Public Health Problem in India. 2024. p. 191–201.
52. Peeriga R, Shiek Arabath SAM, Manubolu K, Thelappilly BB, Yarlagadda LC. Insilico assessment of phytoconstituents in *myxopyrum smilacifolium* blume against arthritis. Biomed Pharmacol J. 2024;17(1):235–241.
53. Manubolu K, Balagani PK, Gope ER, Peeriga R, Sridevi AR. Unlocking the potential of aquasomes: A comprehensive review on innovative nanocarriers in drug delivery and beyond. Int J Chem Biochem Sci. 2023;24(6):405–410.
54. Manubolu K, Peeriga R, Bonthu MG, Gope ER, Kadirvel D. Evaluation of anti-inflammatory activity of *Millingtonia hortensis* leaf extract. Int J Chem Biochem Sci. 2023;24(6):380–385.
55. Peeriga R, Chandrasekhar KB. Comparative study of anti-inflammatory activity of petroleum ether extract of *myxopyrum smilacifolium* blume and ethanolic leaf extract of *pamburus missionis* swingle. J Pharm Sci Res. 2017;9(6):955–957.
56. Peeriga R, Manubolu K (2025). Design strategies for waste reduction and enhanced recyclability in pharmaceutical packaging. In: Yingngam, B., Aslam, M.S., Haghi, A.K. (eds) Sustainable Pharmaceutical Product Development and Optimization Processes. Springer, Singapore.
57. Manubolu K, Peeriga R, Chandrasekhar KB. A Short Guide to Clinical Pharmacokinetics. 1st ed. 2024. Springer.Singapore.
58. Manubolu K, Peeriga R (2025). Ecodesign principles. In: Yingngam, B., Aslam, M.S., Haghi, A.K. (eds) Sustainable Pharmaceutical Product Development and Optimization Processes. Springer, Singapore.

4 Artificial Intelligence and Machine Learning in Drug Discovery

Krishnaveni Manubolu, Talamanchi Balakrishna, Gorintla Sai Supraja, Venkateswara Rao Javvaji, Shaik Rasheed, and Kishore Kumar Kadimpati

Introduction

Artificial Intelligence

Definition

Computer Science is the study of designing machines that can perform tasks that are thought to require human intellect. Examples include speech recognition, natural language interpretation, and problem solving [1].

Types of AI

NARROW AI

Weak AI is built for specific applications such as chatbots, voice assistants, like Siri or Alexa, and recommendation engines, such as those used by Netflix or Amazon. It does not have general cognitive capabilities and only performs a task within a narrow context.

GENERAL AI

This imaginary type of AI is called artificial general intelligence, or AGI (Strong AI). It may perhaps be able to do all those cognitive tasks which an actual human being can. It still remains a long-term, idealistic goal.

Machine Learning

Definition

ML, a branch of AI, that involves the study of various statistical models and algorithms that enable computers to examine, comprehend, and make judgements based on data [2]. ML systems work better by extracting patterns and insights from past data, as opposed to following explicit instructions shown in Figure 4.1.

DOI: 10.4324/9781003564041-4

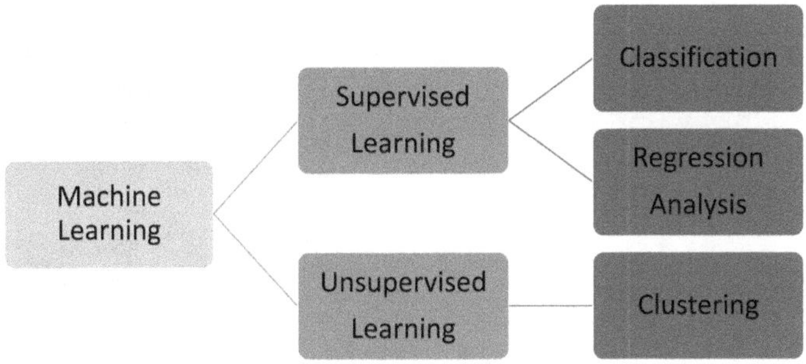

Figure 4.1 Types of ML.

Types of ML

SUPERVISED LEARNING

Labeled data is used for training the algorithm with a known desired output. Through these data, the system learns to map the input to the corresponding outputs and then applies this knowledge to make predictions on new but unknown data. Some examples include regression—for example, property price prediction—and classification, for example, spam detection in emails.

UNSUPERVISED LEARNING

Common approaches have focused on unlabeled data, asking the computer to discover structures or patterns without giving it a set result. Common methods include clustering and dimensionality reduction (e.g., principal component analysis).

REINFORCEMENT LEARNING

It trained the algorithm to make decisions based on some reward for acceptable behavior and a penalty for inappropriate behavior in some sequence. It is used immensely in robotics, games, autonomous systems, etc. An application of reinforcement learning is a robot navigating through a maze, for example [3].

Overview

This has developed computers to use AI, do pattern recognition, language understanding, and make decisions. All these require human intelligence, and the computer does all this by installing technological breakthroughs that allow computers to replicate human cognitive function shown in Figure 4.2.

ML, on the other hand, is a subfield of AI that builds methods allowing the computer to analyze, understand, and predict data. ML systems improve performance automatically through data-driven pattern identification with little or no explicit programming.

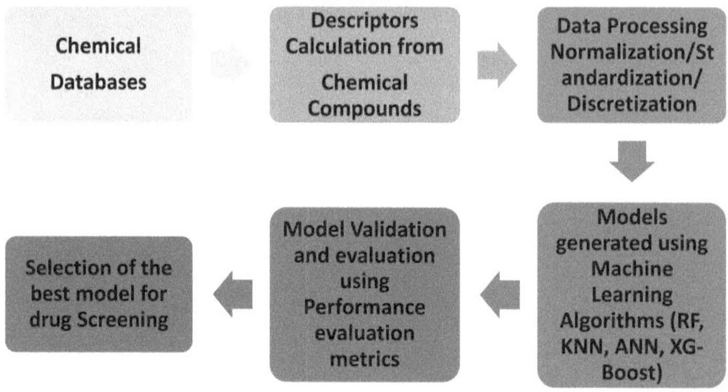

Figure 4.2 Flowchart for ML.

AI and ML have various applications across very diversified sectors. The medical profession deals with the improvement of diagnostic instruments and, therefore, customized medicines. It applies to the financial sector in algorithmic trading and fraud detection. It includes inventory control and personalized recommendation in the retail industry [4]. Transportation-related applications involving AI and ML include driverless autos and optimal routes.

However, there are problems with these technologies: they cannot radically minimize the algorithmic biases of the data, and difficulties ensuring the privacy of the data, and providing understandable and accessible models. The future studies will focus on further improving algorithms, merging AI/ML and breakthroughs in quantum computing and the Internet of Things, and establishing ethical guidelines in their deployment.

The Evolution of Drug Discovery: From Traditional Methods to AI-powered Techniques

Oral Delivery

The most commonly used method is by taking pills and capsules through the oral way as well as allowing the drug to be absorbed in the gut.

Controlled Release

It will be the time-release pharmaceutical formulations that would achieve a progressive release of the medicament.

Delivery Through Injection

Intravenous (IV): In this technique, the medicine is delivered straight to the bloodstream. It tends to act within a few minutes. Subcutaneous and intramuscular injections give a gradual release that is more reliable than an IV injection.

Topical Administration

Creams and Ointment: Given via topical means for some form of dermatosis.

Transdermal Patches

Controlled Release: Medications are delivered through the skin with the expectation that they will act systemically.

Inhalation

Nebulizers and Aerosols: Medicine is directly provided to the lungs.

Transition to AI-based Approaches

Predictive Modeling: AI-computing systems scour vast amounts of information, identify and predict which of all possibilities could be an effective treatment.

Molecular Docking: AI predicts how molecules, which constitute drugs, interact with the targets in a medicine to make drug development more efficient [5].

Personalized Medicine

Patient Stratification: Based on genotypic, environmental, and behavior-related data, AI can provide treatment based on the needs of the patient.

Adaptive Dosing: Dosage is so adjusted in real time through ML algorithms according to the patient's record.

Smart Drug Delivery Systems

It produces nanoparticles, among other things, and allows for high precision delivery of drugs to specific tissues or cells. "Responsive systems" are AI-controlled delivery systems that release medicine to a certain physiological indicator.

Optimized Clinical Trials

Recruitment and Design: With predictions of results and conditions changed, AI recruits volunteers and designs studies much better.

Improved Pharmacovigilance

AI tracks and analyzes data to detect adverse medication effects before they even happen.

Data from varied sources will be reviewed in depth as an avenue to improve the safety and efficacy profiles.

Manufacturing and Supply Chain Efficiency

Process Optimization: AI ensures that processes in pharmaceuticals occur efficiently and uniformly.

Logistics Management: AI predicts demand and supply chain control for minimum wastage and timely delivery.

How AI and ML Are Revolutionizing Drug Development

Drug Discovery: AI, as well as its subset of ML, interprets the vast chemical and biological data to find potential therapeutic candidates [6]. This process can expedite many drug discovery stages at their early stages by predicting how different compounds may interact with biological targets using these algorithms. They can identify interesting properties of compounds existing in giant molecular libraries that might otherwise be overlooked by traditional methods shown in Figure 4.3.

Predictive Modeling: Pharmacokinetics—the way a drug is absorbed, distributed, metabolized, and eliminated—will be predicted with the help of ML models, as well as pharmacodynamics—the way a drug affects the body—for new drugs. Helps in developing drugs with fewer side effects and high efficacy.

Personalized Medicine: AI can tailor therapy to individual patients based on lifestyle and environmental exposure factors and genetics. ML algorithms open doors to more precise, individually suited, and therefore effective treatment plans based on which individuals are likely to benefit from a given medicine.

Clinical Trials Optimization: AI and ML are employed to develop clinical studies that are more efficient by selecting the best applicants, forecasting their reactions, and streamlining trial procedures [7]. For example, AI can evaluate data regarding patients to determine which set of patients is most likely to benefit from specific medication, resulting in a higher probability of a successful study.

Drug Repurposing: AI can also be applied in finding new uses for already-approved drugs. AI systems can discover possible new uses or indications for licensed medicines by analyzing current data, which could be faster and cheaper than finding a new medicine from scratch.

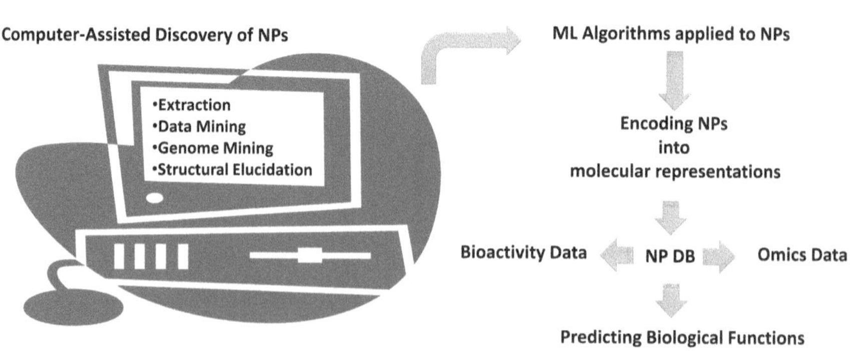

Figure 4.3 AI and ML of drug discovery.

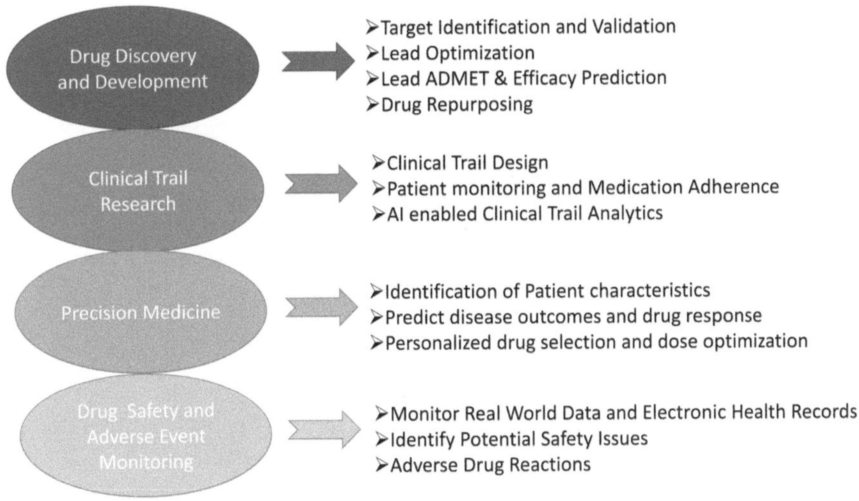

Figure 4.4 AI and ML in revolutionizing the drug development.

Biomarker Discovery: The outputs generated through the utilization of AI and ML in the discovery of new disease biomarkers may herald the dawn of customized medicines. These tools can identify patterns of biomarkers related to particular disease states or response to therapy by analyzing omics data, including genomics, proteomics, etc.

Data Integration and Analysis: AI facilitates the integration and analysis of large volumes of data generated in the drug development process much more efficiently [8]. Data collected from clinical trials, patient files, literature, and experimental outcomes provide insights inaccessible through conventional techniques.

Simulations and Virtual Screening: AI-driven simulations and virtual screening can be utilized by researchers in testing hypotheses digitally or screening drugs before actual trials. This, therefore, means that not many compounds have to be synthesized and tested in laboratories.

Prediction of Safety and Toxicity: With historical data on drug interactions and side effects, ML algorithms can identify potential safety concerns and adverse effects of newly synthesized drugs. This happens to be a much earlier stage in drug development, where possible problems will be identified (Figure 4.4).

How AI Technologies Transforming Drug Discovery

Accelerating Drug Discovery and Development

Predictive Modeling

Example: For example, AI algorithms can predict how active the compounds would be biologically, as well as the potential of the compounds as drugs. The process

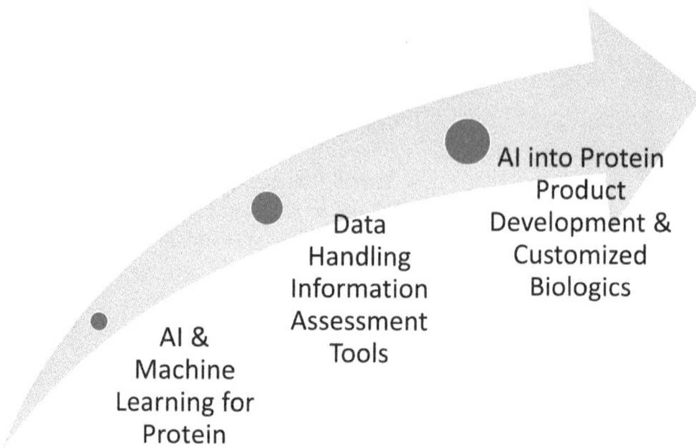

Figure 4.5 AI in transforming drug discovery.

performed by ML models can predict how new compounds would interact with target proteins, considering the data from previously conducted experiments shown in Figure 4.5 [9].

Impact: It reduces the number of compounds that would otherwise have to be tested experimentally and should enhance the speed of early-stage drug discovery.

AI algorithms can predict the biological activity of compounds along with their drug candidate potential. ML models use data from previous experiments to predict how new compounds might interact with target proteins.

Virtual Screening

Example: Virtual screening based on AI can be applied for screening candidates for potential new drugs, as it simulates the interaction of the drug molecule with the target proteins. Algorithms scan large libraries of chemicals to find those that look most promising.

Impact: Saves highly expensive time and effort, as much less physical screening needs to be done

Enhancement in Drug Design and Optimization

Generative Models

Example: Generative adversarial networks (GANs) and other AI algorithms learn from existing data in generating novel drug-like compounds. The potential new chemical compound proposed by these models may be potentially effective at some particular targets [10].

Impact: Enhance the process of finding newer drugs by making an extensive search in the molecular space.

De Novo Drug Design

Example: Extends the scope of discovering new drugs by exploring the molecular space in a much wider extent.
Impact: AI systems formulate new drugs on demand from the drawing board with raw information about the desired properties and biological target. This approach is feasible toward models optimizing molecules for higher efficacy and better tolerance.

Target Identification and Validation

INTEGRATION OF BIOLOGICAL DATA

Example: AI combines genomics, proteomics, and other omics technologies to screen for potential drug targets. AI finds new associations between genes, proteins, and diseases through simple analysis of complex data [11].
Impact: Identify novel targets and provide insight into their role in the disease mechanism

GENE EXPRESSION ANALYSIS

Example: AI algorithms analyze gene expression profiles relevant to biomarker identification and the potential therapeutic target. ML models can identify complex patterns in large gene expression datasets.
Impact: Better validation of targets and enables tailoring drugs for particular patient populations.

Drug Repositioning

Known Drug Repositioning

Example: AI makes use of the data of drugs already accumulated to identify new indications for the drugs that are already approved. For example, an AI can associate drugs that are prescribed for one disease and benefit in another disease.
Impact: Reduces the time required to develop new indications and reduces the risk associated with the development of a drug.

Predictive Analytics

Example: AI models predict the response of individual patients to various treatments based on their genomic and clinical data. Such AI models could be applied in tailoring drug therapies.

Clinical Trial Optimization

Example: AI optimizes clinical trial design since it identifies cohorts of appropriate patients and predicts the output for each clinical trial conducted. Algorithms screen the history over time of each clinical trial, thereby increasing the efficiency and success rate of trials.

Impact: It enhances the chances of clinical trials being successful with reduced input time and cost in clinical development [12].

Enhancement of Drug Safety as well as Predictions of Toxicity

Toxicity Prediction Models

Example: Algorithms AI predict the future potential toxicity of the newly synthesized compounds. They study past toxicity data as well as molecular features to predict future patterns of toxicity. The models trace possible dangerous side effects before they reach the clinical trials.

Impact: This decreases the risk of side effects and simultaneously enhances drug safety at the same time.

Pharmacovigilance

Example: AI-based systems track post-marketing data of adverse drug effects and isolate it for comprehensive analysis. Extracted from social media and medical records with the help of Natural Language Processing (NLP) techniques.

Impact: Adds further to safety monitoring of drugs, and makes identification of potential safety issues at a highly initial stage.

High-throughput Data Analysis

Example: AI makes use of large amounts of data through high-throughput studies, for example, protein assays as well as genome sequencing. In this manner, scientists can get useful information from complicated datasets.

Impact: It enhances better-informed decisions in drug development as well as accelerates the assessment of information.

Real-time Data Integration

Example: AI brings in real-time information across various sources from electronic health records to wearables. This can be used for real-time updates of drugs with respect to safety and efficacy.

Impact: This enables more flexible trial designs and much more flexible responses to new data.

Data-driven Drug Discovery

This has brought a sharp change in the discovery, development, and new drugs by the pharmaceutical industries based on the application of big data and ML. Data-driven drug discovery is called that kind of information here. Based on complex algorithms and tremendous amounts of data sourced from different applications,

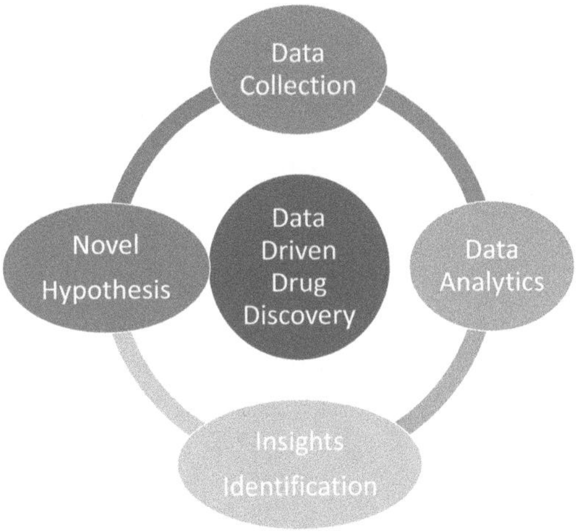

Figure 4.6 Data-driven drug discovery.

it gives meaning to that kind of information as it guides every step of the drug discovery process.

Understanding Data-driven Drug Discovery

Data-driven drug discovery refers to the systematic application of data analytics toward the identification of potential candidates for medication, prediction of their behavior, and optimization for their use in clinics. Thus, data-driven approaches prove more accurate and effective routes toward drug discovery than traditional routes, which are still dependent on experimental trial and error. Rather, data-driven approaches rely on computer capacity in evaluating vast datasets shown in Figure 4.6 [13].

Big Data's Role in Drug Discovery

Huge forms of data, in that regard, encompass within themselves wide varieties of big data in drug discovery, as shown in Figure 4.7.

Omics Data

Genomics: Genomic sequencing data have thrown up potential therapeutic targets as well as the genetic basis of many disorders. Big data analytics helps identify gene expressions, regulatory circuits, and mutations implicated in the processes underlying illness.

Proteomics: The complete complement of proteins produced by an organism, or proteomes, that represent the activities, interactions, and variations of proteins, can provide major datasets, which are indispensable in dissecting disease pathways and identifying candidate therapeutic agents.

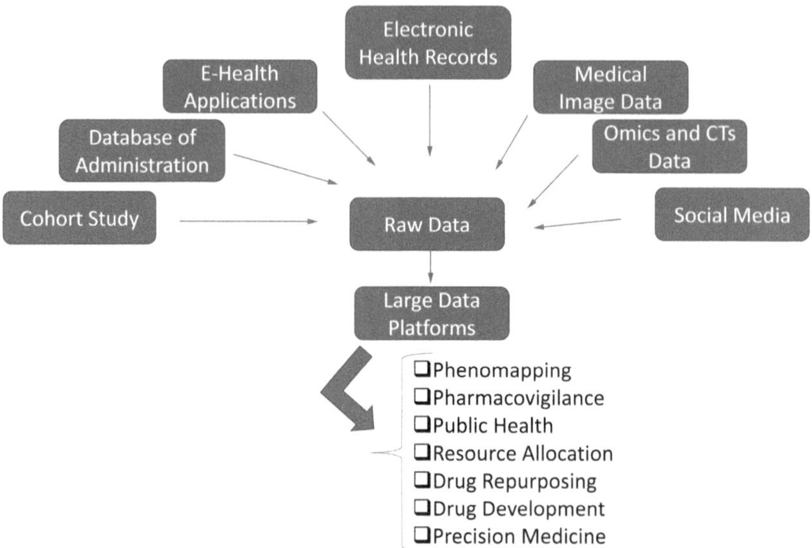

Figure 4.7 Large data for drug discovery.

Transcriptomic: Gene expression profiles can be deduced from RNA transcripts with potential transcriptomic information, and the information might be very helpful in determining how diseases interfere with the cellular functions [14].

Clinical Data

EHRs: EHRs hold records of history of patients, treatment results, and adverse reactions. The private nature of drug reactions derived from such analysis supports personalized medication.

Clinical Trials Data: Such data may even contain the details regarding demographics of patients, patient safety, and the efficacy of drugs. Thus, it may then be possible to identify trends and connections that might not otherwise be perceived by the use of big data analytics while applying conventional analysis of data.

Real-world Data

Patient Registries: Those databases collect outcomes of patients to be further analyzed in order to provide a better understanding of the drug's safety profile and long-term effectiveness.

Wearable Devices: Wearable health-monitoring devices can actually provide a timeline of real-time insights into how patients' health indicators change, which would be used to combine drug discovery with treatment efficacy monitoring.

Chemical Data

Compound Libraries: Hundreds of compounds made available for study and comparison all at once to assist in finding new therapeutic opportunities in the chemical compound databases that have included, right from the outset, both structural information and biological activity.

High-throughput Screening (HTS) Data: HTS screens a very large number of chemicals for their biological activities; this generates huge amounts of data. This makes the determination of active chemicals and the understanding of structure–activity correlations easier [15].

ML in Drug Discovery

ML plays a vital role in the processing and analysis of the huge volumes of data generated during the drug development process, shown in Figure 4.8. Other important applications of ML include:

Target Identification and Validation

PREDICTIVE MODELING

ML algorithms will analyze biological pathways and omics data to predict possible therapeutic targets. For instance, ML models can identify new therapeutic targets for intervention by training against known target-disease pairings.

Network Analysis: This uses ML to analyze the network of protein-protein interaction networks to identify key nodes or targets involved in disease processes

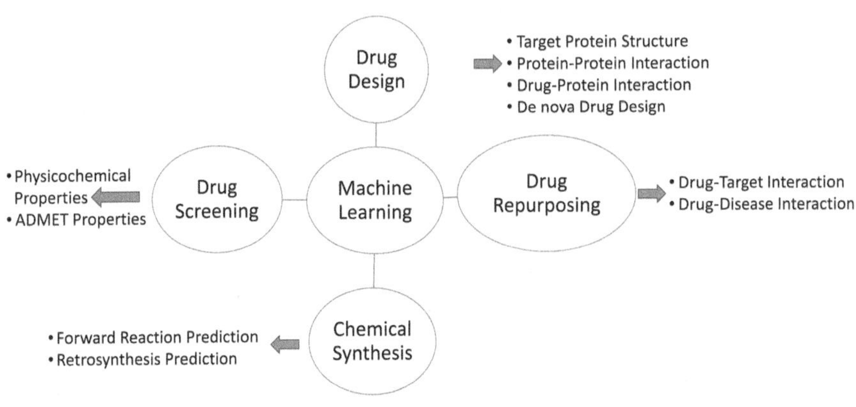

Figure 4.8 ML in drug discovery.

and inform a decision-making process on which of these targets would be the best drug development targets.

Lead Compound Identification

Virtual Screening: It has drastically reduced the number of chemicals that require experimental testing by developing ML models to predict the probability of the chemical compound binding with any given protein.

De Novo Drug Design: These are termed variational autoencoders or Generative Adversarial Networks (GANs). Variational Autoencoders (VAEs) or GANs are types of generative models that learn the properties of existing drugs and generate new compounds with similar attributes.

Drug Repurposing

Pattern Recognition: ML algorithms evaluate the trends of available drug and disease data so that this can help predict novel therapeutic applications of already-approved drugs. This is very important whenever the identification of a cure for a rare or newly discovered disease is being established.

Similarity Analysis: ML could find structural or functional relations that may exist between apparently unrelated drugs, thereby possibly opening new avenues of therapy for drugs already approved.

ADMET Prediction

ADMET includes Absorption, Distribution, Metabolism, Excretion, and Toxicity. These ML models will be able to screen out poor profiles for such drug candidates early in the discovery phase by predicting their pharmacokinetic and toxicological characteristics. Known datasets of chemicals with their ADMET characteristics will serve as the training ground for these models.

Toxicity Prediction: The chemical structure data is analyzed using the ML models so that possible harmful effects of substances being interacted with by the researchers could be precluded.

Personalized Medicine

Patient Stratification: Clinical and genetic data are analyzed by ML algorithms to identify patient groupings most likely to benefit from some course of therapy, thereby enabling more personalized treatment modalities [16].

Biomarker Discovery: Biological markers and ML models in the discovery of biomarkers help in the development of personalized treatment programs to predict patient responses to drugs.

Benefits of Data-driven Drug Discovery

Enhanced Efficiency

- Faster Discovery: The incredible velocity of big data and ML makes it possible to automate big data, accelerating the drug development process, potentially with a shortened timeline from target identification to discovery of lead compound.
- Cost Reduction: The drug development cost can be reduced in general by data-driven approaches that eliminate the costly experimentation.

Improved Accuracy

- Predictive Power: The ML models increase the accuracy of drug effectiveness, safety and patient response prediction; hence, enhanced decisions are made during the early stages of the drug discovery process [17].
- Precision Medicine: Data-driven methodologies may enable the creation of treatments that target more specific treatment conditions. These also enhance patient outcomes and the probability that clinical trials may turn out to be positive.

Discovery of Novel Insights

- Uncovering Hidden Patterns: Use of ML may help in finding new therapeutic targets or pharmacological targets because it is easier to discover patterns and relationships that might be elusive or impossible with other methods.
- Drug Repurposing: Data-driven approaches can discover new uses for existing drugs that have already been approved, providing a faster and therefore less expensive route to drug development

Challenges in Data-driven Drug Discovery

Data Quality and Integration

- Heterogeneity of Data: The combining of data gathered from various sources, including genetic, clinical, and chemical data, is challenging due to the differences in the format, scales, and standards.
- Data Quality: The quality of input data determines how accurate ML models are. Because of the existence of noisy, biased, or incomplete data, sometimes inaccurate predictions come out.

Interpretability and Transparency

- Black-box Models: Most ML models, and certainly deeper learning models, act like "black boxes," meaning we cannot really appreciate how they are reaching

specific types of predictions [18]. This lack of transparency may become an obstacle to the model's uptake in the clinical setting and its eventual regulatory approval.
- Model Validation: These learning machine models must be applied in the process of drug development, having validity and reliability across multiple datasets and contexts.

Ethical and Regulatory Considerations

- Data Privacy: Research based on medication and data from patients is associated with problems of confidentiality and safety in data handling. The GDPR should therefore be respected.
- Algorithmic Bias: If the training data are riddled with historical biases, then these ML models could produce biased outputs, which may have ethical implications, especially in personalized medicine.

Future Directions

Integration with Experimental Approaches

- Hybrid Models: Hybrid approaches of experimental validation using CRISPR gene editing, HTS combined with ML models might enhance these predictions further and accelerate the discovery of new drugs.
- Real-time Data Integration: Input of live data from patient monitoring systems, wearable technology, and many more will be fed into the data-driven drug discovery in the future. This will be directly sending constant input for the model improvement.

Advances in ML

- Explainable AI: More transparent and comprehensible ML models will be crucial in terms of building regulatory clearances and clinician and researcher trust.
- Federated Learning: This method solves the problem of privacy in handling big data while working because ML models can learn from decentralized data without any movement or sharing of data needed [19].

Collaborative Platforms

- Open-source Data Sharing: Collaboration platforms that encourage data sharing and group analysis will accelerate drug discoveries; thus, scientists around the world will be able to contribute to and benefit from shared data and models.
- Cross-disciplinary Collaboration: Increased collaborations among the data scientists, biologists, chemists, and doctors will help in solving complex problems in future for data-driven drug discovery.

Predictive Modeling in Drug Discovery: Enhancing Accuracy and Efficacy

Predictive modeling is one of the important applications of AI and ML in drug discovery, as it particularly enhances the efficacy and precision with which the process of drug development is conducted. Large amounts of data processed through complex algorithms reduce the time and costs associated with drug development and increase the probability of clinical trials succeeding as well as aid in decision-making.

What Is Predictive Modeling in Drug Discovery?

Predictive modeling is the prediction of the response or behavior of biological systems, chemicals, and possible therapeutic alternatives by using computer models. These are past data-based models to predict any kind of outcomes that include how a drug may be absorbed, distributed, metabolized, and excreted from the body, and its toxicity, collectively known as pharmacokinetics

Predictive Modeling Plays a Role in Multiple Stages of Drug Discovery

Target Identification and Validation

Predicting Drug-Target Interactions: AI models help predict the likeliest targets for further research and development by projecting how well a drug candidate will bind to a target protein.

Off-target Predictions: Prediction models predict drug-protein interactions which could be nonintentional and which, in turn, can give rise to unwanted effects. An early warning of such off-target effects would also permit researchers to dabble with the medication to enhance specificity

Identify Lead Compound

Virtual Screening: Large libraries of chemical compounds are visually screened using predictive algorithms for identifying compounds with high potential that are most likely to associate with a compound of interest. This process significantly reduces the laboratory testing required for chemicals [20].

Quantitative Structure–Activity Relationship: Quantitative Structure–Activity Relationship (QSAR) models help identify the best lead candidates as they predict the biological activity of a compound based on its structure.

ADMET Prediction: ADMET profiles of potential drugs are estimated by predictive models. Prior to entering clinical trials, this aids in optimizing medication candidates to improve their safety and efficacy.

Physiochemical Property Prediction: The models predict the physical and chemical properties a drug molecule would have to possess in order to perform well, such as solubility, stability, and permeability.

Biomarker Discovery: Predictive models therefore open up the possibility for attaining customized treatment plans by identifying biomarkers that can forecast how different patient groups are going to respond to a medication.

Patient Stratification: AI algorithms predict which patient, based on the information culled from genetic, proteomic, and clinical data, will most benefit from a given treatment and thus improve treatment results as well as lower the failure rate of trials [21].

Accuracy and Effectiveness Through Prediction Modeling

Some of the ways in which predictive modeling enhances drug discovery are as follows:

Advanced Decision making

Evidence-based Insights: In drug discovery, it is the evidence-based insight drawn from predictive models that guides and directs decisions. The research scientists are able to focus more on the most promising candidates and approaches as the predictive model can make very accurate predictions regarding the outcome [22].

Minimization of Risk: Predictive models minimize the risk of late-stage failures that are expensive and time-consuming. Predictive models enable one to predict potential risks like toxicity or poor pharmacokinetics.

Quickness in Drug Development

Fast Screening: A predictive algorithm would be able to speed the screening of significant chemical libraries significantly; therefore, this could remarkably cut the time necessary to identify potential drug candidates' promising prospects in lead discovery.

Economical Resource Usage: Predictive modeling allows just the allocation of funds and time based upon ranked prospects of drugs and targets.

Higher Strike Rates

Higher Predictive Accuracy: The AI and ML models created have higher prediction accuracy, which in turn promotes the possibility of attaining a successful process in developing medication.

Adjustability and Generalizability: The regular update of predictive models with new data enhances their accuracy. This versatility ensures that the models will always be applicable in different instances of new findings.

Cost Saving

Reduced Cost of Experiments: Predictive modeling, especially during the early stages of drug development, prevents the need for costly and tiring in vitro testing by predicting results in silico.

Reduced Clinical Trial Failures: Predictive models help reduce the failure rates of clinical trials, one of the costliest phases of the drug development process; these occur more as a result of better selection of the drug candidates [23].

Challenges and Future Directions

The advantages of predictive modeling in drug development are above-mentioned; however, the downside is that

Data Quality and Availability

Incomplete or Biased Data: The amount of completeness and quality of the data through which they are trained, therefore, completely ascertains the predictability presented by these predictive models. Incomplete or skewed and noisy data may lead to inaccurate predictions.

Data Integration: Differences in data formats, sizes, and standards make it difficult to combine data from several sources, such as omics data and clinical data.

Model Interpretability

Black-box Models: Very often, the complex prediction models and especially the so-called deep learning models become "black boxes," not fully understanding what happened in the decision-making process. In such a case, transparency will be devastating regarding the acceptance of such models for application in drug development.

Regulatory Challenges: The regulatory environment carefully observes the use of AI-driven prediction models in drug discovery, while putting special emphasis on interpretability and c of the models.

Generalizability

Overfitting: Sometimes, predictive models return good results for known data but not quite as good for fresh, unknown data, as a result of overfitting to the training set. Generalizations of such models are necessary, therefore, to be useful in drug discovery [24].

Ethical Considerations

Predictive algorithms will end up producing a biased prediction if the data used in training is biased as a result of prejudices that were possibly held earlier. This would culminate in ethical implications, mostly from the perspective of personal treatment.

Future Directions

Integrative Experimental Techniques: The predictive modeling needs to be able to integrate into the techniques of validation at an experimental level, which also include CRISPR-based editing of genes and HTS in order for the drug development process to be accelerated.

Advances in AI and ML: With more advancements in AI and ML, we expect to see more accurate and interpretable prediction models and models of prediction that set a higher bar than before in drug development.

Collaborative Platforms: New co-operative systems that would accelerate drug discovery by making data sharing, real-time feedback from experimental outcomes, and predictive modeling. Identification in drug development accelerates the search for new treatments and increases the accuracy of such efforts. Below is how AI is used in each of the critical stages.

Target Identification in Drug Discovery

It has to do with a process wherein one identifies a molecule that can be a protein, usually related to a given disease and can be modulated by a drug to create a therapeutic effect.

Data Mining and Integration: Large amounts of biological data, in the fields of genomics, proteomics, transcriptomics, and metabolomics, could be mined for potential drug-target discovery using AI algorithms, more so with ML models [25]. The datasets could include the data of clinical trials and patient details, such as those available at the Cancer Genome Atlas.

Pattern Recognition: An illustration of how AI, in particular deep learning, can pattern from biological data that a human researcher cannot, including the AI being able to recognize certain gene mutations or protein expressions associated with illnesses and thus are now potentially possible therapeutic targets.

Predictive Modeling: AI algorithms predict the probability of efficacy by focusing on specific substances by ranking targets as the likelihood it would be that predicted targets would yield the successful creation of a drug through relying on historical data generated by drugs developed in the past.

Network Analysis: The AI technologies can be utilized in analyzing protein-protein interaction networks and other biological networks for significant hubs or nodes through which the illness is developed. These usually present a good drug target.

Great scientific literature could be mined and assimilated by the use of NLP in order to get information regarding potential targets. The reference listing for selected proteins/genes/pathways associated with the disease may also be retrieved by the help of NLP for accelerating the process of target identification apart from above-mentioned techniques.

Target Validation in Drug Discovery

The process of verifying that altering a target has a therapeutic impact on the ailment under consideration is known as target validation, shown in Figure 4.9.

In Silico Validation: This is mainly performed by artificial models of biological systems as utilized for the prediction of the consequence of the modification of a target on the clinical course of a disease. These models are primarily in the form

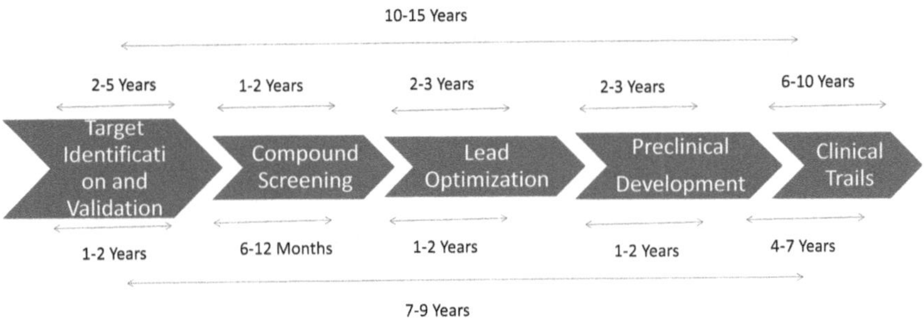

Figure 4.9 Time period required for AI applications.

of computations, mimicry of the biological process, and drug-target interactions of the disease models [26].

Drug-target Interaction Prediction: Predictions of drug-target affinity or, rather, the potential for an interaction to produce a desired therapeutic effect are made by AI models based on deep learning and reinforcement learning. Large collections of documented drug-target interactions are trained on these models.

Gene Editing Technologies: AI provides designs for CRISPR-Cas9 studies of gene knockdown or knockout experiments to confirm the involvement of a target gene in a given disease. AI can predict outcomes of gene editing and provide the best approaches to validate a target.

Omics Data Integration: AI merges data from several omics for validation of objectives. The transcriptomic information, that is, the gene expression, and the proteomic information, that is, the levels of proteins, can be combined to validate whether a target is involved in the disease process or not.

Biomarker Discovery and Validation: AI identifies and validates the presence of biomarkers associated with safety, treatment efficacy, and target engagement. In cases where a drug is not acting upon its pharmacological target as intended, the presence of some biomarkers can serve as a proxy.

Predicting Off-target Effects: Using this information, AI models also predict potential off-target effects by studying the chemical and structural properties of suggested drugs as compared to well-known off-target interactions. This proves that a target might be modified without unwanted side effects.

Benefits of AI in Target Identification and Validation

Speed and Efficiency: AI can identify and validate drug targets more quickly than traditional approaches because it can process and analyze enormous volumes of data much more quickly.

Cost Reduction: AI lowers the cost of drug development by early screening for less promising targets and precise prediction of possible targets.

Improved Accuracy: With the ability of AI to integrate and evaluate many datasets, the possibility of effective drug development increases, thereby leading to the refining of drug target selection and validation [27].

Personalized Medicine: AI aids in the identification of targets unique to each patient, opening the door for personalized medicine strategies that customize medications based on each patient's genetic profile.

Challenges and Concerns Target Identification and Validation

Data Quality: In case the correctness and completeness of the input data are concerned, effective AI-based target identification and validation will be dependent on that. The Predictions may go wrong with incorrect data.

Interpretability: It might be difficult to read AI models, especially when deep neural networks become so complicated to understand why a given target was selected or verified.

Ethical and Legal Issues: AI in drug development and its allied application raises moral and legal questions, especially regarding algorithmic bias, data privacy, and the transparency of AI decision-making processes.

ML Algorithms for Drug Screening and Optimization

As computers can learn directly from the data provided, rather than having to be explicitly programmed, they can predict or make decisions because of the algorithms used in ML. ML algorithms are broadly categorized into four types that are related to the type of learning paradigm that they indulge in—supervised learning, semi-supervised learning, unsupervised learning, and reinforcement learning. The following is a general overview of the most commonly used ML algorithms along with general information about how they are usually applied.

Supervised Learning Algorithms

The supervised learning systems emanate from labeled datasets wherein the input is paired with its proper output. The problem is to find the correct mapping that could be applied to new, unseen data, but which hasn't been demonstrated beforehand.

Linear Regression

Type: Regression

Application: A continuous output variable is predicted by considering the correlation between the input characteristics. Often used for forecasting trends, prices, and other numerical quantities.

Logistic Regression

Type: Classification

Application: used for classification problems where the outcome is binary (yes/no, true/false), like spam detection or sickness diagnosis.

Decision Trees

Type: Classification and Regression
Application: Divides input data into decision branches and makes judgments from those features so that one can predict the outcome. Helpful for work like sickness diagnosis and credit scoring.

Support Vector Machines (SVMs)

Type: Classification
Application: Finds the best boundary, or hyperplane, that separates different classes of data points. Find applications in text categorization, bioinformatics, and image classification.

K-Nearest Neighbors (KNN)

Type: Classification and Regression
Application: Classify a data point according to the majority class amongst its KNNs. Uses in anomaly detection, pattern recognition, and recommendatory systems.

Random Forest

Type: Classification and Regression
Application: an ensemble method that improves on the predictive accuracy through assembling many decision trees. Used for tasks like predicting a stock price, risk assessment, and feature selection.

Gradient Boosting Machines

Type: Classification and Regression
Application: constructs a highly accurate prediction model by sequentially adding multiple weak learners (such as decision trees). Often used in structured data models that win competitions.

Unsupervised Learning Algorithms

Unsupervised learning algorithms, mainly used for finding latent patterns or natural structures in the data, analyze and build a model based on data that does not require any kind of labeled responses.

K-Means Clustering

Type: Clustering
Use: Groups data into K different clusters depending upon the similarity between features. Used for client grouping, picture compression, and market segmentation.

Hierarchical Clustering

Type: Clustering

Application: It produces a dendrogram hierarchy that is used in visualizing the linkages of data. In hierarchies in classification, gene expression analysis, and social network analysis.

PCA

Type: Dimensionality Reduction

Application: It decreases the dimension of the data while retaining the maximum amount of volatility. It is applied for feature extraction, noise reduction, and visualization of the data.

T-distributed Stochastic Neighbor Embedding

Type: Dimensionality Reduction

Application: Maps high-dimensional data into a lower-dimensional space to see it; this method is often used to explore and visualize clusters in data.

Autoencoders

Type: Dimensionality Reduction and Feature Learning

Application: Neural network that can reconstruct input data after being encoded in a form that has a lower dimension. Dimensionality reduction, picture denoising, anomaly detection.

Semi-supervised Learning Algorithms

In cases where it becomes challenging or expensive to gather the labeled data, semi-supervised learning utilizes both labeled and unlabeled data for training.

Self-training Algorithms

Type: Classification

Application: Refine accuracy by iteratively labeling the data using the model, since the model is trained on recognized data. Used in scenarios with a small amount of labeled documents, such as in text categorization.

Generative Models (e.g., Gaussian Mixture Models)

Type: Classification and Clustering

Application: models the joint distribution of inputs and outcomes using partially labeled data to make predictions. applied in bioinformatics, semi-supervised image classification, and voice recognition.

Reinforcement Learning Algorithms

Reinforcement learning algorithms learn new skills by interacting with their environment, receiving feedback in the form of rewards or penalties, and modifying their actions to maximize the total number of rewards.

Q-Learning

Type: Model-free Reinforcement Learning
Essentially, Application: learns which policy is best to make decisions and which actions are most valuable in what states. Applied in Autonomous Systems, Robotics, and Gaming AI.

Deep Q-Networks

Type: Deep Reinforcement Learning
Application: Employs deep neural networks as well as Q-learning to deal with high-dimensional state spaces. applied in the more involved decision-making activities, autonomous vehicles, and game playing.

Policy Gradient Methods

Type: Model-free Reinforcement Learning
Usage: Optimizes the decision-making policy of the agent specifically and is applicable in continuous action spaces. Used in advanced strategic games, robotic control, and finance.

Actor-critic Methods

Hybrid Reinforcement Learning

Type: Hybrids
Application: a combination of both policy-based and value-based approaches by using an actor model in action selection and a critic model in action evaluation. Used in trading algorithms, adaptive systems, and real-time strategy games [28].

Deep Learning Algorithms

Multilayered neural networks or "deep networks" are a subset of ML algorithms used to learn hierarchical representations of data.

Convolutional Neural Networks

Type: Supervised Learning
Application: Primarily used for processing image and video-related applications, this is to be applied to object detection, facial recognition, and picture classification.

Recurrent Neural Networks:

Type: Supervised Learning
Application: It is suitable for the sequential data process as the algorithm fits very well for tasks like time-series forecasting, voice recognition, and language modeling.

Long Short-term Memory Networks

Supervised Learning

Application: a type of RNN that can track long-range dependencies in sequence data. Used in speech synthesis, predictive maintenance, and machine translation.

GANs

Type: Unsupervised Learning
Application: Comprises two networks that fight against each other—the discriminator and the generator—and is widely used to generate very plausible text, audio, and images.

Transformers

Type: Supervised Learning
Application: Largely used in natural language processing operations, for example, language modeling, text summarization, and translation. For example, models such as GPT and BERT are transformer-based.
AI-aided drug design: This is one of the most innovative approaches being adopted in the drug discovery process, which allows a drug to be researched and developed fully with the aid of AI. AI technologies are introduced at all stages of processes-from the initial discovery of molecules to the release of a drug, which enhances prospects for success, reduces costs, and increases efficiency. How AI is revolutionizing the design of medicines—from molecules to the market—is elaborated upon as follows [29].

Molecule Identification and Design

De Novo Drug Design

AI Techniques: Generative models are employed to generate novel chemical compounds that are supposed to possess desired biological properties. GANs and VAEs are some of those architectures.
Applications: The models increase the chemical space available for drug development because they yield entirely new compounds that would not appear in a library of known chemicals.
Benefits: With AI-driven de novo design, researchers can explore new chemical entities that possess specific features appropriate for interference with target biological processes.

Virtual Screening

AI Techniques: Huge chemical libraries are scanned to find out candidates for drugs using ML models such as Random Forests, SVMs, and deep neural networks.

Applications: Predictive AI algorithms pick out compounds to further research based on their anticipated biological activity, toxicity, and pharmacokinetic properties.

Advantages: The virtual screening accelerates early stages of drug development significantly by eliminating costly and time-consuming physical screens.

Lead Optimization

ADMET Property Prediction

AI Techniques: ADMET properties are predicted by supervised learning type prediction models to estimate the ADMET properties of the drug candidates [30].

AI algorithms incorporate all the past data of other drugs which were built in the past and apply that to predict which compounds will most likely work based on the targeting compounds. Such measures can be prioritized according to each predicted target with its chances of eventually turning out to be a drug.

Applications: Through the prediction of metabolism or toxicity liability, these models guide lead compound optimization by focusing on the changes to enhance drug-like properties.

Benefits: AI-driven predictions help avoid failures at a later stage in the design cycle because these ADMET-related problems are encountered early in the process.

Structure–Activity Relationship Modeling

AI Methods: Regression models comprising QSAR models are used to understand the relationship between chemical structure and biological activity.

Usage: Structure–Activity Relationship (SAR) models guide the changes that enhance the structures for safer, more effective, and selective drugs.

Advantages: SAR modeling rapidly accelerates the lead optimization that includes practical knowledge of the effects of chemical changes in drug activity.

Preclinical Development

Biomarker Identification

AI Techniques: ML algorithms assess genomics, proteomics, and other omics data for biomarkers that predict treatment responses or disease progression [31].

Applications: Preclinically, this is being used for disease condition traceability, therapy prediction, and patient stratification.

Benefits: The drug biomarker discovery using AI has brought more targeted drugs, developing and adapting the treatment of drugs more precisely.

Toxicology Prediction

AI Techniques: Deep learning-based models predict the safety features of new drug molecules based on the historical toxicology data.
Applications: AI-based models predict drug-drug interactions, potential off-target liabilities, and organ-specific toxicities.
Benefits: Identification of toxicological risk at an early stage improves the safety profile of new drugs, which reduces the chances of undesirable outcomes during later stages.

Clinical Trials

Patient Recruitment and Stratification

AI Techniques: ML algorithms and NLP review clinical data and electronic health records to identify qualified participants for clinical trials.
Applications: With such genetic profiling or features of an illness, AI can also match patients to relevant clinical trials to enhance the efficiency and outcomes of such studies.
Benefits: Optimizing the recruitment and classification of patients shortens the trial duration and increases the possibility of proving medication efficacy [32].

Trial Design Optimization

AI Techniques: In the improvement of the design of clinical studies, including the dose regimens, selection of outcomes, and randomization of patients, AI models mimic many situations for a clinical trial.
Applications: With AI-driven clinical study design, one can identify the best tactics to reduce risks and have a higher probability of getting regulatory clearance.
Benefits: AI-boosted clinical studies are even more successful, cost-effective, and time-efficient.

Regulatory Approval

Regulatory Submission and Review

AI Techniques: AI can help in processing and analyzing such data for regulatory filings to conform with legal standards and predict possible questions the regulatory body might have.
Applications: Clinical trial data can be represented and structured using NLP and ML models for faster review.
Benefits: AI allows better, more complete proposals to be made, which, in turn, may improve the speed of regulatory clearance [33].

Post-market Surveillance

AI Techniques: ML algorithms follow the actual data from social media, electronic health records, and others after a medicine has been introduced to detect ADRs.

Applications: AI systems would be able to spot potential problems sooner and more correctly than traditional methods.

Benefits: The enhanced post-market surveillance would be able to detect problems that would require immediate response and avoid endangering the patient in the future.

Launch in the Market and Beyond

Market Strategy and Demand Forecasting

AI Technologies: Predictive analytics and ML algorithms enable predictions of demand and sales pattern analysis, patient demographics, and market data to improve market strategy.

Applications: Pharmaceutical companies can implement product launch strategies, pricing plans, and logistics of distribution more strategically with AI.

Benefits: Accurate demands and targeted marketing techniques maximize the commercial potential of a drug while ensuring adequate supply for it.

Patient Compliance and Personalized Therapy

AI Techniques: AI-enabled wearables along with mobile phone applications monitor and track patient compliance for therapy and allow for personalized health information.

Applications: These devices enhance patient involvement, maximize treatment efficiency, and present current information to health care providers

Benefits: Enhanced patient compliance results in better health outcomes while also sustaining the long-run viability of newly introduced medicine.

Ethical Considerations and Regulatory Analysis of AI in Drug Development

It could change the face of the pharmaceutical industry due to cost saving, faster drug development, and exploration for therapeutic directions unthought-of hitherto [34]. However, there are a number of ethical issues pertinent to AI-based drug development.

Some of the Issues that Are Listed Below

Ethical Issues

Bias and Fairness

Data Bias: AI models tend to have a quality that results from the data it was trained by. So if the biased training data sets are taken, it will then propagate the ones that are currently in practice or exaggerate them into existence. This, therefore, may make the formulation of particular medications not very effective or toxic in other population sections.

Algorithmic Transparency: The nature of AI algorithms as black boxes makes it difficult to understand how decisions are being made, and this raises ethical questions about the principles of accountability and trust.

Informed Consent and Data Privacy

Patient Data: AI in drug discovery often uses huge datasets, such as genetic data and medical records. Important ethical issues include obtaining patient consent for data usage and protecting patient privacy [35].

Identification: De-identified data can potentially be re-identified; thus, leading to a probable violation of privacy.

Effect on Labor

Job Displacement: There are ethical concerns with the implications on the labor force as some jobs that were once carried out by human investigators are now automated. This can lead to unemployment or a change in employment.

Accessibility and Fairness

Global Inequities: The benefits from the discovery of AI-based medicines are not likely to come to all populations equitably. The least benefits are going to reach low and middle-income countries.

Price of New Medicines: This speed at discovering new medicines is going to cost them, which will keep them out of the pockets of most who would actually use the drugs [36].

Human Overdrive

Decision-making: I can monitor drug development, but I should be under human surveillance to ensure that ethical issues are addressed within any decision made, especially when it is regarding patient safety and clinical trials.

Regulatory Approaches

Validation and Quality

Model Validation: FDA and EMA demand that regulatory agencies should validate the AI models used in drug discovery to ensure safety, efficacy, and reliability [37].

Quality Standards: The pharmaceutical industry requires developing standards in the use of AI in drug development for the sake of homogeneity and safety.

Regulatory Guidelines

Evolving Regulations: Since AI in drug development is at an early stage, the laws that regulate it likewise keep on changing; for this reason, agencies shall have to evolve or alter new regulations that deal particularly with the challenges AI introduces, like an intelligent measure of quality for medication candidates created by AI.

Approval Processes since AI results are different from the regular processes in nature and speed, they could challenge the existing approval processes. The approvals and timelines may need to be readjusted by the regulatory bodies.

Data Governance

Data Sharing and Security: There is an urgent need for regulatory bodies to provide specific guidelines relating to data exchange and security involving AI. That would mean crossing borders in streams of data, especially since companies are geographically scattered around the borders, as drug research programs are [38].

Ethics in the Use of AI: The regulating bodies may have to impose regulations that ensure the moral use of AI to avoid misuse or unethical drug discovery processes.

Post-market Surveillance

Surveillance for AI-discovered Drugs: The AI-generated drugs have to be followed even further and continuously during rollout from licensing to ensure not only that they remain safe but also that they prove to be effective in real life. That may require novel surveillance methods fitted to the deployment of AI-generated therapies.

Collaboration with AI Developers

Public-Private Partnerships: It may require regulatory agencies to be closer working in collaboration with academic institutions, pharmaceutical enterprises, and AI developers, such that the AI technologies are conceived and implemented toward public health objectives.

Exscientia and DSP-1181: The First AI-designed Drug

Overview

In a collaborative effort to treat OCD, UK-based AI-driven drug Development Company, Exscientia, has collaborated with Sumitomo Dainippon Pharma to develop DSP-1181 as a potential therapeutic candidate.

Usage of AI

Design of Drug: Exscientia designed DSP-1181 using its AI platform. Thus, AI derived and optimized new chemicals according to specific biological targets of OCD by screening a huge chemical space [39].

Time to Discovery: It cut the traditional 4–5 years of identifying a drug and designing it to 12 months using the AI approach.

Outcome

DSP-1181 was the first fully AI-designed drug advanced into clinical trials in humans in the year 2020. This is simply great what AI brings to the process, making it much shorter in discovering drugs and producing new treatments.

In Silico Medicine and New Fibrosis Treatment

Overview

Idiopathic pulmonary fibrosis (IPF) is one of the chronic and potentially fatal lung diseases. In silico Medicine, a biotech company with a focus on AI in drug discovery, applied an AI platform to discover novel medication candidates for IPF [40].

AI Application

Target Identification: The AI of In silico identified new biological targets linked to IPF by analyzing multiomics data, including transcriptomics, proteomics, and genomes.
Compound Generation: The AI system synthesized and optimized novel small compounds that may act on these targets for developing the potential treatment options.
Validation: Promising results were shown by the preclinical animals when the drugs generated by the AI system were validated in the experiment.

In silico showed how AI could shave off all the time from discovering a target to achieving preclinical validation in just 18 months by doing it all at once. Now that the lead chemical has gotten into the preclinical stage, future clinical studies can be performed [41].

Atom Wise and ALS Therapy

Overview

The AI-driven drug discovery startup Atomwise collaborated with several academic institutions in search of potential treatments for the debilitating neurological disease known as ALS, or amyotrophic lateral sclerosis.

AI Application

Virtual Screening: Atom screened millions of chemicals atom-wise with the help of its AI technology, Atom Net. The task given to the AI was to identify compounds that can bind to a specific protein target associated with ALS.

Compound Selection: A small number of very promising candidates were left on the short list for additional testing after the AI model estimated the binding affinity and drug-likeness of possible compounds.

Outcome

In preclinical models, the efficacy of AI-selected drugs shows a promising outcome and has thus created more interest and research. The process adopted by Atomwise is one of the most brilliant examples through which AI can efficiently screen massive chemical libraries to look for new therapeutic options, especially for challenging diseases such as ALS [42].

Benign AI and Baricitinib on COVID

Background

There is a London-based AI startup called Benevolent AI that capitalized on existing approved drugs for repositioning and discovery of potential treatments for the COVID-19 pandemic in its early stages.

AI Use

Drug Repurposing: Benevolent AI identified drugs already known for repurposing in treating COVID-19 from humungous biological data through their AI platform. The AI system initially oriented itself toward the drugs that may block SARS-CoV-2, the virus responsible for COVID-19, from entering the body.

Identification of Drug Baricitinib: The AI identified the drug Baricitinib, which is approved for use with a drug initially in the treatment of rheumatoid arthritis, as a potential COVID-19 drug through its anti-inflammatory properties and antiviral entry into host cells.

Outcome

The FDA immediately cleared Baricitinib for use within COVID-19 clinical studies and issued an Emergency Use Authorization (EUA) [43]. It was one of the select few drugs that could be applied with a high degree of effectiveness to treat COVID-19, therefore embodying AI's capacity to quickly repurpose existing medicines for new treatments.

GSK and AI for Target Identification

Overview

To enhance the discovery of potential drugs, GlaxoSmithKline (GSK), which is one of the world's largest pharmaceutical companies, formed a partnership with an AI-Start-up company known as Insilico Medicine.

AI Implementation

The following are the details of new targets that came from the humongous data set of proteomics and genomics; new targets which would otherwise have been passed over during the traditional approach were revealed through AI.

Collaboration: The information derived by the AI was useful in focusing targets and accelerating drug discovery because the targets found were appended to GSK's list of drugs being developed.

As a result of the partnership between GSK and Insilico Medicine, many new therapy targets emerged; some are currently under investigation in pre-clinical and clinical studies. This is an excellent example of how fruitful AI can be for new target identification in drug-development in the case of complex diseases.

Deep Mind and Protein Folding (Alpha Fold)

Introduction

Deep Mind is an AI research laboratory that belongs to Alphabet, and it has designed an AI system that makes accurate predictions about the shapes of proteins. Because the shape of a protein determines its function as well as how it would interact with any potential medications, protein folding is a very important step in developing a new drug [44].

Application of AI

Inferred Protein Structure from its Amino Acid Sequence: Alpha Fold uses deep learning to predict the 3D structure of proteins based on amino acid sequences. Accurate protein structure prediction is important for an understanding of causes of disease and designing efficacious medications.

Acceleration of Drug Development: Because Alpha Fold's predictions give detailed structural information guiding target validation and drug design, new drug development has been accelerated in crucial ways.

Result

This came at the time when Alpha Fold demonstrated structural biology as having finally changed the game, in terms of accurately and amazingly good predictions to win the CASP Critical Assessment of Protein Structure Prediction competition. Predictions of this system are already used within several drug discovery projects, helping researchers design ever-more targeted treatments.

Application in Drug Design and Optimization

Lead Identification

Virtual Screening: AI rapidly screens huge chemical libraries for possible lead compounds, which reveal potential pharmaceutical activity [25]. On the basis of predicted binding affinities in these chemicals toward the target protein, ML algorithms narrow down the candidates that need further exploration.

Ligand-based Drug Design: Based on chemical structure and activity data derived from known ligands, AI models are able to predict the activity of novel molecules, thus discovering new leads with comparable or even better qualities.

Lead Optimization

Predicting ADMET Properties: Since the AI capability also predicts the ADMET properties of the lead compound, the attributes may be optimized early during the drug development process. It thus lowers the chances for late-stage failure due to toxicities or improper pharmacokinetics.

Multiobjective Optimization: AI will be useful in optimizing simultaneously potency, selectivity, solubility, and safety of a lead compound by screening the vast chemical space and identifying the ideal ratio between these properties.

DTIs Prediction

ML Models: Huge databases of known drug targets may computationally be interrogated with AI systems to predict the bio-target drug interactions. This helps find new possibilities for treatments or repurpose existing drugs in unexplored markets [45].

Network-based Strategies: AI may analyze biological networks to predict the interaction of a given drug with other components of biological systems and hence potential therapeutic opportunities as well as possible off-target effects.

Compound Property Prediction

The main thing is that AI may be used to predict multiple chemical properties, which are inevitable and critical for drug development and determination, such as solubility, stability, or reactivity. Such predictions would help in the designing of drugs that would have a higher possibility of success upon undergoing clinical trials.

QSAR Models: AI develops QSAR models that predict the actions of a chemical compound from its molecular structure. Such models further explain the relation of molecular structures to biological functions, which results in inventing more potent drugs [46].

Drug Repurposing

Creation of New Applications for Known Compounds AI can analyze very huge sums of biological data to discover identifications of potential new uses of established pharmaceuticals. Reworked drugs can take extensive amounts of time and many valuable resources that might be assigned to developing drugs because of already being evaluated for both safety and efficacy at many levels.

Integration of Omics Data: AI will predict new therapeutic targets for already existing drugs by integrating omics data such as genomics and proteomics toward the development of innovative therapy of complex disorders [27].

Predictive Modeling of Clinical Outcomes

Predictive Patient Response: AI can predict the response of the patient population to a medicine based on lifestyle, genetic, and environmental characteristics. This creates further scope for development in the personalized medicine domain along with the identification of biomarkers for patient stratification in clinical studies.

Optimization of Clinical Trials: AI can be used to develop better clinical trials by predicting results, identifying the appropriate patient populations, and optimizing dosing regimens.

Automation of Medicinal Chemistry

Automated Synthesis Planning: AI can really help organic chemists plan synthetic routes to potential drug candidates with the most practical and effective pathways. This reduces the time taken to synthesize and evaluate new chemicals.

Automated HTS: HTS is also enhanced through AI-driven automation that enables fast, accurate detection of potential drug candidates by screening thousands of compounds in the shortest possible period.

Drug Formulation and Delivery

Optimization of Drug Formulations: Using AI, chemical stability, bioavailability, and solubility can be predicted in different delivery methods to optimize medication formulations. This ensures the final medicine product is safe, effective, and easy to manufacture [47].

This would design drug delivery systems where AI would predict how the drugs interact with those systems as well as how they would be released inside the human body. It may probably develop advanced means of medication delivery, for instance, controlled-release formulations or nanoparticles.

In silico toxicology: The AI models may predict at the early stages of drug discovery that the chemical compound could be toxic, thus minimizing the chance of late-stage failures. Predicts the compound's potential for causing adverse effects based on its structure.

Off-target effects: The AI enabled the designing of safer drugs with fewer surprises by predicting possible off-target interactions that may cause adverse effects.

Challenges and Limitations of AI in Drug Discovery

In all certainty, ML and AI technologies shall promise great potential to improve drug development in the pace of discovery, costs, and results. However, several issues and constraints must be approached in order to maximize the advantages of current technologies [48, 49].

Data Quality and Availability

Data Scarcity: There is a scarcity of high-quality labeled datasets for training AI/ML models. It is usually very difficult to obtain when it comes to rare diseases or novel therapeutic targets, thereby limiting the amount of accuracy with which the models can predict the future.

Data Heterogeneity: The drug discovery data is obtained through diverse sources, ranging from electronic medical records and chemical libraries to clinical trials and genetic data. Due to its heterogeneity, it's generally tricky to integrate or align the information for the effective training of AI/ML models [50].

Data Bias: The AI/ML models might make biased or less generalizable predictions if the training data is skewed, for instance, over-representing certain populations or medication classes, which may lead to outcomes worse than optimal, or exacerbate existing health inequalities.

Validation and Generalization

Overfitting: Though the AI/ML models would do quite well on training data, they will not generalize to fresh, untested data. This is a very serious issue for drug development since the models may overfit certain datasets and completely fail in practical settings.

Validation: Verification of AI/ML models on a large scale is extremely difficult, as in the case of such biologically complex systems and unprecedented pharmacological targets. Ideally, for being exercised, therefore, in actual life use cases, they must make outputs reproducible in dependence upon different scenarios and their corresponding datasets [51].

Interoperability with Existing Workflows

Resistance to Change: Traditionally anchored researchers might be resistant to integrating AI/ML into traditional flows for drug development. Slower changes might occur due to the unwillingness of people to accept insights from AI concerning validity concerns.

Workflow Compatibility: The architecture of AI/ML tools must integrate with the existing computation and experimental practices. It is no easy job to coordinate the chemists, biologists, pharmacologists, and the AI specialist since they belong to different fields with different views.

Ethical and Legal Challenges

Patient Privacy: AI/ML models generally need large sets of patient data, raising privacy and security issues about the data. Insights into how to protect patient data and anonymize it are therefore important, especially when transferring such information across borders or companies.

Intellectual Property: With AI/ML applications in drug discovery, intellectual property rights are in question. For example, the intellectual property of a medicine is relatively uncertain if it is detected by an AI model, especially when many parties are involved with the process [52, 53].

Bias and Fairness: Ensuring that AI/ML models are fair and do not introduce current biases is an ethical challenge, though especially crucial in drug development, because biased models might lead to biased access to new treatments or even worse than optimal effects for certain population groups.

Computational Intensity

Resource-intensive: Both training and inference require a large amount of computing resources by AI/ML models, especially deep learning models. It is challenging for small research groups or businesses due to the limited access to high-performance computer resources.

Scalability: The other major challenge in the field of drug development is the scalability of AI/ML models. Biological systems are complex, and large chemical spaces often don't adjust well to any small model. Scalable algorithms should be developed that can handle huge datasets within a reasonable time and give accurate predictions [54].

Biological Complexity

Biological systems: Biological systems are very complex due to their large interdependent parts and feedback mechanisms. It is difficult for AI/ML models to encode this complexity and reduce the resulting system into a simpler form, leading to a prediction that has a chance of not being true.

Unknown Mechanisms: Still, our knowledge of biological functions limits current AI/ML models. Application of models in drug discovery can be jeopardized if these pathways are not properly understood, since they rarely predict outcomes accurately.

Reproducibility and Robustness

Reproducibility Crisis: Another major issue with the AI/ML models that really plagues drug development is the lack of reproducibility. Differences in outcomes might arise from variability in model performance across different datasets, experimental settings, or even random training seeds.

Noise Robustness: Biological data is generally noisy, and AI/ML models should be able to be robust to it for providing reliable predictions. One major problem in that regard is ensuring that models can generate accurate predictions even in the presence of noisy data [55].

Ethical Use of AI/ML

AI-driven Experimentation: There are several questions that arise concerning whether human researchers using AI and ML should design and optimize experiments [56, 57]. There is an immediate need to ensure that AI complements human abilities rather than replacing them, and that it is introduced in tandem with appropriate ethical considerations when applied for research purposes.

Impact on Drug Prices: Even though AI/ML would allow the cost of drug discovery to come down, there are concerns that the benefit of such savings would not reach the customers in specific, especially the life-saving drugs. Ethically, therefore, one must ensure that drugs developed with the support of AI should be at reasonable prices to the consumers.

Opportunities of AI and ML in Drug Discovery

There are numerous opportunities in drug discovery with AI and ML, as they can revolutionize pharmaceutical research at various stages of drug development. The novelty of these technologies is not only to increase productivity or reduce costs, but also to come up with new medicines never seen before.

Boosting Medication Discovery: The time to get from target identification to lead compounds may be cut down dramatically by scanning the large datasets using AI/ML and quickly finding potential drug candidates. This is especially useful when responding to the emergence of new health dangers such as pandemics [58–63].

De Novo Drug Design: AI-driven models may create new, desirable molecular structures from scratch, avoiding the need for time-consuming trial-and-error procedures and accelerating the development of new medications.

Cost Reduction

Reduced R&D Costs: AI and ML have the potential to significantly lower research and development costs by automating labor-intensive operations and increasing the effectiveness of drug discovery procedures. This is especially helpful in the normally expensive early stages of drug research.

Predictive Toxicology: During the early development stage, AI/ML models may predict a compound's toxicity, thereby reducing the chances of late-stage failures that can be expensive and wasting resources on less viable candidates.

Precision Medicine

Personalized Drug Design: AI/ML enables the creation of personalized medications by evaluating genetic, environmental, and lifestyle data to customize drug design for specific patients. This strategy can increase therapeutic efficacy and reduce side effects by focusing medicines on certain patient subgroups [64–66].

Biomarker Discovery: The use of AI and ML can lead to finding biomarkers that may denote how a patient would respond to a particular medication; this could help with matching patients and the generation of personalized treatment. This can lead to better results in precision medicine and more powerful therapies.

Improved Predictive Modeling

Drug-target Interaction Prediction: High-accuracy predictions of drug-biotarget interactions may be made by AI/ML models, which speed up the process of identifying potential candidates and cut down on time wasted on fruitless searches.

ADMET Prediction: AI/ML can help optimize drug candidates before clinical trials by predicting the characteristics of Absorption, Distribution, Metabolism, Excretion, and Toxicity (ADMET) of drugs, thus enhancing the safety and efficacy profiles.

Improved Data Usage

Big Data Integration: AI/ML may integrate and analyze large volumes of data from many sources, such as literature, electronic health records, and omics data (genomics, proteomics). This detailed data analysis might offer new insights and propose new therapeutic targets.

Real-world Evidence: AI/ML may evaluate clinical and patient data as well as other RWD for assisted drug development and discovery. This will enhance clinical trial designs and allow new therapeutic applications of already approved drugs [67, 68].

Drug Repurposing

Identifying New Indications: AI/ML can recognize new therapeutic indications for approved drugs by assessing the available data of drugs, thus causing more rapid and cost-effective drug development processes. The approach has previously been utilized to cure diseases such as COVID-19.

Predictive Analysis: Researchers can predict off-target effects and even new uses for existing drugs with the help of AI/ML, thus increasing the therapeutic application and providing a new treatment option.

Optimization of Clinical Trials

Automation and Efficiency Gains

Automation of Drug Synthesis: AI/ML designs and performs chemical synthesis routes for drug candidates, therefore increasing productivity and reducing the time to synthesize new molecules.

HTS: Use of AI/ML to speed up procedures for HTS that may considerably hasten early-stage drug development by rapidly evaluating a large number of compounds to identify those with the most promising activity.

Improving Teamwork and Knowledge Collaboration

AI/ML-powered collaboration tools: AI/ML may further accelerate the pace of drug discovery by offering opportunities for scientists from multiple institutes and universities to share data and learnings across different collaborations.

AI/ML will follow patterns and trends between various studies; hence, information will be shared, ensuring efficiency in the process of drug development and not attempting to make the process redundant.

Polypharmacology: AI and ML development of drugs by modulating several pathways or receptor targets shows particular effectiveness in the treatment of complex diseases arising out of many biological activities.

Regulatory Support

Regulatory Submissions Support: Thus, AI/ML is expected to support regulatory submission preparations with such automated data analyses and reporting, improving and reducing the time needed to review submissions for regulations.

Post-market Surveillance: AI/ML continues to automatically scan the data for any unforeseen undesirable events while ensuring the drugs are safe and effective.

New Mechanisms

Identification of New Biological Pathways: Analyzing big data with the use of AI/ML will disclose new biological processes and pathways, which can open new vistas for therapeutic intervention.

Target identification: AI/ML can study genomic and proteomic data to identify new targets for pharmacology, creating medications that bind to new targets and fulfilling unmet medical needs.

Conclusion

The bright horizon of AI and ML in drug discovery: At every turn, AI and ML are making the process of drug development more accurate and swift. Traditionally, this is a very expensive and time-consuming process; the whole process of drug development requires time-consuming procedures for screening hundreds of chemicals and interpreting complicated biological data. AI and ML are trying to tackle these challenges by automating and optimizing many steps in the process of discovery.

Accelerated Identification of Drug Candidates: AI and ML systems can identify potential drug candidates much faster compared to traditional methods by processing large volumes of data. These algorithms identify the right cocktail of chemicals interacting well with certain disease targets through a deep analysis of patterns in both biological and chemical data. This helps speed up early-stage drug discovery by allowing researchers to focus on more promising candidates.

AI and ML have thus improved predictive modeling through sophisticated algorithms simulating and predicting how the medications will react in the body. Such models predict interactions of medicines, side effects, and effectiveness, and therefore decrease the necessity of doing multiple animal tests and lower the failure rates in the final stages of medication creation. It thus requires such predictive capabilities so that medication development is optimally done, ensuring that only the best candidates reach clinical trials.

AI and ML have transformed the landscape in the design of clinical trials by evaluating patient data to find eligible candidates and predict their reactions to treatment. This results in studies that are more effective and individualized while cutting down on the time and expense needed to identify volunteers and oversee trials. AI-powered solutions could also monitor real-time progress of clinical trials, and, where possible, identify problems early and adapt to these with further adjustments to improve outcomes.

AI and ML have, to a great degree, facilitated the advanced integration of different data types: genomic, proteomic, and clinical. In some sense, this interconnection of databases has endowed researchers with the capability for greater insight into the processes of a disease and identification of new targets of therapy. This approach is all-encompassing, offering new and advanced understandings of complicated diseases and helping in the process of targeted, more efficient treatment.

Drug Repurposing: Drug repurposing could be another area where AI and ML can be used; it includes an investigation into already approved drugs for their possible applications. ML algorithms scour existing drug data to find new indications for either drugs that are still in development or for those that have already received approval. Using this approach can greatly shorten the time to market new therapies using current safety and effectiveness data.

Improved Efficiency and Cost Reduction: By automating monotonous tasks and enhancing various stages of the drug discovery process, AI and ML can reduce overall costs and minimize the time it takes to bring a medicine to market. Processing and analyzing large amounts of data quickly and accurately lowers the risk of costly errors and increases the overall efficacy of the drug development process.

In conclusion, AI and ML technologies are revolutionizing drug discovery: speeding up drug development through better accuracy and efficiency. They enhance processes, allow for customized treatment plans, and boost prediction ability.

References

1. Vrontis D, Christofi M, Pereira V, Tarba S, Makrides A, Trichina E. Artificial intelligence, robotics, advanced technologies and human resource management: A systematic review. Int J Human Res Manag. 2022;33:1237–1266.
2. Howard J. Artificial intelligence: Implications for the future of work. Am J Ind Med. 2019;62:917–926.
3. Arinez JF, Chang Q, Gao RX, Xu C, Zhang J. Artificial intelligence in advanced manufacturing: Current status and future outlook. J Manuf Sci Eng. 2020;142(11): 142.
4. Nath A, Khandelwal A, Kanojia A, Minocha I, Niyogi R. Design and implementation of an intelligent cab service system. *2017 Tenth International Conference on Contemporary Computing (IC3)*. IEEE; 2017. p. 1–6.
5. Abduljabbar R, Dia H, Liyanage S, Bagloee SA. Applications of artificial intelligence in transport: An overview. Sustainability. 2019;11:189.
6. Begoli E, Bhattacharya T, Kusnezov D. The need for uncertainty quantification in machine-assisted medical decision making. Nat Mach Intell. 2019;1:20–23.
7. Abasolo JM, Gomez M. MELISA: An ontology-based agent for information retrieval in medicine. *Proceedings of the 1st international workshop on the semantic web (SemWeb2000)*. 2000. p. 73–82.
8. Abdel-Karim BM, Pfeuffer N, Hinz O. Machine learning in information systems - a bibliographic review and open research issues. Electron Mark. 2021;31(3):643–670.
9. Agerfalk PJ. Artificial intelligence as digital agency. Eur J Inf Syst. 2020;29(1):1–8.
10. Arnott D, Pervan G. A critical analysis of decision support systems research. J Inf Technol. 2005;20(2):67–87.
11. Zachi I. Attia, Suraj Kapa, Francisco Lopez-Jimenez, Paul M. McKie, Dorothy J. Ladewig, Gaurav Satam, Patricia A. Pellikka, Maurice Enriquez-Sarano, Peter A. Noseworthy, Thomas M. Munger, Samuel J. Asirvatham, Christopher G. Scott, Rickey E. Carter & Paul A. Friedman. Screening for cardiac contractile dysfunction using an artificial intelligence-enabled electrocardiogram. Nat Med. 2019;25:70–74.
12. Yuichi Mori, Shin-ei Kudo, Masashi Misawa, Yutaka Saito, Hiroaki Ikematsu, Kinichi Hotta, Kazuo Ohtsuka, Fumihiko Urushibara, Shinichi Kataoka, Yushi Ogawa, Yasuharu Maeda, Kenichi Takeda, Hiroki Nakamura, Katsuro Ichimasa, Toyoki Kudo, Takemasa Hayashi, Kunihiko Wakamura, Fumio Ishida, Haruhiro Inoue, Hayato Itoh, Masahiro Oda, and Kensaku Mori, Real-time use of artificial intelligence in identification of diminutive polyps during colonoscopy. Ann Intern Med. 2018;169:357.
13. Ramesh A. Artificial intelligence in medicine. Ann R Coll Surg Engl. 2004;86:334–338.
14. Steels L, Brooks R. The Artificial Life Route to Artificial Intelligence: Building Embodied, Situated Agents. Routledge; 2018.
15. Abagyan R, Totrov M, Kuznetsov D. ICM–a new method for protein modeling and design: Applications to docking and structure prediction from the distorted native conformation. J Comput Chem. 1994;15(5):488–506.
16. Ain QU, Aleksandrova A, Roessler FD, Ballester PJ. Machine-learning scoring functions to improve structure-based binding affinity prediction and virtual screening. Wiley Interdiscip Rev Comput Mol Sci. 2015;5(6):405–424.
17. Artursson P, Karlsson J. Correlation between oral drug absorption in humans and apparent drug permeability coefficients in human intestinal epithelial (caco-2) cells. Biochem Biophys Res Commun. 1991;175(3):880–885.
18. Bengio Y. Learning Deep Architectures for AI. Norwell: Now Publishers Inc.; 2009.
19. Polina Mamoshina, Marina Volosnikova, Ivan V. Ozerov, Evgeny Putin, Ekaterina Skibina, Franco Cortese, Alex Zhavoronkov. Machine learning on human muscle transcriptomic data for biomarker discovery and tissue-specific drug target identification. Front Genet. 2018;9:242.
20. Ganesh GS, Kolusu AS, Prasad K, Samudrala PK, Nemmani KVS. Advancing health care via artificial intelligence: From concept to clinic. Eur J Pharmacol. 2022;934.

21. Vamathevan J, Clark D, Czodrowski P, et al. Applications of machine learning in drug discovery and development. Nat Rev Drug Discov. 2019;18:463–477.
22. Taylor L, Nitschke G. Improving deep learning with generic data augmentation. Proc IEEE Symp Comput Intell (SSCI 2018). Piscataway, NJ, USA: IEEE Inc.; 2019. p. 1542–1547.
23. Schraagen JM, van Diggelen J. Expertise at Work. Cham, Switzerland: Palgrave Macmillan; 2021. p. 149–175.
24. Karimian G, Petelos E, Evers SMAA. The ethical issues of the application of artificial intelligence in healthcare: A systematic scoping review. AI Ethics. 2022;2:539–551.
25. DiMasi AJ, Grabowski HG, Hansen RW. Innovation in the pharmaceutical industry: New estimates of R&D costs. J Health Econ. 2016;47:20–33.
26. Fleming N. How artificial intelligence is changing drug discovery. Nature. 2018;557:55–57.
27. Mak KK, Pichika MR. Artificial intelligence in drug development: Present status and future prospects. Drug Discov Today. 2019;24(3):773–780.
28. Fuster V, Bhatt DL. AI in cardiovascular medicine. Nat Rev Cardiol. 2018;15:197–198.
29. Topol EJ. High-performance medicine: The convergence of human and artificial intelligence. Nat Med. 2019;25(1):44–56.
30. Andre Esteva, Brett Kuprel, Roberto A. Novoa, Justin Ko, Susan M. Swetter, Helen M. Blau & Sebastian Thrun Dermatologist-level classification of skin cancer with deep neural networks. Nature. 2017;542:115–118.
31. Rajpurkar P, Irvin J, Zhu K, et al. CheXNet: radiologist-level pneumonia detection on chest X-rays with deep learning. *arXiv Prepr arXiv171105225.* 2017.
32. Yu KH, Beam AL, Kohane IS. Artificial intelligence in healthcare. Nat Biomed Eng. 2018;2:719–731.
33. Harari YN. 21 Lessons for the 21st Century. Spiegel & Grau; 2018.
34. Schwab K. The Fourth Industrial Revolution. Crown Business; 2016.
35. Brynjolfsson E, McAfee A. The Second Machine Age: Work, Progress, and Prosperity in a Time of Brilliant Technologies. W.W. Norton & Company; 2014.
36. Russell S, Norvig P. Artificial Intelligence: A Modern Approach. 3rd ed. Pearson; 2010.
37. Goodfellow I, Bengio Y, Courville A. Deep Learning. MIT Press; 2016.
38. LeCun Y, Bengio Y, Hinton G. Deep learning. Nature. 2015;521:436–444.
39. Silver D, Huang A, Maddison CJ, et al. Mastering the game of Go with deep neural networks and tree search. Nature. 2016;529:484–489.
40. Bostrom N. Superintelligence: Paths, Dangers, Strategies. Oxford University Press; 2014.
41. Badano, A. In silico imaging clinical trials: cheaper, faster, better, safer, and more scalable. Trials **22**, 64 (2021)
42. Bajwa J, Munir U, Nori A, Williams B. Artificial intelligence in healthcare: transforming the practice of medicine. 2021.
43. Bhattamisra SK, Banerjee P, Gupta P, Mayuren J, Patra S, Candasamy M. Artificial intelligence in pharmaceutical and healthcare research. 2023.
44. Chanana SA-O, Thomas CA-O, Zhang F, Rajski SA-O, Bugni TA-O. Automated hierarchical clustering and principal component analysis of large metabolomic datasets in r. Meta. 2020;10(7):297.
45. Paul SM, Mytelka DS, Dunwiddie CT, Persinger CC, Munos BH, Lindborg SR, Schacht AL. How to improve R&D productivity: The pharmaceutical industry's grand challenge. Nat Rev Drug Discov. 2010;9:203–214.
46. Van de Waterbeemd H, Gifford E. ADMET in silico modelling: Towards prediction Paradise? Nat Rev Drug Discov. 2003;2:192–204.
47. Yang X, Wang Y, Byrne R, Schneider G, Yang S. Concepts of artificial intelligence for computer-assisted drug discovery. Chem Rev. 2019;119:10520–10594.
48. Eder J, Sedrani R, Wiesmann C. The discovery of first-in-class drugs: Origins and evolution. Nat Rev Drug Discov. 2014;13:577–587.

49. Brown D. Unfinished business: Target-based drug discovery. Drug Discov Today. 2007;12:1007–1012.
50. Hsu YH, Yao J, Chan LC, Wu TJ, Hsu JL, Fang YF, et al. Definition of PKC-α, CDK6, and MET as therapeutic targets in triple-negative breast cancer. Cancer Res. 2014;74:4822–4835.
51. Chen B, Butte A. Leveraging big data to transform target selection and drug discovery. Clin Pharmacol Ther. 2016;99:285–297.
52. Kodama K, Horikoshi M, Toda K, Yamada S, Hara K, Irie J, et al. Expression-based genomewide association study links the receptor CD44 in adipose tissue with type 2 diabetes. Proc Natl Acad Sci USA. 2012;109:7049–7054.
53. Zhu Z, Zhang F, Hu H, Bakshi A, Robinson MR, Powell JE, et al. Integration of summary data from GWAS and eQTL studies predicts complex trait gene targets. Nat Genet. 2016;48:481–487.
54. Van Dam S, Võsa U, van der Graaf A, Franke L, de Magalhães JP. Gene Co-expression analysis for functional classification and Gene-disease predictions. Brief Bioinform. 2018;19:575–592.
55. Petyuk VA, Chang R, Ramirez-Restrepo M, Beckmann ND, Henrion YR, Piehowski PD, et al. The human brainome: Network analysis identifies HSPA2 as a novel Alzheimer's disease target. Brain. 2018;141:2721–2739.
56. Lee S, Zhang C, Liu Z, Klevstig M, Mukhopadhyay B, Bergentall M, et al. Network analyses identify liver-specific targets for treating liver diseases. Mol Syst Biol. 2017;13:938.
57. Zou Q, Li J, Song L, Zeng X, Wang G. Similarity computation strategies in the microRNA-disease network: A survey. Brief Funct Genomics. 2016;15:55–64.
58. Chen X, Xie D, Wang L, Zhao Q, You ZH, Liu H. BNPMDA: Bipartite network projection for MiRNADisease association prediction. Bioinformatics. 2018;34:3178–3186.
59. Atmakuri LR, Peeriga R, Begum S, Vallamkonda B, Baratam A. Novel bioanalytical LC-MS/MS method for determination of metoprolol in human plasma. J Appl Pharm Sci. 2024;14(12):131–138.
60. Peeriga R, Venkata Bangaru GK. Implementation of the POCSO act in schools. In: Child Sexual Abuse: A Public Health Problem in India. Springer publications, Singapore 2024. p. 391–413. Springer Publications, Singapore.
61. Peeriga R, Yarlagadda LC, Alla NR. Protection of children from sexual exploitation. In: Child Sexual Abuse: A Public Health Problem in India. 2024. p. 191–201. Springer Publications, Singapore.
62. Peeriga R, Shiek Arabath SAM, Manubolu K, Thelappilly BB, Yarlagadda LC. Insilico assessment of phytoconstituents in *myxopyrum smilacifolium* blume against arthritis. Biomed Pharmacol J. 2024;17(1):235–241.
63. Manubolu K, Balagani PK, Gope ER, Peeriga R, Sridevi AR. Unlocking the potential of aquasomes: A comprehensive review on innovative nanocarriers in drug delivery and beyond. Int J Chem Biochem Sci. 2023;24(6):405–410.
64. Manubolu K, Peeriga R, Bonthu MG, Gope ER, Kadirvel D. Evaluation of anti-inflammatory activity of *Millingtonia hortensis* leaf extract. Int J Chem Biochem Sci. 2023;24(6):380–385.
65. Peeriga R, Chandrasekhar KB. Comparative study of anti-inflammatory activity of petroleum ether extract of *myxopyrum smilacifolium* blume and ethanolic leaf extract of *pamburus missionis* swingle. J Pharm Sci Res. 2017;9(6):955–957.
66. Peeriga R, Manubolu K (2025). Design strategies for waste reduction and enhanced recyclability in pharmaceutical packaging. In: Yingngam, B., Aslam, M.S., Haghi, A.K. (eds) Sustainable Pharmaceutical Product Development and Optimization Processes. Springer, Singapore.
67. Manubolu K, Raveesha P, Chandrasekhar KB. A short guide to clinical pharmacokinetics. 1st ed. 2024. Springer. Singapore.
68. Manubolu K, Peeriga R (2025). Ecodesign principles. In: Yingngam, B., Aslam, M.S., Haghi, A.K. (eds) Sustainable Pharmaceutical Product Development and Optimization Processes. Springer, Singapore.

5 Structure-Based Drug Design and Fragment-Based Drug Discovery

Lakshmana Rao Atmakuri, Raveesha Peeriga, Gope Edward Raju, Srikanth Pottendla, Marapatla Shiny, and Amala Masa

Introduction

Structure-Based Drug Design (SBDD) and Fragment-Based Drug Discovery (FBDD) are among the most effective approaches that the modern drug discovery pipeline has to offer. It is quite rational and is based on the presence of the 3D structure of biological targets, usually proteins or nucleic acids, to design small molecules capable of influencing the target's activity [1].

Structure-based Drug Design

SBDD is a molecular modeling and chemical synthesis method introduced in the 1980s to design small molecules that can reproduce the effects of a series of compounds interacting with target macromolecules with known 3D conformations. It enables the design of molecules that influences the biological activity of the target depending on the shape and chemical context of its active site or receptor binding pocket [2]. (Figures 5.1 and 5.2).

Key Principles of SBDD

3D Structure of the Target

For SBDD, it is possible to identify the most accurate initial step in the technique, the acquisition of highly detailed data of the target biomolecule. This can be done using X-ray crystallography, NMR spectroscopy or using Cryo-electron microscopy (Cryo-EM). When experimental data cannot be procured, computational predictions like homology modeling can be used [3].

Binding Site Identification

Once one is sure of the structure of the target, the next thing is to determine which part of the protein gets bound to small molecules—ligands. Such binding sites are almost always situated at active or allosteric sites of the protein on the protein's surface [4].

DOI: 10.4324/9781003564041-5

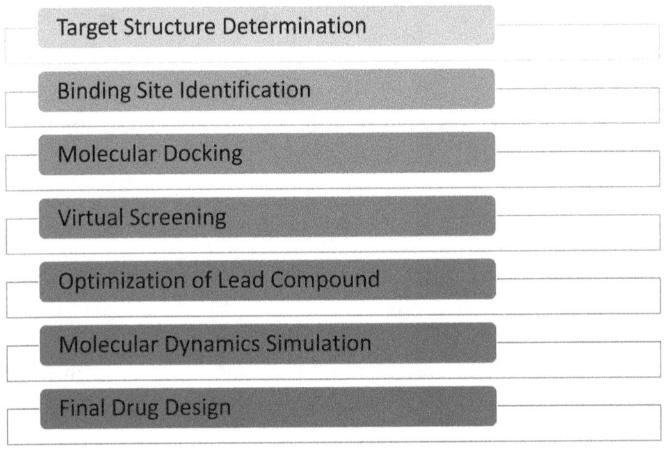

Figure 5.1 Steps involved in sequential drug design.

Molecular Docking

Molecular docking is a computational strategy that estimates the orientation/interaction of small molecules or drug-like compounds to the target binding sites. Docking algorithms position a compound into the target's binding pocket and rate the binding energy of the interaction to predict its relative strength of binding and hence rank molecules for further testing [5].

Virtual Screening

Virtual screening employs computerized approaches to filter out large numbers of compounds likely to interact with the target. This makes it an effective means of ranking compounds for further experimental testing [6].

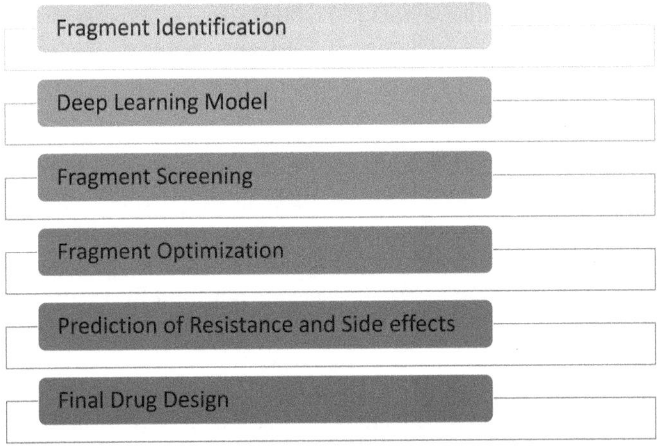

Figure 5.2 Steps involved in FBDD.

Lead Optimization

Following the initial recognition of a promising lead, it optimizes the compounds in terms of their ability to interact with the target, their selectivity for that target and their pharmacokinetic and toxicology profiles. This process generally comprises structure–activity relationship (SAR) analysis [7].

Advantages of SBDD

Precision: SBDD affords an opportunity to design molecules directly at the target, free from any off-target side effects, hence improving the therapeutic value of the final product.
Speed: Attached tools help in the faster development and analysis of new drug prospects.
Cost-efficiency: Compared to screening of large compound libraries, SBDD is time-saving, given that it is utilized to screen fewer and more structurally diverse libraries of compounds.

Fragment-based Drug Discovery

FBDD is an orthogonal drug discovery strategy to discover small and low molecular weight chemical fragments with low affinity for a biological target. These fragments are then elongated or further connected to other, even more powerful drug-like substances. The success is because FBDD affords lead chemical entities that bind an amino acid sequence or amino acid targets in a systematic, efficient manner, particularly in hard targets in which conventional drug design strategies may not work sometimes [8].

Key Principles of FBDD

Fragment Libraries

FBDD begins with the accumulation of a small but diverse resource of small chemical fragments with low molar mass (150–300 Da) and low molecular complexity. It is of a low interaction type with the required target but in certain manners [9].

Fragment Screening

This fragment library is then screened for fragment that binds to the target, and the hits are formed in this stage. The binding of the fragments is relatively gentle, occurring in the micromolar to millimolar ranges. Some common methods for binding and structural determination are NMR spectroscopy, X-ray crystallography and Biacore optical biosensor or Surface Plasmon Resonance (SPR) [10].

Fragment Linking and Growing

Identified weakly binding fragments may be linked or grown the first time that they are identified in order to enhance further the drug-like character of the fragment, described fragment growth as the addition of functional groups that enhance the interaction of the compound with the target molecules and fragment linking as a process of combining two fragments that have an affinity to proximal target regions [11].

Structure-Based Optimization

If an identified binding amine is available, molecular docking, MD simulations and other related computational strategies are employed to design improved binding interactions and split the amine fragments into even more effective drug-like compounds [12].

Fragment Merging

Molecular tag joining involves attaching different scaffolds of two or more fragments that interact with unique subsites of the target binding domain. The application of this strategy leads to the establishment of new scaffolds with higher binding constants [13].

Advantages of FBDD

- Higher Hit Rates: The simplicity of fragments allows FBDD to achieve a higher hit rate than traditional high-throughput screening (HTS).
- Access to Novel Chemotypes: With limited access to chemical space, traditional libraries often do not contain compounds appropriate for biomedical discovery, and the likelihood of discovering unique drug leads is high with FBDD.
- Efficiency in Targeting Challenging Proteins: FBDD is particularly useful for targeting difficult, previously intractable targets, such as protein-protein interactions (PPIs) or protein conformational change (Table 5.1).

Table 5.1 Comparison of SBDD and FBDD

Aspect	*SBDD*	*FBDD*
Starting point	3D structural data of a macromolecule (typically a protein)	Low molecular weight fragments with minimal structural complexity
Binding affinity	High-affinity leads (typically in the nanomolar to picomolar range)	Low-affinity fragments (typically in the micromolar to millimolar range)
Molecular size	Larger drug-like molecules (typically > 300 Da)	Smaller fragments (150–300 Da)
Optimization process	Lead optimization through SAR and docking	Fragment optimization through linking, growing, and merging techniques
Target suitability	Best suited for targets with well-defined binding sites	Ideal for complex or difficult targets, including PPIs
Development speed	Faster for targets with known structural information	Faster for screening large fragment libraries
Chemical diversity	Dependent on the diversity of compound libraries	Relies on the diversity and simplicity of fragment libraries

Techniques of SBDD and FBDD

SBDD and FBDD are two emerging methods in drug discovery and design. Small molecules or fragments, which act as agonists or antagonists to modulate the function of their biological targets, i.e., usually proteins, rely on a fairly reasonable degree of estimation of how these corresponding targets are formed in their natural environment, i.e., structure.

Key Concepts in SBDD

Target Structure Determination

The first step of SBDD is to identify the secondary structures of the target macromolecule, like protein or nucleic acid, for which techniques like X-ray crystallography, Nuclear Magnetic Resonance (NMR) spectroscopy, or Cryo-EM are used [14].

Binding Site Identification

And after the 3D structure of the target is modeled, the researchers look for potential binding sites, such as a pocket or groove on the protein, where small molecules will bind. Target sites may be active sites or active sites, which are regions responsible for enzymatic activity or allosteric sites, which control the protein's activity when a molecule binds to it [15].

Molecular Docking

The process of molecular docking as the method of predicting how a drug-like molecule (ligand) interacts with the protein target. The purpose is to find the molecules that fit the binding pocket extremely well and interact with it by the binding energy or the docking score.

Virtual Screening

Virtual screening is the computational process of assessing vast compound archives against the binding site of a target in order to discover lead compounds. This approach is performed with two techniques, either ligand based or structure based [16].

Optimization of Leads

After discovering such a lead through the above said promising lead molecules, there are strategies like fragment-based lead optimization and SAR analysis, where the lead molecule can be optimized for potency, selectivity, and pharmacokinetic profile.

MD Simulations

It is used to analyze changes in the motion of atoms in a protein throughout time, information that can be used to better understand conformational changes that affect drug binding. Further, these simulations prove useful in enhancing the docking predictions, thus extending the prospect of identifying tertiary or temporary binding sites [17].

Key Concepts in FBDD

Fragment Library

Here, we identify very small molecules that bind only weakly to the target and then optimize them into highly potent drug leads. This approach is different from conventional HTS of large libraries that usually require large and complex compounds in the initial stages [18].

Fragment Screening

Fragment screening is a process in which the fragments of the target protein are checked for binding by techniques like NMR spectroscopy, X-ray crystallography, or SPR. A relatively low affinity is allowed, yet their interaction with the target yields valuable information concerning the target's binding site.

Fragment Linking

This can then be repeated using chemical links (or growth) to add linked fragments with weak, yet highly selective binding to other parts of the target binding site to form bigger and more influential molecules. The individual fragments can be joined or optimized so that they fit more nicely into the binding pocket [19].

Fragment Growing and Merging

In fragment growing, further chemical groups are incorporated to the fragment to extend the time that the molecule interacts with the target. These groups add to the binding site so that better interaction can occur. The fragment merging involves two fragments where each can only bind to its distinct region in the binding site, and join the two fragments to form an even larger new portion.

Structure-based Optimization

Once a fragment is bound to a target, docking, MD and SAR analysis are done in SBDD techniques to enhance and make the fragment more potent and drug-like. Occasionally, it might need the alteration of the fragments to increase the number of anchors and improve ADMET properties [20–30].

Fragment Linking with Scaffold Hopping

Scaffold hopping is a method of identifying two fragments that bind to the same target in two different scaffolds, then connecting them together into a single scaffold. Such mechanisms can then produce new, more efficient drug leads with a unique mode of action.

Key Techniques and Tools in SBDD and FBDD

Computational Tools

Several software tools exist in SBDD, and some of these include AutoDock, Genetic Optimization for Ligand Docking (a molecular docking software) (GOLD), and Dock. For accurate compound virtual screening in FBDD, some bioinformatics tools like Fast Rigid Exhaustive Docking (a docking tool by OpenEye) (FRED) or PyRx are available.

Biophysical Techniques

For the evaluation of the binding interactions in both SBDD and FBDD techniques, SPR and isothermal titration calorimetry are employed.

X-Ray Crystallography and NMR Spectroscopy

Molecular imaging approaches such as X-ray crystallography and NMR spectroscopy are essential in both rational and FBDD, since the structure of native proteins and their complexes with ligands must be known.

Ligand Efficiency Metrics

The evaluation of the degree to which a compound interacts with the target in terms of the size of the compound is done by Lipophilic ligand efficiency and ligand efficiency.

Case Studies in SBDD and FBDD

SBDD and FBDD techniques have proved useful in the synthesis of several drugs, particularly for diseases that are difficult to cure at first instance. In the remainder of this chapter, we describe a few case studies illustrating how these techniques can be used in real-world drug discovery.

Case Study 1: Imatinib - SBDD for Targeted Cancer Therapy

Target: BCR-ABL Tyrosine Kinase
Therapeutic Area: Cancer (Chronic Myelogenous Leukemia [CML])

Imatinib is one of the best examples of other resistance-source connected in targeting cancer by SBDD. It was developed as BCR-ABL tyrosine kinase inhibitors for CML cancer, which is incited by the BCR-ABL fusion protein. The swap between the DNA of the BCR gene and the ABL gene results in the ABL kinase remaining active all the time to encourage cell division.

SBDD Process

Structural Insight

SBDD was used in the design of a molecule that would selectively block the aberrant functioning of the BCR-ABL fusion protein. Information on the 3D structure of the ABL kinase domain was gained by performing X-ray crystallography. The structure unveiled a kinase pocket by which ATP attaches to initiate kinase activity. Perhaps, if a molecule is shaped to meticulously nestle in the kinase pocket, it would inhibit it from functioning properly.

Design and Optimization

Imatinib was intended to fit into the ATP binding site of the ABL kinase, thus culminating in the inhibition of the kinase activity. SAR analysis was also performed to increase Event-Related Potential (brain response measured using EEG (ERP))'s binding affinity and selectivity toward BCR-ABL relative to other kinases further.

Outcome

There was empirical evidence that Imatinib sufficiently and effectively targeted CML, for it selectively fought the BCR-ABL fusion protein without endangering other body cells. It was of great value in treating CML, raising the survival rates considerably.

Significance

Imatinib is arguably one of the greatest hallmarks of targeted cancer therapy, and for the first time, SBDD proved itself as most effective in designing drugs with respect to molecular targets. It is a small molecule that was the first of the Tyrosine Kinase Inhibitors (a class of cancer drugs) (TKIs) to be used clinically and set the stage for other targeted anticancer agents.

Case Study 2: Dorzolamide—Structure-Based Drug Discovery for Glaucoma Treatment

Target: Carbonic Anhydrase II
Therapeutic Area: Ophthalmology (Glaucoma)

Dorzolamide belongs to the class of carbonic anhydrase inhibitors and is used to manage the diseases which cause the elevation of intraocular pressure, glaucoma, and open-angle glaucoma in particular, as elevated pressure can result in optic nerve damage and vision loss.

SBDD Process

Target Identification

Carbonic anhydrase II (CA-II) is primarily responsible for modulating the formation of aqueous humor, a fluid located in the eye responsible for intraocular pressure. Inhibition of CA-II synthesis may help decrease this fluid production and thus reduce the Intraocular Pressure (IOP).

Structure Determination

Employing X-ray crystallography, the author was able to determine the structure of carbonic anhydrase II, identifying the structure of its active site. This information was important for the development of inhibitors capable of attaching to the enzyme and thereby inhibiting it.

Drug Design

Dorzolamide was designed based on the structure of carbonic anhydrase and was optimized to fit into the active site, bind with the enzyme tightly and selectively. The unique part of this molecule is the sulfonamide moiety, which binds very tightly at the active site through the interaction with the zinc ion and thus inactivates the enzyme.

Outcome

It has been mapped as a potent inhibitor of CA II and is among the first carbonic anhydrase inhibitors prescribed for glaucoma in the topical form. It is employed in cases where improvement of aqueous humor outflow cannot be obtained with beta-blockers.

Significance

This case study shows how SBDD can be applied to designing drugs for diseases including glaucoma that result from the specific inhibitory treatment of a molecule of interest; carbonic anhydrase II in this instance.

Case Study 3: Vemurafenib, Marketed as Zelboraf—A Case Study on the Role of SBDD for Targeted Cancer Therapy

Target: BRAF (B-Raf Proto-Oncogene, Serine/Threonine Kinase (a gene involved in cell growth signaling)) V600E Mutation
Therapeutic Area: Cancer (Melanoma)

Vemurafenib is an orally administered small-molecule BRAF kinase inhibitor targeted for the treatment of metastatic melanoma with the BRAF V600E mutation that is found in approximately 50% of metastatic melanomas. BRAF is actually a kinase which fits into the MAPK signaling pathway, which helps to determine the level of cell proliferation.

SBDD Process

Structure Determination

The formation of BRAF and the ATP-binding was determined by means of X-ray crystallography. The conformation of this mutative variant of the protein was also analyzed, and the binding pocket of the V600E mutant protein differs from that of BRAF by a little bit.

Design of Inhibitor

Here, SBDD was applied to identify small molecules that would selectively bind to the mutated BRAF V600E protein. The idea was to create a molecule that fits into the ATP binding site and selectively blocks the activity of the mutated BRAF without interfering with the wild-type protein.

Outcome

The study further reveals Vemurafenib to be effective in the treatment of patients with BRAF V600E-positive melanoma. It considerably increased the overall survival and was endorsed by the FDA in 2011 for the management of metastatic melanoma.

Significance

Vemurafenib is a classic example of how, from an early start, SBDD could effectively develop highly specific drugs selective for certain mutations, thus being a marked progress in the treatment of melanoma and advancing other targeted therapies in cancer treatment.

Case Study 4: Finding Entinostat—FBDD for Epigenetic Treatment of Cancer

Target: Histone Deacetylase (HDAC)
Therapeutic Area: Cancer

Entinostat is an orally bioactive HDAC inhibitor used in cancer treatment. HDACs are proteins that function as acetylases or deacetylases, incumbent on histones and, in this manner, on gene expression. HDACs can be targeted to reverse the epigenetic changes that transform tumor suppressor genes to taking on a silent status.

FBDD Process

Fragment Screening

The synthesis of Entinostat was initiated from the FBDD. HTS was imparted a fragment library to successfully shortlist the small molecules that could bind to the active site of HDAC enzymes.

Fragment Identification

Those fragments that had a relatively low affinity for the enzyme were analyzed by a variety of methods, such as NMR spectroscopy and X-ray crystallography. These fragments were then optimized to enhance their selectivity and potency for HDAC.

Fragment Growing and Linking

After recognizing initial fragments, these fragments were grown by attaching functional groups that would improve the fit to the target's binding pocket, also investigated the possibilities of linking the fragments in order to raise potency.

Outcome

The last of the drugs studied was Entinostat, which was found to be a potent HDAC inhibitor that had been used in experimental animal models as well as in phase I/II cancer therapy trials. It is currently still in trial studies to be used alongside other cancer treatments.

Significance

This case study demonstrates how it is possible to employ FBDD to maximize lead compounds for targets that are challenging to drug using lead discovery techniques that are conventional, like the case with HDAC. It also put the emphasis on the role of epigenetic drugs to help with cancer, even as their use is more extensive than initially expected, it remains an area of particular significance.

Integration with Computational Methods in SBDD and FBDD

SBDD and FBDD are two critical methods in drug discovery that depend on computational techniques to enhance the drug design process. Computational methods not only help in the discovery and design of drugs, but also help to understand the nature of small molecules and their targets. Since the advent of computational tools, there has been a revolution and improvement in the results yielded by both SBDD and FBDD.

This integration can be broadly categorized into the following aspects:

Computational Methods in SBDD

SBDD is constructed depending upon the availability of a high-resolution 3D structure of the target, usually a protein or nucleic acid. It will be seen that computational methods are employed at multiple or indeed successive phases of the design process, from target identification to lead optimization.

Key Computational Methods Used in SBDD

Molecular Docking

Molecular docking is the primary function of SBDD. It is a process of using computation to estimate the orientation and conformation of small molecules to the target protein's active site. The docking algorithms produce several conformations of the ligand and rank them in terms of their presumed binding energy with the target.

Applications: Virtual Screening and Lead Optimization
Software Tools: AutoDock, Docking (DOCK), Gold, FlexX

MD Simulations

MD simulations describe protein flexibility and conformational motion as well as protein-ligand complex structures over time. A major advantage of MD is that it allows the study of the interaction between a ligand and its target at the atomic level, considering the time dependence of the process.

Applications: BAE, Investigation of protein-ligand interactions
Software Tools: GROMACS, AMBER, CHARMM.

Quantitative Structure–Activity Relationship

QSAR models employ statistical tools to relate the molecular descriptor of a compound to its biological activity. Computer applications in the design allow the estimation of the changes in the potency and other characteristics of the lead compounds after modifying their structural formulas.

Applications: Prediction of biological activity and lead optimization
Software Tools: MOE, ChemOffice, Dragon

Free Energy Calculations

Several programs for free energy calculations including thermodynamic integration and molecular mechanics Poisson–Boltzmann surface area predict the binding free energy of the ligand to the target. Using these approaches, potential ligand-target binding affinity changes due to alterations in the ligand or target structure may be predicted.

Applications: Binding Affinity Prediction, Lead Optimization
Software Tools: Amber, GROMACS, Schrodinger.

Virtual Screening

Virtual screening is more of docking a large collection of compounds against a desired protein to obtain hits. By employing a ligand-based approach, where known active compounds are an essential part of the calculation or a structure-based approach, in which the target protein structure is required for the calculation.

Applications: Hit identification, also known as lead discovery, is the process of identifying a molecule to further optimize for effectiveness against the target.
Software Tools: ZINC, MolPort, eDrug3D

Computational Methods in FBDD

FBDD begins by first identifying small chemical fragments that may be used to find new drugs. It is essential because the computational methods serve to determine efficiently, at least, the search for initial and optimized fragments, as well as processes of expanding these fragments into high-potential drug candidates.

Key Computational Methods Used in FBDD

Fragment Docking

Fragment docking is employed to fit small, low molecular weight fragments into the binding sites of targets. Unlike the conventional docking being the one, which handles large molecules, fragment docking encompasses the placement of fragment molecules into targeting sites in a bid to study noncovalent, weak binding.

Applications: Fragment Library Screening, Selecting the Right Fragment Binding
Software Tools: AutoDock, Glide, FlexX

Fragment Growing and Linking

Fragment growing and linking are employed to improve fragments' performance by increasing fragments' size to fit better the binding pocket or joining fragments that bind to two near regions of the target protein's active site.

Applications: Fragment developing, fragment concatenation
Software Tools: LigBuilder, RosettaLigand, Schrodinger's Maestro

Structure-based Fragment Optimization

Once fragments are identified, other SBDD tools such as molecular docking and MD simulations are employed in designing more fragment based, larger and potent compounds which will have optimized binding trends as well as improved drug-like properties such as solubility and pharmacokinetic properties.

Applications: Lead Optimization and Selectivity
Software Tools: Schrodinger, Discovery Studio, AutoDock

Virtual Fragment Screening

Structure-based virtual screening involves the use of computer software to virtually evaluate libraries of small chemical fragments against a target protein. This enables researchers to quickly shortlist potential fragment hits in advance of physical screening.

Applications: First Orbit Propose the Fragments, Second Confirmation the Hit
Software Tools: ZINC database, e.cite, Open Eye.

Free Energy Perturbation and MD

In FBDD, free energy perturbation (FEP) and MD simulations are employed to improve the accuracy of the binding affinity estimates and alignment of the fragment interactions. These methods mimic the manner by which slight alterations of the structure of a fragment influence the binding energy and, therefore, efficacy of a drug.

Applications: Performance Enhancement of Fragments for Fragment Library, Fragment Growth
Software Tools: GROMACS, AMBER, OpenMM

Applications

Application area	*SBDD*	*FBDD*
Target types	Best suited for targets with well-characterized, known 3D structures (e.g., enzymes, receptors).	Effective for difficult or poorly characterized targets (e.g., PPIs, challenging enzymes).
Drug discovery speed	Faster for targets with known structural information.	Can be faster for difficult targets or when the 3D structure is unavailable.
High-affinity lead discovery	Ideal for discovering high-affinity leads (nM to pM range) based on detailed structural data.	Generally begins with low-affinity fragments (μM to mM range), which are later optimized.

(*Continued*)

Application area	*SBDD*	*FBDD*
Target-specific drug development	Effective for developing drugs targeting specific sites on the protein (e.g., active sites, allosteric sites).	Used for identifying hits for less-specific targets, such as allosteric sites, PPIs, or previously undruggable targets.
Lead optimization	Focuses on optimizing drug leads through SAR analysis, molecular docking.	Fragment optimization involves linking or growing fragments to enhance potency and specificity.
Complex targets	Works well for targets with defined binding pockets or clear active sites.	Particularly useful for targets lacking defined binding pockets or for complexes like PPIs.
Biological pathways	Used in targeting well-known pathways with validated structures.	Suited for targeting complex and novel pathways that have not been previously targeted.
Drug-receptor interaction	Helps optimize drug-receptor interactions using the known receptor structure and docking models.	Focuses on fragment-screening to identify weak-binding fragments which are later optimized for stronger interactions.
Allosteric modulation	Can be used to design allosteric modulators by targeting alternate binding sites.	Ideal for discovering allosteric inhibitors by identifying binding sites not involved in the active site.
Chemotherapy and cancer therapy	Widely used in designing targeted therapies for cancer, e.g., kinase inhibitors, monoclonal antibodies.	Can be applied to develop cancer drugs by targeting undruggable proteins and PPIs.
Antibiotic development	Used for designing antibiotics by targeting specific bacterial enzymes or receptors.	Effective in the discovery of antibiotics by targeting complex or previously resistant microbial proteins.
Neurodegenerative diseases	Applied in designing drugs for diseases like Alzheimer's, Parkinson's by targeting specific proteins involved in neurodegeneration.	Used to discover small molecules for neurodegenerative diseases, particularly for protein aggregates and misfolded proteins.

Conclusion

SBDD and FBDD are two tremendous tools which have become new milestones of modern drug discovery, and the two methods have similar characteristics. This is because SBDD depends on the high-resolution 3D structural information to design larger molar (up to high affinity) for the known binding site of proteins of targets whose structures are characterized. Contrarily to the second approach, in FBDD we begin with small, weakly binding fragments, as the concept most derived from statistical dense sampling which is then boosted via such strategies as fragment linking and fragment growing to produce potent drug leads particularly when targeting difficult and complex biological targets that other methods cannot effectively tackle. Altogether, these approaches make it possible for researchers to tackle many types of diseases like cancer, infectious diseases, neurological diseases and cardiovascular disease, as well as many other unmanageable biological questions. By such a method combination, drug discovery is faster, more efficient, and it will, consequently, bring about more effective and more selective therapies.

References

1. Kuntz ID, Oatley SI, Stern JL. Computational methods for the design of molecules that bind to biological macromolecules. Science. 1982;257(5062):1078–1082.
2. Kitchen DB, Decornez H, Nivon L. Docking and scoring in virtual screening for drug discovery. Nat Rev Drug Discov. 2004;3(11):939–949.
3. Xie L, Zhang Z, Liu S. Structural bioinformatics and computational drug discovery. J Med Chem. 2011;54(22):7437–7450.
4. Lam LK, O'Neill MJ. Identifying potential binding sites in protein targets for drug discovery. Curr Drug Discov Technol. 2005;2(2):135–141.
5. Sanner MF. Python: A programming language for software integration and development. J Mol Graph Model. 1999;17(1):57–61.
6. Macalino SJY, Lee CS, Lee KW. Virtual screening for drug discovery: An overview of methods and applications. Front Pharmacol. 2015;6:94.
7. Ertl P, Kümmerer M. Fragment-based drug design: From ligand binding to structure-based optimization. Nat Rev Drug Discov. 2007;6(7):576–587.
8. Haan JC, Gupta SP. Fragment-based drug discovery: A literature update. Future Med Chem. 2013;5(10):1133–1150.
9. Durrant JD, Sanner MF. Fragment-based drug discovery: The importance of molecular fragments in drug discovery. Future Med Chem. 2011;3(10):1235–1245.
10. Teague SJ, O'Connell T. The role of molecular shape in drug discovery. J Med Chem. 1999;42(8):1031–1043.
11. Hartshorn MJ, Brouwer H. Fragment-based drug discovery: A new approach to building lead molecules. J Med Chem. 2007;50(13):3097–3106.
12. Hopkins AL, Groom CR. The druggable genome. Nat Rev Drug Discov. 2002; 1(9):727–730.
13. Turner MT, Morrison MA. Fragment-based drug discovery: Insights into recent advancements and future directions. Drug Discov Today. 2014;19(3):311–318.
14. Sharma V, Kumar P. Fragment libraries and fragment-based drug discovery. Drug Dev Res. 2009;70(6):297–306.
15. Blundell TL, Kipling D. Fragment-based screening for drug discovery. Nat Rev Drug Discov. 2010;9(11):897–903.
16. Crowther JW, Williams AP. Fragment-based drug discovery. J Med Chem. 2011;54(14):4986–5000.
17. McGovern SL, Hsieh W. Fragment-based screening of chemical libraries. Nat Rev Drug Discov. 2003;2(9):734–739.
18. Macalino SJY, Tan YL. Fragment-based drug discovery: A new approach to hit identification. Curr Med Chem. 2017;24(18):1904–1915.
19. Kooistra AJ, Stouten PF. Fragment-based drug design: From fragments to leads. Drug Discov Today. 2009;14(19-20):895–901.
20. Winter JL, Xie Z. Fragment-based drug discovery for novel and difficult targets. Nat Rev Drug Discov. 2014;13(9):708–719.
21. Atmakuri LR, Peeriga R, Begum S, Vallamkonda B, Baratam A. Novel bioanalytical LC-MS/MS method for determination of metoprolol in human plasma. J Appl Pharm Sci. 2024;14(12):131–138.

22. Peeriga R, Venkata Bangaru GK Implementation of the POCSO act in schools. In: Child Sexual Abuse: A Public Health Problem in India. Springer publications, Singapore. 2024. p. 391–413. Springer Publications, Singapore.
23. Peeriga R, Yarlagadda LC, Alla NR. Protection of children from sexual exploitation. In: Child Sexual Abuse: A Public Health Problem in India. Springer publications, Singapore. 2024. p. 191–201. Springer Publications, Singapore.
24. Peeriga R, Shiek Arabath SAM, Manubolu K, Thelappilly BB, Yarlagadda LC. Insilico assessment of phytoconstituents in *myxopyrum smilacifolium* blume against arthritis. Biomed Pharmacol J. 2024;17(1):235–241.
25. Manubolu K, Balagani PK, Gope ER, Peeriga R, Sridevi AR. Unlocking the potential of aquasomes: A comprehensive review on innovative nanocarriers in drug delivery and beyond. Int J Chem Biochem Sci. 2023;24(6):405–410.
26. Manubolu K, Peeriga R, Bonthu MG, Gope ER, Kadirvel D. Evaluation of anti-inflammatory activity of *Millingtonia hortensis* leaf extract. Int J Chem Biochem Sci. 2023;24(6):380–385.
27. Peeriga R, Chandrasekhar KB. Comparative study of anti-inflammatory activity of petroleum ether extract of *myxopyrum smilacifolium* blume and ethanolic leaf extract of *pamburus missionis* swingle. J Pharm Sci Res. 2017;9(6):955–957.
28. Peeriga R, Manubolu K. (2025). Design strategies for waste reduction and enhanced recyclability in pharmaceutical packaging. In: Yingngam, B., Aslam, M.S., Haghi, A.K. (eds) Sustainable Pharmaceutical Product Development and Optimization Processes. Springer, Singapore.
29. Manubolu K, Peeriga R, Chandrasekhar KB. A short guide to clinical pharmacokinetics. 1st ed. 2024. Springer. Singapore.
30. Manubolu K, Peeriga R (2025). Ecodesign principles. In: Yingngam, B., Aslam, M.S., Haghi, A.K. (eds) Sustainable Pharmaceutical Product Development and Optimization Processes. Springer, Singapore.

6 Chemical Biology Approaches in Drug Discovery

Raveesha Peeriga, Krishnaveni Manubolu, Shaik Sabreen, Sajja Jayanth Babu, Nagul Meeravali Shaik, and Saidatri Arige

Introduction

Modern drug discovery requires a powerful interdisciplinary field known as chemical biology, which brings together chemical and biological sciences to become the backbone of modern treatment development. Research investigators benefit from the scientific unification of chemistry and biology because it enables them to study disease mechanisms better while identifying fresh therapeutic possibilities [1]. The prevailing drug discovery approaches have primarily used phenotypic screening and target-based testing methods, which end in identifying promising compounds that prove ineffective due to poor specificity and potency requirements. The combined framework of small-molecule chemistry with biological knowledge through chemical biology offers researchers superior control to explore complex cellular events and illnesses. The following section explains how chemical biology operates in today's drug discovery practice while showing the benefits against conventional processes and describing chemical probes along with tool compounds and target deconvolution principles [2].

Figure 6.1 illustrates chemical biology strategies that drive drug discovery by using probes and tool compounds to identify targets and validate them along with screening methods to find active compounds and elucidating target mechanisms to develop better drugs.

The Role of Chemical Biology in Modern Drug Discovery

The discipline of chemical biology connects chemistry and biology with pharmacology as it forms at their interdisciplinary crossroads [3]. Short chemical compounds serve as research tools that investigate biological systems, therefore helping scientists identify diseases at their molecular level and new drug targets. More specific drug developments become achievable by uniting chemical tools with biological systems.

Modern drug discovery depends on disease molecular comprehension for the development of therapeutic solutions. Traditional drug discovery methods begin with high-throughput screening (HTS) for lead compound identification before conducting optimization of pharmacokinetics properties as well as activity and

DOI: 10.4324/9781003564041-6

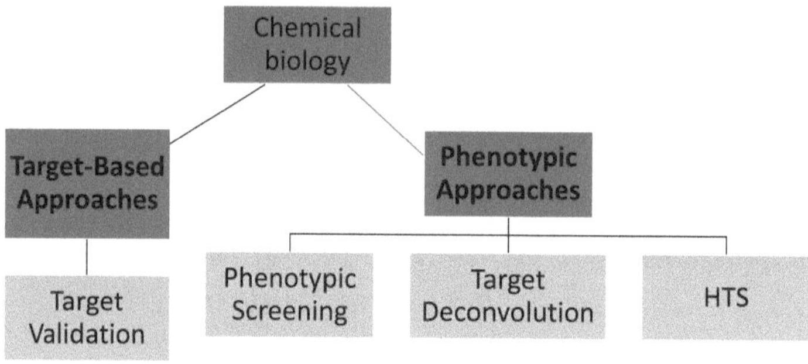

Figure 6.1 Chemical biology approaches in drug discovery.

selectivity. Long durations and exorbitant costs characterize this drug development process since numerous candidates fail late in development because of their poor specificity along with toxicity and inadequacy in clinical trials.

Chemical biology uses small molecules as specific chemical probes to tackle biological interaction challenges [4]. Small-molecule chemical probes allow investigators to identify new targets, explain biological pathways, and understand potential drug candidate mechanisms. The use of chemical tools in chemical biology lets drug discovery focus on developing specific compounds which attach to disease-relevant targets rather than performing only phenotypic screening.

The ability of chemical biology to connect experimental drug discovery with complex biological systems stands as its main benefit. Through the use of small molecules, chemical biologists can examine diseases at their molecular level by controlling targeted proteins or biological pathways. The ability to understand disease mechanisms at a molecular level enables better design of specific treatments that become crucial during the personalized medicine movement.

Advantages of Chemical Biology Approaches Over Traditional Methods

The integration of chemical biology into drug discovery offers several significant advantages over traditional methods, such as phenotypic screening and target-based approaches (Figure 6.2).

The figure emphasizes four essential benefits of chemical biology in drug discovery, as it enables more precise disease protein targeting and novel target discovery through chemical probes and mechanism understanding that produces effective, tailored therapies.

Precision and Specificity

The major advantage of chemical biology lets scientists create customized molecules which precisely hit particular proteins or biological pathways. The drug discovery process through traditional phenotypic screening evaluates multiple cellular

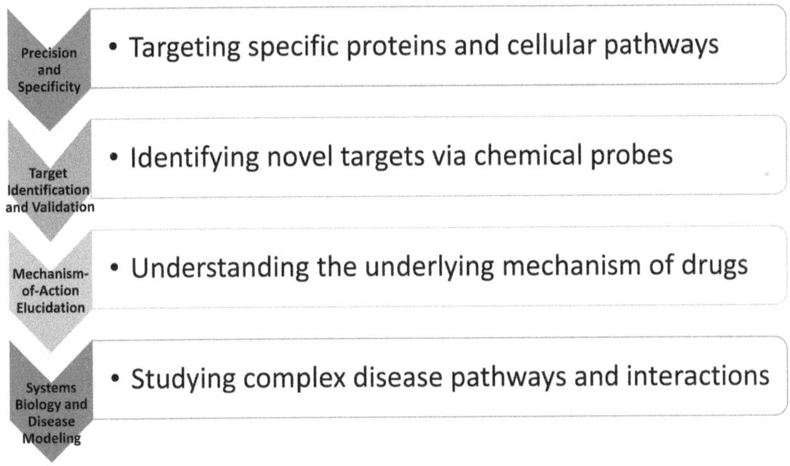

Figure 6.2 Advantages of chemical biology in drug discovery.

examples for compounds which transform disease-related characteristics [5]. This strategy produces appealing candidates but produces compounds which tend to interact with different targets and transmit harmful side effects.

Chemical biology gives researchers the ability to develop precise chemical probes which bind only to defined targets. This inquiry tool allows scientists to examine protein functionality inside living cells, thereby revealing disease-linked information that leads to medical developments of precise pharmacological treatments. The research on the family of proteins known as kinases employed selective chemical probes to investigate these proteins in living cells. Medical scientists employed small molecule-based targeting mechanisms to generate kinase inhibitors which serve as disease-targeting drugs for cancer therapy as well as other medical treatments.

Target Identification and Validation

The major benefit of chemical biology involves discovering and validating fresh drug targets. The target-based approach in traditional drug discovery begins with disease-related target speculations to determine compounds which can bind to these targets [6]. If successful through prior knowledge-based approaches, this method depends strongly on disease mechanism understanding yet ignores possible unexplored target candidates.

The ability of chemical biology to use probes limitlessly to investigate proteomic targets enables researchers to discover previously undiscovered targets. Scientists use chemical proteomics to discover new disease targets for cancer and neurological disorders, and infectious diseases through small molecule measurement and protein identification of drug-like compound interactions [7]. The probes permit target validation because they enable the assessment of biological changes resulting from target modifications in living cellular environments.

Mechanism-of-action Elucidation

Drug therapeutic functionality together with side effect management requires a full comprehension of drug activity mechanisms. Standard drug discovery research uses a process of random testing where compounds are applied to different disease test systems for response evaluations. Every measured effect from testing compounds fails to identify how these compounds produce their outcomes [8].

Through chemical exploration, scientists can measure small-molecule process mechanisms by using targeted probes which affect precise cellular protein functions and signaling pathways. Such methods allow scientists to discover disease-related molecular targets together with disease-related cell pathways and explain compound mechanisms at the basic level [9]. Chemical probes facilitate the identification of proteins that lead to chemotherapy drug resistance, thus helping researchers develop anti-resistant medications which enhance therapeutic success.

Systems Biology and Disease Modeling

Through its unique target study capabilities, chemical biology advances the systems biology approach that investigates disease-caused interactions between biomolecules and proteins and genes. Scientists apply chemical probes to disrupt certain cell pathways, which they can observe affecting the entire biological system [10]. Researchers gain complete disease mechanism insights while developing new therapeutic targets that evade detection using traditional research methods through this approach.

Chemical biology explores biological complexes between oncogenes and tumor suppressors, as well as signaling molecules which operate in cancer cells through research examples. The manipulation of biological pathways through small molecules within chemical biology research has resulted in the development of new therapeutic strategies to fight cancer along with other diseases [11].

Figure 6.3 demonstrates how chemical biology improves drug development by enhancing target specificity and uncovering new targets and revealing deeper mechanisms, which result in better efficiency of drug discovery processes.

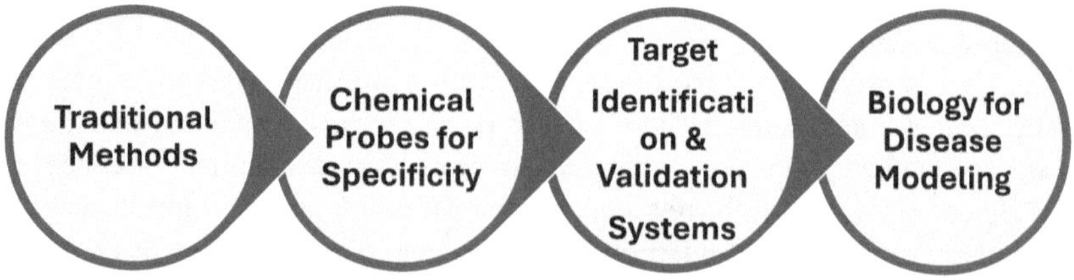

Figure 6.3 Chemical biology vs traditional methods.

Key Concepts in Chemical Biology: Chemical Probes, Tool Compounds, and Target Deconvolution

Several key concepts are central to the field of chemical biology, each playing a crucial role in drug discovery. These include chemical probes, tool compounds, and target deconvolution, which are discussed below (Figure 6.4).

Chemical Probes

Research scientists use small chemical probes as tools to recognize particular biological targets for studying their disease functions. The main purpose of chemical probes differs from drugs as the compounds function exclusively as laboratory tools for biological research and target identification [11, 12].

Chemical probes function as binding components that researchers utilize to examine modification pathways of particular biomolecules, including proteins. A chemical probe can block a specific enzyme responsible for disease pathway activities, so researchers can analyze what happens to the disease process when enzyme blockage occurs. The discovery and development of numerous new therapeutic targets as well as advanced medical treatments for various diseases, became possible through chemical probe applications [13].

Tool Compounds

Drug discovery applications make use of tool compounds as small molecular structures that serve to evaluate biological systems and validate therapeutic targets. Additional properties distinct from chemical probes enable tool compounds to function beyond their basic probe capabilities. These properties include longer actions and better cell penetration. The main function of tool compounds is to prove

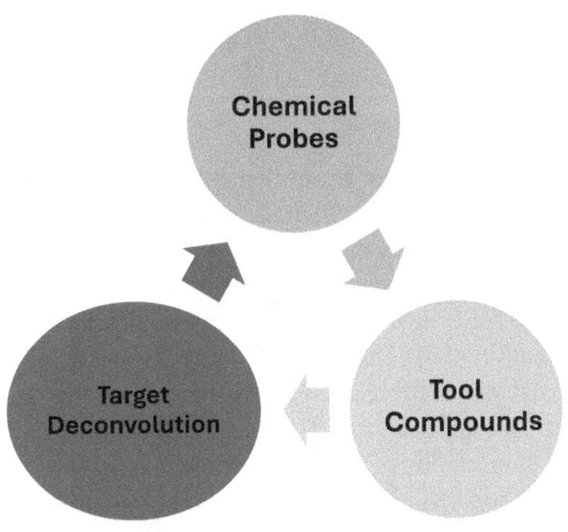

Figure 6.4 Key concepts in chemical biology.

target validity through observations that adjusting the target with a small molecule will generate detectable changes in disease states.

Tool compounds enable researchers to verify disease relevance of targets by acting on the target through genetic screens using additional validation methods. Tool compounds can undergo improvement processes to transform into therapeutic agents that advance from research tools to future clinical candidates [14].

Target Deconvolution

The figure explains the three core elements of chemical biology, which include chemical probes as well as tool compounds and target deconvolution. The strategies display their utility for drug discovery research by permitting investigators to conduct pathway studies and evaluate treatment targets, and detect essential molecular interactions for therapeutic development. The target deconvolution process allows scientists to discover new drug targets together with information about molecular disease pathways. Researchers gain improved understanding of therapeutic potential and optimize clinical properties through the identification of which targets a compound engages with [15].

Drug discovery has experienced a revolution through chemical biology because it allows scientists to find therapeutic agents with enhanced specificity through systematic development. The combination of chemical probes with tool compounds and target deconvolution strategies through chemical biology helps researchers study complex disease-related biological systems to discover new therapeutic targets, which allows for the development of more effective drugs. The interdisciplinary field keeps advancing while providing new discovery possibilities for medicine and deeper knowledge of disease processes. Food and Drug Administration places high expectations on chemical biology because this rapidly evolving field is certain to become more vital for producing the next generation of therapeutic agents that will improve treatment options across multiple diseases.

Chemical Probes and Tool Compounds

The discovery of drugs in modern times depends heavily on chemical probes and tool compounds because these substances help scientists explore biological operations and confirm prospective treatment targets. Scientists design these molecules to connect with particular biomolecules consisting of proteins, as well as enzymes and nucleic acids, to investigate disease functions and identify new therapeutic targets for drug creation [16]. The research tools known as chemical probes and tool compounds exist with different objectives together with distinct construction methods and functional applications. This part discusses the definitions of chemical probes and tool compounds and their importance alongside differences between them as well as selection criteria and optimization strategies. It provides case examples that demonstrate the application of these tools to target kinases and epigenetic modulators.

Definition and Importance of Chemical Probes in Drug Discovery

Chemical probes function as small molecules that specifically engage biological targets, particularly proteins and enzymes, while controlling their functional activities in order to study disease causes. Research tools make up the primary usage of chemical probes because they help scientists investigate cellular processes as well as signaling pathways and disease mechanisms, rather than serving therapeutic purposes. Target identification and validation as well as disease understanding at the molecular level depend on their existence [17].

The examination of diseases at their fundamental operational level becomes possible with chemical probes. A chemical probe that focuses on signaling proteins enables researchers to understand how these proteins influence cellular mechanisms such as proliferation and apoptosis, as well as immune responses. Scientists can identify new therapeutic targets through pathfinding processes and enhance treatment development when they disrupt molecular targets via chemical probes [18].

Temperature-dependent probes have become necessary for drug discovery research because they provide better methods to examine drug targets both efficiently and precisely. Biological system complexity decreases when researchers use targeted molecular modifications to study disease mechanisms. This approach brings deeper insights into diseases [19].

Differences Between Tool Compounds and Chemical Probes

While both tool compounds and chemical probes are used in drug discovery and biological research, they differ in their specific functions and design criteria.

- Chemical probes represent small molecules which exist primarily for biological investigation purposes because they assess particular protein functions or pathway activities. Although these compounds are optimized for target specificity and strength and mechanism assessment, they do not require therapeutic optimization [19]. The wide spectrum of biological studies utilizes chemical probes for protein-protein interaction investigations and functional genomics evaluations, and systems biology research.
- Tool compounds function as biological modulators through small molecules, yet their main goal is to establish therapeutic value for designated molecular targets [20]. Tool compounds show therapeutic value among researchers who choose them because they modify target activity, like how actual medicines function. The compounds advance through sequential optimization for effectiveness and pharmacokinetic properties and safety before preclinical trials help drug development initiatives.

Tool compounds differ from chemical probes since their primary functions serve opposite purposes. The main function of chemical probes is to study molecular targets and biological pathways, while tool compounds evolve with therapeutic intent that leads to additional modifications for clinical use.

Selection Criteria for Effective Probes and Tool Compounds

Effective tool compounds and chemical probes need selection as the core foundation for successful drug discovery research. Various factors must be taken into account for selecting or developing new probes alongside tool compounds:

Selectivity and Specificity

Chemical probes together with tool compounds need to demonstrate fine discrimination when interacting with biological targets. The objective remains to avoid unwanted interactions with targets aside from the intended one to prevent misleading results alongside toxicity risks. The desired outcome of high selectivity makes compounds connect primarily to their intended target, so scientists can obtain dependable data about target functions [21].

Research teams increase selectivity through structure-based drug design, which utilizes target protein 3D structures for creating compounds that can specifically bind to a particular site. Experimental data quality depends on how selectivity matches between the probe and the tool compound.

Potency

Rational chemical probes alongside tool compounds need high target affinity for them to appropriately modulate their targets at reduced concentrations. The compound's potential to deliver its desired action to its target serves as its potency measure. Probes need to demonstrate high potency because the molecule has to deliver its intended effect while diluted in experimental solutions. Involvement of tool compounds depends heavily on potency because low drug concentrations are necessary to reach therapeutic effects during preclinical testing or human clinical trials.

Mechanism of Action

Research teams need to understand probe and tool compound mechanisms before selecting them for their investigations. The selection of chemical probes depends on their target-specific modulation capabilities, and researchers must establish complete information about how probes bind to their targets [22]. Tool compounds need characterization based on their impact on biological systems because they replicate therapeutic drug effects within biological systems.

Chemical Stability

Research teams need to understand probe and tool compound mechanisms before selecting them for their investigations. The selection of chemical probes depends on their target-specific modulation capabilities, and researchers must establish complete information about how probes bind to their targets [23]. Tool compounds need characterization based on their impact on biological systems because they replicate therapeutic drug effects within biological systems.

Pharmacokinetics

The clinical success of tool compounds depends heavily on pharmacokinetic properties because these molecules belong to category that requires preclinical and human trial applications. Poor PK properties including unfavorable absorption and distribution together with metabolism and excretion (ADME) profiles make tool compounds ineffective in achieving their target both inside and outside of a living organism [23, 24].

The figure depicts essential approaches for optimizing chemical probes regarding their selectivity and specificity. The process focuses on structure-based design in combination with fragment-based screening techniques while accounting for target class and mechanism to generate potent and selective probes that are suitable for biological use [25].

Designing and Optimizing Probes for Specificity and Selectivity

The design of chemical probes requires a careful balance between potency, specificity, and selectivity. To achieve the desired characteristics, researchers must consider several strategies:

Figure 6.5 depicts essential approaches for optimizing chemical probes regarding their selectivity and specificity. The process focuses on structure-based design in combination with fragment-based screening techniques while accounting for target class and mechanism to generate potent and selective probes that are suitable for biological usc [26].

Case Examples: Probe Compounds Targeting Kinases and Epigenetic Modulators

Kinase Inhibitors as Chemical Probes

Enzymes from the kinase category control cellular functions while regulating cell division, metabolism, and apoptosis. The regulation of kinase activity becomes dysfunctional in many disease cases, featuring cancer among them. Chemical probes that target kinases played a vital role in understanding kinase functions and produced various approved therapeutic kinase inhibitors [26–28].

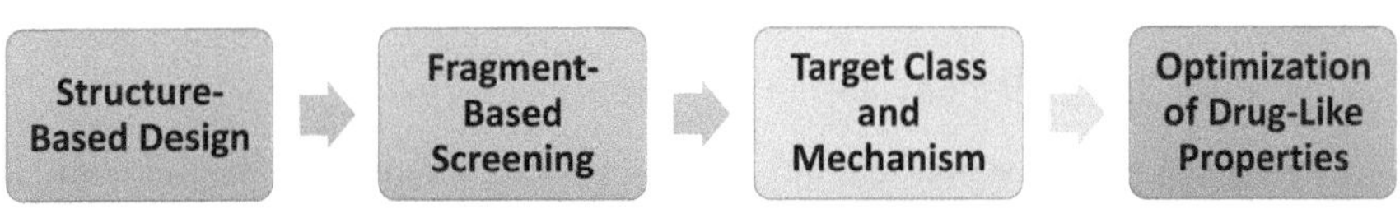

Figure 6.5 Optimizing chemical probes for specificity and selectivity.

Imatinib (Gleevec) started life as a tool compound to assess BCR-ABL kinase activity in chronic myelogenous leukemia (CML) patients, but it advanced to become a standard therapeutic drug. The research team optimized Imatinib to connect specifically with the BCR-ABL fusion protein because this protein causes uncontrolled CML cell growth. Understanding the drug-kinase bond interactions was possible through the use of chemical probes, which helped optimize the process [29].

Epigenetic Modulators as Probes

Enzymes from the kinase category control cellular functions while regulating cell division, metabolism, and apoptosis. The regulation of kinase activity becomes dysfunctional in many disease cases, featuring cancer among them. Chemical probes that target kinases played a vital role in understanding kinase functions and produced various approved therapeutic kinase inhibitors [27, 28].

Imatinib (Gleevec) started life as a tool compound to assess BCR-ABL kinase activity in chronic myelogenous leukemia (CML) patients, but it advanced to become a standard therapeutic drug. The research team optimized Imatinib to connect specifically with the BCR-ABL fusion protein because this protein causes uncontrolled CML cell growth. Understanding the drug-kinase bond interactions was possible through the use of chemical probes, which helped optimize the process [30].

The drug discovery process depends heavily on chemical probes as well as tool compounds because they are fundamental research tools. Research scientists benefit from chemical probes to better explore disease mechanisms, besides using tool compounds for determining therapeutic targets and developing new drugs. Researchers advance disease treatment discovery through compound selection and optimization for precise functions and responsive power, thereby generating trustworthy data.

Target Deconvolution Strategies

Drug discovery researchers need to establish molecular targets of small molecules because this enables them to understand both the mechanism of action and therapeutic effects. Multiple target interactions of many compounds produce either unintended effects or unanticipated therapeutic responses. Borderline Discrimination comprises methods that determine which specific biomolecules primarily interact with therapeutic agents or drugs to disclose their biological actions and create new, improved therapeutic agents [30–32]. The following section details the necessity of target deconvolution along with the implemented strategies and demonstrates their applications within oncology and infectious disease research.

The Need for Target Deconvolution in Drug Discovery

The discovery of new medications requires target identification and validation processes as initial critical steps during early development. A compound which interacts with multiple proteins through a biological system becomes challenging to identify the specific molecular targets affecting its therapeutic outcomes [33]. Biological systems display such complexity because their various interconnected elements lead to effects on the compound's effectiveness and safety output.

Target deconvolution is essential for a few key reasons:

1 Deconvoluting a compound's targets leads to better comprehension of its biological mechanism through Mechanisms of Action understanding. Research success depends on target discovery since it helps scientists understand how the drug interacts with its biological pathways, essential to both safety assessment and effectiveness evaluation.
2 Scientists enhance drug selectivity when they specify precise target proteins because they can reengineer their compounds to choose their specific targets without activating different proteins. The selection process of molecular targets helps both decrease drug adverse effects and enhance therapeutic results.
3 Target deconvolution provides an opportunity to identify alternative medical applications for drugs that already exist at pharmaceutical companies. Research success depends on identifying which molecular structures a drug compound connects with in the body.

Target deconvolution represents an essential procedure in the drug discovery framework because it helps researchers understand drug-target interactions, which supports the development of more effective therapy strategies (Figure 6.6).

Target deconvolution serves as a key process for drug discovery, according to this illustration. Target deconvolution serves crucial purposes for understanding how drugs function while helping developers improve selectivity and security and enabling drug rebirth. Target deconvolution serves as an essential method to determine exact drug-target connections, which creates highly efficient yet safe medical therapies.

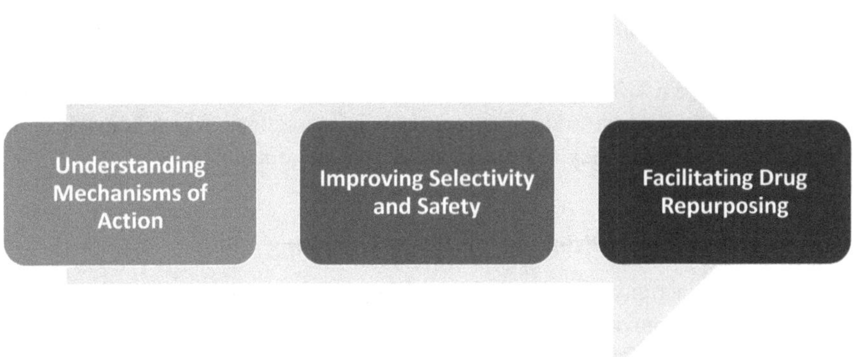

Figure 6.6 Importance of target deconvolution in drug discovery.

Affinity-based Approaches for Target Identification

The identification of targets for drug discovery utilizes affinity-based techniques as one of its primary methods in wide practice. Small-molecule binding specificity allows researchers to exploit these interactions when searching for proteins binding to their targets.

Affinity chromatography stands as the most frequently used affinity-based methodology. The method employs liquid moving across a column that contains small molecules attached to a solid support to catch target molecules present in lysate solutions. A filtrate containing bound proteins stays on the ligand while all noninteracting proteins get washed out. The laboratory uses mass spectrometry to analyze the proteins that get released from the column, followed by extensive characterization to study their contributions toward the biological functions of the target compound [34].

The advanced proteomic method known as affinity-based proteomics combines mass spectrometry with affinity enrichment technologies to identify and quantify protein targets. This approach was described in detail by Subhash V. Mocholi36. Affinity probes connected to specific tags serve as tools for capturing drug-target proteins and determining their identity. The approach generates a complete view of drug target networking and clarifies the foundation of therapeutic interactions [35].

Example: Affinity-based Proteomics for Target Deconvolution

The research of kinase inhibitors demonstrates a typical case of how affinity-based proteomics works in target deconvolution. The drug target category of kinases maintains crucial functions during disease development, not only for cancer but also for many other illnesses [36]. Through affinity-based proteomics, researchers have identified the particular set of kinases that various small molecules target. The BET family of proteins, which regulates epigenetics, have been examined through affinity-based proteomic approaches through BET inhibitors as per research [37]. The identification process of multiple cellular pathways has become possible through these inhibitors, leading to improved knowledge about their impact in cancer treatment.

The technique of affinity-based proteomics enables researchers to study small-molecule inhibitor-kinase and regulatory protein interactions, which helps develop drugs with greater accuracy and enhances therapeutic outcomes.

Activity-based Protein Profiling for Target Discovery

The strategy of activity-based protein profiling (ABPP) provides researchers with great power to deconvolute targets. The research approach ABPP uses small molecules to build covalent bonds with target protein active sites [38]. The probes include reactive groups that allow binding to nucleophilic residues inside enzyme active sites, which act as reaction-based protein labels.

The ABPP methodology allows one to identify modified proteins through mass spectrometry since it reveals which proteins have bound to the probe molecules. The identification of active proteins together with their cellular functions becomes possible through this technique because it detects the active protein form and its process engagement.

ABPP serves as a method which assists identification of serine hydrolase targets because these enzymes perform crucial functions in cellular signaling, lipid metabolism, and inflammation processes [39]. The application of ABPP with particular activity-based probes has enabled researchers to detect numerous proteins connected to disease mechanisms, which now directs investigations into potential therapeutic drugs for treating neurological conditions and cancer.

Chemoproteomics Approaches and Thermal Proteome Profiling

The tool ABPP functions as a highly effective process for target deconvolution. ABPP employs chemical probes through active site binding of target proteins to achieve analysis goals [40]. These probes contain reactive groups that bond covalently with the nucleophilic residues found in enzyme active sites, which leads to labeling of proteins in their active state.

Mass spectrometry enables the identification of proteins that interact with the probe through covalent bonds to show which compounds have become modified by the labeling agent. Studying enzymes together with other proteins that exhibit catalytic properties becomes possible through this approach since it reveals which active protein form performs cellular work.

The ABPP method helps detect the target proteins of serine hydrolases, particularly because this enzyme family controls cellular signaling and lipid breakdown and inflammatory activity [41]. Researchers utilize specific activity-based probes through ABPP to detect proteins related to disease processes that now serve as potential drug candidates for treating neurological diseases and cancer [42].

Complementary Methods: CRISPR and RNAi in Target Identification

- The target identification process benefits from the combination of chemical proteomics techniques like affinity-based methods and ABPP together with genetic methods, including clustered regularly interspaced short palindromic repeats (CRISPR) and RNA interference (RNAi) [43].

The CRISPR/Cas9 system performs exact genome modifications that help scientists disable specific genes. The method enables target deconvolution through its ability to detect genes whose knockout makes a drug inactive. The target genes that result in CRISPR-modified cells losing drug efficacy reveal information about the drug's mechanism of action.

The specific genes become dormant through small interfering RNAs (siRNAs) in RNAi processes. The method of target knockdown using RNAi works in a fashion similar to CRISPR for investigating cellular responses under different drug treatment conditions. Genetic alteration via this method aids scientists in gaining knowledge about which proteins play a role in drug action.

Case Studies: Successful Target Deconvolution in Oncology and Infectious Diseases

Target deconvolution has led to several breakthroughs in oncology and infectious disease research:

1 The investigations of cancer targets through target deconvolution techniques served as a notable instance in oncology. Scientists used chemoproteomics and CRISPR screening methods to deconvolve the targets of the breast and ovarian cancer medication Olaparib45. The research outcome showed that PARP1 functions as the primary target, while new proteins associated with DNA damage repair were identified. The analysis of these interactions enabled doctors to optimize therapeutic approaches while identifying new targets as treatment markers for selecting appropriate patients.
2 Infectious diseases research using ABPP technique identified P. falciparum histone deacetylases to serve as drug targets in malaria [44]. Target deconvolution analysis revealed particular parasite proteins that caused antimalarial drug resistance thus assisting in developing the following generation of treatment options.
3 Target deconvolution stands as an important drug discovery method which helps scientists reveal molecular targets and their corresponding effect mechanisms. Researchers utilize premium models of proteomics such as ABPP alongside chemoproteomics and affinity-based proteomics as well as CRISPR and RNAi to fully investigate drug interactions within biological networks. Several cancer and infection disease cases indicate how these methods boost pharmaceutical research speed and produce better healthcare results while minimizing adverse effects windfall.

Applications in Understanding Disease Mechanisms

The application of chemical probes together with tool compounds through chemical biology methods has transformed our ability to understand complex disease mechanisms. These tools make precise pathway modulation possible, which enables scientists to dissect and understand complex biological processes of different diseases [44–46]. Research investigations of disease pathways in oncology, neurodegenerative diseases, and infectious diseases have become possible through the use of chemical probes and tool compounds. The subsequent part examines the important function of chemical probes in disease mechanism comprehension as well as their specific disease investigation applications along with real-world illustrations of their impact.

Using Chemical Probes to Study and Dissect Disease Pathways

Chemical probes that are small molecules or compounds study the functionality of biological targets, especially proteins, by attaching to them and probing them inside cellular environments. The probes possess a particular design for modifying target protein activity, which allows scientists to study resulting effects and detect downstream consequences. Chemical probes enable precise temporal and spatial control over protein manipulation in order to fully examine disease-related protein functions [47].

Probes designed for oncogenic proteins in cancer studies enable researchers to control these proteins for investigating their contribution to tumor development along with cancer progression. The examples include kinases, epigenetic regulators, and tumor suppressors [48]. Research teams can study cancer origin mechanics through protein manipulation for cell division and survival and the examination of migration and metastasis events.

The progression of Alzheimer's disease and Parkinson's disease receives vital insight through chemical probes that focus on enzymes and receptors involved with disease progression. Amyloid-beta plaque generation in Alzheimer's disease can be studied through beta-secretase and gamma-secretase enzyme probes because they enable researchers to understand molecular processes and plaque-related pathology.

Mechanistic Studies in Oncology, Neurodegenerative Diseases, and Infectious Diseases

Researchers utilize chemical probes specifically for disease mechanistic studies because they provide insights into disease development at a molecular scale. The identification of new therapy targets remains essential because research using disease mechanisms helps discover drug development possibilities. The following section demonstrates multiple uses of chemical probes in oncology treatments alongside their implementation for studies in neurodegenerative diseases and infectious diseases.

Oncology

In oncology, chemical probes are widely used to dissect the molecular mechanisms that drive cancer development and progression. Cancer cells often harbor mutations in oncogenes—genes that promote uncontrolled cell growth. For example, kinase inhibitors, which are small molecules designed to inhibit specific kinases, have been used to study the roles of key signaling pathways, such as the PI3K/Akt/mTOR pathway and the MAPK pathway, in cancer [48, 49].

Case Study: Kinase Inhibitors in Oncology

The development of Imatinib (Gleevec) as a kinase inhibitor for the BCR-ABL kinase demonstrates a remarkable use of chemical probes in oncology at 51. The targeted chemical inhibitor Imatinib blocks BCR-ABL while selecting that abnormal fusion protein in leukemia cells, which causes uncontrolled cell growth. Understanding oncogenic pathways including the BCR-ABL-driven signaling cascade in CML became possible through Imatinib alongside other kinase inhibitors used by scientists. Scientists have gained knowledge about tumor growth signaling pathways through the development of kinase inhibitors, which target receptors like EGFR and VEGF (vascular endothelial growth factor) in addition to Imatinib (Gleevec) in tumors [50, 51].

Kinase inhibitors have also been instrumental in identifying new biomarkers and patient stratification strategies, enabling more targeted and personalized therapies in cancer treatment.

Neurodegenerative Diseases

Studies of neurodegenerative diseases depend on chemical probes because they uncover the contribution of proteins tau and amyloid-beta and alpha-synuclein to disease development pathways. Beta-secretase inhibitors serve as chemical probes to enable studies of amyloid precursor protein APP proteolytic cleavage that results in amyloid formation in Alzheimer's disease patients [52].

Case Study: Chemical Probes in Alzheimer's Disease

The examination of amyloid-beta plaque prevention through BACE1 enzyme suppression has been conducted through research utilizing beta-secretase (BACE1) chemical probes aimed at this APP-cleaving enzyme. BACE1 inhibitor studies within preclinical models have revealed vital information about the connection between amyloid-beta protein and cognitive decline together with brain damage. Tool compounds aimed at blocking tau aggregation and alpha-synuclein aggregation in Parkinson's disease serve as research tools to examine protein misfolding and aggregation processes vital for these diseases [53].

Infectious Diseases

Research on infectious diseases depends on chemical probes that assist scientists in identifying crucial proteins which enable pathogens between the biological life cycles of bacteria, viruses and parasites. Chemical probes have been employed to investigate Plasmodium proteins for new treatment targets in malaria research. Chemical probes support research of viral protein-host cell interaction studies in cases like HIV infection [54].

Case Study: Probes in Malaria Research

Studies about the Plasmodium falciparum parasite responsible for malaria represent one application of chemical probes within infectious disease research. Research teams have discovered new antimalarial therapy targets by using chemical probes that target Plasmodium essential survival enzymes like proteases and kinases. These probes play a critical role in studying parasite drug resistance development as well as preventing existing medications from facing resistance, such as chloroquine, contributing to new inhibitor discovery [55].

Research on HIV/AIDS resulted in antiretroviral therapies due to tool compounds which prevent protease and reverse transcriptase enzyme operations. Through utilizing chemical probes, scientists have been able to plot viral replication stages while finding critical enzymes for blocking, which resulted in the development of combined therapies that effectively treat HIV infection.

Leveraging Tool Compounds to Reveal Disease Mechanism Insights

In addition to chemical probes, tool compounds serve as specific protein modulators that enhance disease mechanism discovery. The selection priority of tool compounds directs their utilization as probes for specific protein study within complicated biological environments.

Chromatin-modifying enzymes face activity changes from epigenetic modulators, which make up one category of tool compounds [56]. Researchers use these compounds to investigate how gene expression modifications through chromatin changes contribute to cancer along with neurodegenerative conditions and cardiovascular conditions.

Tool compounds function as identification tools for discovering biomarkers associated with disease progression. Researchers use their understanding of biomolecule interactions to study protein modulation effects on cellular responses and gene activity patterns for disease marker identification.

Applications in Drug Discovery and Development

Drug discovery along with development has established chemical biology as an essential discipline by delivering tools which boost both drug target identification and validation processes and therapeutic compound optimization. The application of specifically designed chemical probes in drug discovery contributes valuable assets to various discovery phases from phenotypic screening until hit identification, drug redefinition, and precision medicine development. The high specificity along with selectivity enabled by chemical probes enables a better understanding of complex disease processes and leads to the discovery of novel therapeutic options. Test cases show how chemical probes contribute to drug discovery during this section of analysis [57].

Chemical Probes in Phenotypic Screening and Hit Identification

Toward the beginning of drug discovery research, phenotypic screening enables scientists to watch cellular biological outcomes during compound treatments using cellular models. Phenotypic screening depends highly on chemical probes because these compounds enable researchers to detect compounds which affect disease-relevant pathways. The investigative tools help scientists study the effects of small molecules on cells through measures of survival, proliferation, differentiation, and death. Screening based on phenotypic effects remains a useful technique, since researchers do not need prior information about which molecule their compounds target [58].

Research teams use chemical probes either to verify molecular targets or to enhance their final optimized versions after screening protocols. The first step in hit identification requires checking numerous compounds against disease phenotype alterations. Following hit identification, chemical probes validate the findings by confirming the targets of interaction for the identified compounds. Laboratory testing validates that detected cellular behavior occurs from target-specific modifications rather than from side effects of the compounds [59].

Case Study: Kinase Inhibitors in Targeted Cancer Therapies

Chemical probes achieve their most successful utilization through phenotypic screening applications, which result in small-molecule kinase inhibitor discovery within oncological research [57]. The enzymes known as kinases control cellular signaling pathways, yet their improper regulation leads to cancer formation along with other diseases. Scientists use chemical probes to discover new kinase inhibitors which target cancer-dominant factors epidermal growth factor receptor (EGFR) and BCR-ABL (a fusion protein linked to chronic myelogenous leukemia). Research probes have enabled scientists to look for inhibitors that stop these kinases, thus leading to medications like Imatinib (Gleevec) to treat patients with CML [60].

HTS Facilitated by Chemical Biology Tools

Through HTS, scientists conduct essential drug discovery analysis that screens extensive libraries of compounds against targets of interest at thousands or millions of rates. Large-scale compound screening becomes more precise and reliable when chemical biology tools and their chemical probes are used to enhance HTS operations. The analytical tools enable researchers to evaluate numerous small molecules within large, diverse libraries to discover compounds that affect the target of interest, thus speeding up lead compound selection.

Variations of chemical probes display high selectivity for binding to receptors and enzymes as well as ion channels before they can alter these protein functions. Compound-target interactions become measurable through the implementation of detection methods such as fluorescence and mass spectrometry, and bioluminescence on large scales. The utility range of chemical probes extends through cell-based assays, which provide real-life cellular conditions for testing compounds to help researchers understand these molecules' effects on cellular activities and disease models.

Example: HTS for Enzyme Inhibition

The development of new drug candidates has greatly benefited from chemical probes designed for protease and kinase, and transcription factor inhibition work in enzyme research. Using HTS with chemical probes, researchers detected protease inhibitors which proved able to block HIV protease effectively during viral replication. The discovery of protease inhibitors became the fundamental element that forms antiretroviral therapy for HIV treatment.

Applications in Drug Repurposing and Rescue with Validated Probes

Existing drugs get examined through drug repurposing strategies because of chemical probes. The approach shortens drug discovery operations through testing current medicines for fresh indications from their initial disease applications. The use of chemical probes enables scientists to discover new possible molecular targets for diseases they had not examined before, leading to previously unknown treatment opportunities.

The exceptional value of chemical probes emerges during drug rescue attempts when researchers try to restore efficiency to drugs rendered useless through drug resistance. Research RCN probes enable scientists to discover resistance mechanisms, allowing them to generate new compounds that outperform current obstacles. The use of specific probe molecules permits screening with resistance-conferring mutations for compounds able to re-sensitize both cancer cells and bacterial strains with viral variants [61].

Case Study: Drug Repurposing for COVID-19

Chemical probes together with chemical biology tools enabled researchers to discover existing drugs that potentially fought against SARS-CoV-2 virus when the COVID-19 pandemic hit. The researchers deployed HTS combined with chemical probes, which focused on viral enzymes like 3CL protease and RNA-dependent RNA polymerase, to discover approved drugs for alternative conditions. The use of chemical biology screening led scientists to discover remdesivir as a promising COVID-19 therapy and earned this Ebola antiviral its emergency use authorization in COVID-19 treatment.

Case Examples: Discovery of Small-molecule Inhibitors in Targeted Therapies

Targeted therapies have proven highly successful after researchers discovered how small-molecule inhibitors function with chemical probes. The treatment of cancer benefits from chemical probes which identify selective inhibitors that block cancer-driving mutations and signaling pathways. Subsequent to its discovery Imatinib proved beneficial in treating patients with CML. The cancer-fighting drug Imatinib focuses exclusively on the BCR-ABL fusion protein that CML patients exhibit. Researchers identified this therapeutic method after using chemical probes which bound to the fusion protein, thus inhibiting its activity to enable an effective CML treatment.

BRAF inhibitors stand among important drugs used for treating melanoma. BRAF V600E mutation causes uncontrolled growth of melanoma cells, so chemical probes deliver small-molecule inhibitors for selective targeting of the mutated

BRAF V600E form. Vemurafenib, one of the inhibitors, has led to improved survival results specifically for patients who have BRAF-mutant melanoma.

Impact on Precision Medicine and Personalized Drug Discovery

Rolling chemical probes into drug discovery processes has revolutionized precision medicine, which creates individualized treatments from genetic profiles and disease characteristics and biological targets. Therapy development benefits from chemical probes because they reveal exact disease-causing molecular pathways, which enables medical teams to produce targeted treatments specifically adapted for individual patients' genetic structures and molecular signatures.

Commercial probes enable researchers to create biomarkers, which demonstrate their capability for patient selection before deciding which therapy will produce maximum benefit. The discovery of unique biomarkers for HER2-positive breast cancer enabled scientists to develop trastuzumab (Herceptin), which has delivered better clinical outcomes to patients bearing this breast cancer subtype. The development of EGFR mutation-targeted probes enabled medical professionals to create treatments against non-small cell lung cancer (NSCLC).

The combination of chemical biology with advanced genomics and patient data allows drug discovery to develop personalized, effective treatments that match individual patients based on their unique genetic and molecular characteristics. The development of drug targets, biomarkers, and therapeutic strategies experiences accelerated discovery thanks to chemical probes, which speed up target validation.

Future Directions and Emerging Trends

Current developments in chemical biology create fresh possibilities to solve obstacles related to drug development and discovery processes. Scientific progress along with emerging technologies will revolutionize disease treatments through chemical biology approaches, particularly for target detection and precision healthcare and complex pathology investigation. Future developments in chemical proteomics are combined with artificial intelligence (AI) and machine learning (ML) integration and the expansion of broad disease target-specific chemical probe libraries.

Advances in Chemical Proteomics for Target Deconvolution

Chemical proteomics represents a major achievement in chemical biology because researchers have been advancing the proficient method for detecting protein targets in their native cellular environment. Chemical proteomics gives scientists the power to study protein-ligand interactions in living cells by using chemical probes, which also helps researchers identify new drug targets and understand complex disease-related signaling pathways. The development of affinity-based methods including chemical cross-linking and ABPP together with thermal proteome profiling (TPP) enables better and more thorough detection of protein targets alongside their interaction networks. This evolving technology shows potential to deliver enhanced knowledge about drug resistance and off-target effects along with multitarget interactions, which will streamline therapeutic strategy development [57].

Integrating AI and ML with Chemical Biology Approaches

Drug discovery will experience a revolutionary shift through the growing relationship between chemical biology and AI together with machine learning systems. The integration of computational tools alongside experimental data through AI and ML enhances chemical probe development speed and optimizes their design as well as compound-target prediction while identifying new drug candidates. AI algorithms learn to forecast small-molecule biological functions through large-scale molecular and biological data analysis, leading to the invention of new compounds as well as target discovery suggestions. The optimization processing capabilities of machine learning models enhance chemical probes by improving their selectivity and pharmaceutical profiles, and specific properties. The combined usage of AI systems with chemical biology produces synergistic effects that decrease the time needed for drug discovery as well as the financial requirements and analytical challenges involved in drug target evaluation [58–71].

Expanding Chemical Probe Libraries for a Wider Range of Disease Targets

Modern drug discovery through chemical probes operates out of restricted libraries that mainly investigate established targets among kinases and enzymes together with GPCRs. The scientific community actively works to expand chemical probe libraries for investigating disease targets that prove difficult to drug and remain understudied. The disease factors include transcription factors and intracellular proteins as well as epigenetic modulators, which are essential for cancer development and control neurodegenerative disorders and autoimmune diseases. Scientists develop probes for hard-to-study disease targets to study mechanisms inaccessible to current methods and discover new possible treatments. Fragment-based drug discovery together with degraders has emerged as a vital synthesis strategy for developing chemical probes, which aim to target multiple molecular pathways more effectively.

Conclusion

Chemical biology research demonstrates future potential to solve complex diseases, which include neurodegenerative disorders and cancer together with infectious diseases. Multiple disease targets formed by intricate molecular networks produce conditions that show complex interactions between various targets within dynamically evolving systems. Research groups will keep using chemical probes along with advanced proteomics approaches to explore complicated biological systems for discovering new diagnostic targets and disease markers. Internal progress in the field will increase our capacity to generate personalized treatments by adapting therapeutic approaches to individual genetic profiles through precision medicine. The development of individualized therapies demands essential chemical biology tools to create treatments that utilize patients' distinct genetic information combined with their disease manifestations and targeted biological entities. Chemical probes that examine disease origins at molecular scales will direct the development of targeted medicine, which produces strong results alongside minimal adverse effects when managing heterogeneous diseases.

The convergence of machine learning with chemical proteomics technology and advanced AI systems together with broadened chemical probe resources establishes chemical biology as the foundational element for future drug development research. The new technological advancements will help researchers understand disease mechanisms better while creating better treatments that match individual patient needs and achieve high precision. The field of chemical biology shows potential to become increasingly important for the solutions of unmet medical needs, which will emerge in the future.

References

1. Smith J, et al. Understanding the role of chemical biology in drug discovery. Nat Rev Drug Discov. 2020;19(8):603–618.
2. Jones T, et al. Applications of chemical probes in cellular signaling research. Cell Chem Biol. 2019;26(6):845–858.
3. Barton A, et al. Chemical biology approaches to study molecular interactions in cell signaling. Nat Rev Drug Discov. 2018;17(4):264–277.
4. Yan X, et al. Chemical probe development for protein-protein interaction targets. Nat Rev Drug Discov. 2020;19(8):504–515.
5. Graham MA, et al. Chemical probes in drug discovery. Nat Rev Drug Discov. 2015;14(12):827–841.
6. Lange MS, et al. Targeting protein kinases with chemical probes. Nat Rev Drug Discov. 2017;16(10):649–664.
7. Svensson AS, et al. Chemical tools for targeted drug discovery. Nat Rev Drug Discov. 2018;17(3):215–229.
8. Balasubramanian K, et al. Chemical biology approaches for drug discovery. Nat Chem Biol. 2015;11(2):109–117.
9. Kapoor R, et al. Target validation using chemical probes. Nat Rev Drug Discov. 2018;17(7):383–395.
10. Li Y, et al. Designing small molecules as tools for studying protein-protein interactions. Nat Chem Biol. 2020;16(1):12–24.
11. Zhao D, et al. The evolving role of chemical probes in drug discovery. Nat Rev Drug Discov. 2019;18(3):181–192.
12. Papp A, et al. Advances in chemical biology for drug discovery. Trends Pharmacol Sci. 2017;38(8):758–770.
13. Fernandez T, et al. Targeted drug discovery through chemical biology. Nat Chem Biol. 2019;15(10):952–965.
14. Yang Z, et al. Small molecules as chemical probes in drug discovery. J Med Chem. 2020;63(5):2456–2469.
15. Zhang L, et al. Chemical proteomics in drug discovery. Nat Rev Drug Discov. 2017;16(2):112–123.

16. Park J, et al. Epigenetic chemical probes in drug discovery. Nat Rev Drug Discov. 2018;17(6):350–362.
17. Reed S, et al. Target deconvolution and the role of chemical probes. Nat Rev Drug Discov. 2019;18(4):210–221.
18. Hernandez D, et al. Chemical biology and its role in modern drug discovery. Trends Pharmacol Sci. 2020;41(7):456–467.
19. Jones P, et al. Understanding chemical probes in drug discovery. Drug Discov Today. 2020;25(1):12–20.
20. Tan K, et al. Chemical biology in cancer research: A step towards precision medicine. Cancer Res. 2017;77(9):2439–2450.
21. Lin H, et al. The role of chemical probes in the investigation of cancer signaling pathways. Cell Chem Biol. 2019;26(7):943–957.
22. Morris S, et al. Small molecule chemical probes in disease research. Nat Rev Drug Discov. 2017;16(6):409–420.
23. Boucher D, et al. Proteomics-based target deconvolution for drug discovery. Nat Chem Biol. 2020;16(6):577–588.
24. Williams M, et al. Chemical proteomics in drug target identification and validation. Curr Opin Pharmacol. 2018;40:99–106.
25. Yang Y, et al. Thermal proteome profiling: A method to study protein-ligand interactions. Nat Protoc. 2020;15(1):99–112.
26. Feng X, et al. CRISPR-based chemical probe development. Nat Chem Biol. 2019;15(7):598–610.
27. Wu X, et al. Chemical probes for epigenetic targets in cancer therapy. Nat Rev Cancer. 2017;17(4):204–221.
28. Muller M, et al. Applications of chemical probes for epigenetic therapy. Cell Chem Biol. 2019;26(5):618–630.
29. He M, et al. The development of chemical probes in neurological disorders. J Med Chem. 2020;63(3):937–954.
30. Lee R, et al. Targeting epigenetic regulators for cancer therapy with chemical probes. Nat Rev Drug Discov. 2018;17(5):356–371.
31. Cho H, et al. Development of small molecule chemical probes in drug discovery. Nat Rev Drug Discov. 2019;18(1):26–40.
32. Green S, et al. Kinase inhibitors in drug discovery. Nat Rev Drug Discov. 2017;16(6):408–419.
33. Vaughan C, et al. Chemical proteomics for target discovery and drug development. Trends Pharmacol Sci. 2017;38(9):740–754.
34. Carter C, et al. New trends in the development of small-molecule chemical probes. Trends Pharmacol Sci. 2020;41(1):28–41.
35. Schmidt E, et al. Therapeutic protein-protein interaction modulators as drug discovery tools. Nat Rev Drug Discov. 2018;17(10):646–662.
36. Turner S, et al. Unlocking drug discovery with small-molecule chemical probes. Trends Pharmacol Sci. 2020;40(12):956–968.
37. Lo Y, et al. Chemical probes for the study of epigenetic regulators. Nat Chem Biol. 2020;16(8):797–808.
38. Miao Z, et al. Chemical biology in drug discovery: From concepts to clinical applications. Nat Rev Drug Discov. 2018;17(3):186–204.
39. Thompson A, et al. Developing chemical probes for immune modulation. Cell Chem Biol. 2019;26(8):1189–1199.
40. Gundry C, et al. Application of chemical proteomics for targeted cancer therapy. Cancer Cell. 2018;33(3):401–415.
41. Alvarez S, et al. Chemical probes for cancer cell signaling. Cell Chem Biol. 2019;26(11):1554–1570.
42. Reeves R, et al. Chemical biology approaches for drug target identification. Trends Pharmacol Sci. 2020;41(4):294–306.

43. Kang J, et al. Target identification with chemical probes in drug discovery. Nat Rev Drug Discov. 2019;18(9):597–610.
44. Zhu J, et al. Chemical biology approaches for cancer target validation. Nat Rev Cancer. 2018;18(2):129–140.
45. Stewart T, et al. Small molecule inhibitors as chemical probes for studying metabolic diseases. Nat Rev Drug Discov. 2020;19(5):285–297.
46. Jones R, et al. Chemical proteomics: A powerful tool for drug discovery. Nat Rev Drug Discov. 2020;19(3):217–232.
47. Wang Y, et al. Chemical biology in neurodegenerative diseases. Nat Rev Drug Discov. 2018;17(11):831–844.
48. Liu J, et al. Chemical probes for targeted therapy in cancer. Trends Pharmacol Sci. 2020;41(7):497–508.
49. Peng Z, et al. Targeted chemical probes for drug discovery. Nat Rev Drug Discov. 2018;17(2):97–112.
50. Zhao H, et al. Small molecules as chemical probes in cancer research. Nat Rev Cancer. 2019;19(5):290–304.
51. Xie H, et al. Therapeutic chemical probes for protein degradation. Nat Rev Drug Discov. 2020;19(6):399–411.
52. Harris R, et al. Chemical probes in metabolic diseases. Trends Pharmacol Sci. 2018;39(10):891–907.
53. Lu Z, et al. Chemical tools for dissecting protein function. Nat Rev Drug Discov. 2019;18(4):235–246.
54. Jackson L, et al. Chemical probes in signal transduction. Nat Rev Mol Cell Biol. 2020;21(3):128–141.
55. Schroder M, et al. Chemical proteomics in drug discovery. Nat Rev Drug Discov. 2019;18(9):589–604.
56. Xu X, et al. Chemical probes for neurodegenerative diseases. Cell Chem Biol. 2018;25(9):1125–1137.
57. Wang F, et al. Development of chemical probes for oncology research. Nat Rev Cancer. 2020;20(4):223–236.
58. Yuan Z, et al. Chemical biology for cancer therapy. Nat Rev Cancer. 2019;19(9):594–607.
59. Ding J, et al. Chemical biology of protein misfolding diseases. Nat Rev Drug Discov. 2020;19(8):469–484.
60. Lu X, et al. Chemical probes for cellular pathways. Nat Rev Drug Discov. 2018;17(8):588–602.
61. Singh S, et al. The application of chemical biology in drug development. Nat Rev Drug Discov. 2019;18(11):663–678.
62. Atmakuri LR, Peeriga R, Begum S, Vallamkonda B, Baratam A. Novel bioanalytical LC-MS/MS method for determination of metoprolol in human plasma. J Appl Pharm Sci. 2024;14(12):131–138.
63. Peeriga R, Venkata Bangaru GK. Implementation of the POCSO act in schools. In: Child Sexual Abuse: A Public Health Problem in India. Springer publications, Singapore, 2024. p. 391–413. Springer Publications, Singapore.
64. Peeriga R, Yarlagadda LC, Alla NR. Protection of children from sexual exploitation. In: Child Sexual Abuse: A Public Health Problem in India. Springer publications, Singapore 2024. p. 191–201. Springer Publications, Singapore.
65. Peeriga R, Shiek Arabath SAM, Manubolu K, Thelappilly BB, Yarlagadda LC. In-silico assessment of phytoconstituents in *myxopyrum smilacifolium* blume against arthritis. Biomed Pharmacol J. 2024;17(1):235–241.
66. Manubolu K, Balagani PK, Gope ER, Peeriga R, Sridevi AR. Unlocking the potential of aquasomes: A comprehensive review on innovative nanocarriers in drug delivery and beyond. Int J Chem Biochem Sci. 2023;24(6):405–410.

67. Manubolu K, Peeriga R, Bonthu MG, Gope ER, Kadirvel D. Evaluation of anti-inflammatory activity of *Millingtonia hortensis* leaf extract. Int J Chem Biochem Sci. 2023;24(6):380–385.
68. Peeriga R, Chandrasekhar KB. Comparative study of anti-inflammatory activity of petroleum ether extract of *myxopyrum smilacifolium* blume and ethanolic leaf extract of *pamburus missionis* swingle. J Pharm Sci Res. 2017;9(6):955–957.
69. Peeriga R, Manubolu K (2025). Design strategies for waste reduction and enhanced recyclability in pharmaceutical packaging. In: Yingngam, B., Aslam, M.S., Haghi, A.K. (eds) Sustainable Pharmaceutical Product Development and Optimization Processes. Springer, Singapore.
70. Manubolu K, Peeriga R, Chandrasekhar KB. A Short Guide to Clinical Pharmacokinetics. 1st ed. 2024. Springer. Singapore.
71. Manubolu K, Peeriga R (2025). Ecodesign principles. In: Yingngam, B., Aslam, M.S., Haghi, A.K. (eds) Sustainable Pharmaceutical Product Development and Optimization Processes. Springer, Singapore.

7 Interdisciplinary Perspectives in Drug Discovery

Krishnaveni Manubolu, Talamanchi Balakrishna, Chandika Naga Veera Venkata Pravallika, K. Ravi Shankar, Lakshman Kumar Dogiparthi, and Sreenivasulu Munna

Introduction

Novel therapeutic agents [1–3] are developed in drug discovery, and chemistry plays a key role in this development. Chemists develop and synthesize new chemicals to increase their potency, selectivity and safety with regard to their target biological activity, emphasizing the better chemical structure of new drug candidates. Analytical methods are developed for the purity and stability of these compounds, and structure–activity relationship (SAR) studies are made on the SAR in order to refine molecules according to their biological activity [4]. This chemical foundation is needed to develop the safe and promising medication candidates.

The field of biology, that is, biology plays its role in disease processes and finds and confirms biological targets [5]. Drug candidates are investigated by biologists for interactions with these targets on the molecular and cellular levels as an attempt to learn more about their mode of action and their therapeutic potential [6]. By performing animal models and cellular assays they look at how chemicals are safe and effective in more crinkly biological systems and provide much needed knowledge about how medicines work in living things.

The main objective of pharmacology is to understand how medications work on patients' bodies. Pharmacologists study interactions between pharmaceuticals and their targets [7] and their mode of action, therapeutic benefits, if any, and implications. Also covered are pharmacodynamics (how medications change the biological systems) and pharmacokinetics (how drugs are absorbed, transported, metabolized, and eliminated). This assessment is to support the development of drug candidates through preclinical and clinical stages, from which is sought the safety and efficacy of the candidates.

Informatics helps improve the drug discovering process by using computational tools for complicated biological and chemical data analysis and integration. It is the application of computational approach in analyzing the biological data that is referred to as bioinformatics, which has been used to uncover biomarker, and potential therapeutic target. As its name implies though, the discipline used to organize and assess chemical data in a way which helps to create and optimize compounds is known as cheminformatics. It includes SARs. Moreover, informatics is the assimilation of information from different sources and use in producing

DOI: 10.4324/9781003564041-7

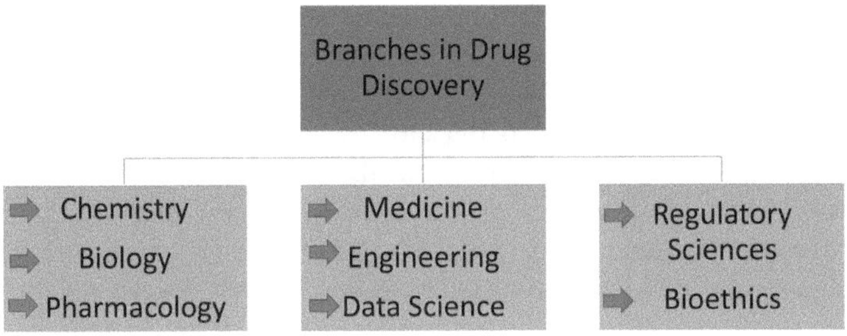

Figure 7.1 Branches in drug discovery.

simulations and predictive models which quicken drug development procedure and make better decisions [8]. The branches in drug discovery are shown in Figure 7.1.

To a large extent, engineering advances drug discovery just by simplifying and improving several steps in the process. Automated high-throughput screening (HTS) technologies quicken the process for identifying potential drug candidates, while the design of drugs improves by predicting molecular interactions through computational modeling and simulations. Improvements in biomanufacturing enhance the complicated manufacture of biologics. Microfluidics provides efficient testing of properties in smaller setups, while engineering breakthroughs in drug delivery systems improve targeted therapy. Machine learning (ML)-based data analytics provide excellent automated forecasts and analysis. All this work combines into one and improves the therapeutic outcomes while speeding up the drug development process and increasing its precision.

Data science, by way of sophisticated analytics and machine learning, is revolutionizing pharmaceutical development through massive data screening, medication interaction simulation, design improvement, and possible biomarker identification. Personalized treatments by a genetic profile advance HTS and go with precise clinical trial administration and individualized medicine. Data science develops drug repurposing as well as side effect prediction to speed up development and increase the efficacy and safety of new therapies [9].

Because they take all kinds of innovative drugs through all regulatory procedures and norms in their entire course of development, regulatory affairs are involved in the whole drug discovery process. Regulatory affairs experts navigate through the maze of complex rules to expedite the authorization process by means of the preparation and submission of required documents to the regulated authorities, like the FDA or EMA. IND submissions are done by these specialists for after-the-fact studies, which ensures that such studies are designed and conducted per regulatory requirements. They also handle inquiries or questions with regulatory agencies. Another crucial and important duty performed by regulatory affairs specialists is keeping up-to-date with changing standards and regulations—this always helps to adapt to and maintain compliance for medication producers. This process finally helps in steering drugs from discovery to market approval and from post-market surveillance. They have the utmost responsibility for adequately ensuring therapy for efficacy and safety.

Drug development relies on bioethics to ensure adherence to ethical standards during any research process and safeguards the welfare and rights of participants and animals. It assures informed consent, prioritizes participant safety, makes reporting of results more transparent, and delegates fair selection of participants and conflict management to bioethics, thereby ensuring drug development processes are conducted responsibly and respectfully without undermining the integrity of the process itself but creating public trust. The combined influence of these areas generates a unified approach to drug discovery where each area offers special angles, approaches, and techniques to devise new treatments that are safe and effective.

In Contribution with Chemistry

The majority of contemporary medical science and therapy is reliant on numerous developments in chemistry and related domains. And today, more than ever, the industry must engage in fundamental chemical research in order to provide solutions, given the rapidly rising number of health issues and the incidence of noninfectious diseases. To guarantee the appropriate development of medications, it is therefore even more crucial for the healthcare sector to stay up to date with the rapidly evolving trends in the chemical sciences. In this way, chemists' roles and contributions are becoming increasingly recognized in the modern period in an effort to enhance the state of healthcare overall.

The chemistry of molecules and their relationship to biological processes are the driving forces behind drug discovery and development. Bio-active compounds are modified from natural products [9] using the classical or traditional procedure used by medicinal chemists. Chemistry is essential to the drug discovery process because it provides the building blocks for the creation of novel therapeutic agents. These are a few significant contributions:

Hit Identification and Optimization

Discovery and improvement of early "hit" molecules with promising medicinal applications [10] is aided by the study of chemistry. Methods are developed by scientists to alter chemical structures to improve potency, selectivity, and pharmacokinetic qualities, e.g., medicinal chemistry and HTS.

Structure–Activity Relationship

Chemists study the way a compound's biological action relates to its chemical structure. Scientists can adjust a variety of molecular components to find and optimize the structural factors that are necessary for a molecule to do its job.

Synthesis of New Compound

Organic synthesis [11] can produce new compounds, including highly specific or not easily obtainable compounds, that were not previously possible. Chemists make these substances and can then test them for safety and effectiveness.

Pharmacodynamic and Pharmacokinetic

In studying drug absorption, distribution, metabolism, and excretion (ADME), chemistry helps us to understand how pharmaceuticals behave in the body. In addition, this means transforming drugs into a form most likely to increase bioavailability and ensure they perform as prescribed.

Formulation Development

Chemists devise diverse medicinal formulations with nothing less than stability, efficacy, and proper administering of the drug. Controlled release technologies also make the medication release slowly over time, which raises the patient adherence and therapeutic results.

Analytical Chemistry

Analytical methods are used by chemists to test pharmaceutical goods to make sure potency, purity and uniformity of pharmaceutical goods and chemists are involved from the beginning to the end of every step in this. These techniques both provide quality control and analysis of drug metabolites for determination of their effect on safety and efficacy.

Computational Chemistry and Modeling

Computer technologies are employed to simulate drug target interactions and to predict the effects of the molecular changes on drug activity by chemists. However, virtual screening methods allow one to easily search through very large chemical libraries to find promising drug ideas [12].

Safety and Toxicology

Chemists perform experiments to determine the toxicity and safety of potential drug candidates and to plan the experiments. It's been done to ensure the drug is safe in clinical trials by studying how medications are metabolized, looking for hazardous metabolites or bad interactions.

Green Chemistry

The environmental friendliness [13] of drug synthesis and manufacturing procedures is improved utilizing aspects of green chemistry. It includes reducing waste, cutting waste, and using sustainable approaches in the research of drugs and improving energy efficiency.

Regulatory Compliance

After all, chemistry makes sure good manufacturing practices and other regulatory criteria are being followed when developing a medication. Compliance is key in order to get regulatory clearances and to get novel medications to the market in a safe and efficient manner.

In Contribution with Biology

Because human biology is so complex, it is a difficult task to develop new safe and effective medications. And the focus has now turned to integrating multiple data types to put together molecular and pathway information for predicting illness outcomes. An explosion of high-throughput data has been generated via systems biology omics-based studies [14]. Further prediction of drug effects in patients will be enabled by better models of human disease biology, including more extensive network-based models that can handle multiple omics data sources and more relevant experimental systems, which will increase the success rate of novel drugs in the clinic and reveal new applications for previously approved drugs.

By increasing our understanding of disease mechanisms from the molecular, cellular, to systemic levels, biology has an indispensable role in drug development by bringing the groundwork for finding and validating new therapeutic targets. Methods from the field of molecular biology, genomics, proteomics, and bioinformatics allow the discovery of genes and proteins implicated in disease, and structural biology and bioinformatics allow the creation of compounds with specific interactions with these targets. Cell biology and pharmacology have produced cellular and animal models to assess the safety and effectiveness of new treatments before they enter—typically years—of clinical trials. Together, developments in systems biology and immunology enable the creation of personalized medicine, allowing for the prediction of drug effects on complex biological networks, as well as the development of individualized treatment plans. Biology is ultimately integral to every step of the drug discovery process, from target identification through safe and effective medicine.

Drug research is a product of several disciplines of biology, each to its own specialization. Several fundamental forms of biology are employed in the process of finding and creating new drugs:

- Molecular biology
- Cell biology
- Biochemistry
- Genomics
- Proteomics

- Structural biology [15]
- Pharmacology
- System biology
- Microbiology
- Immunology
- Toxicology
- Neurobiology
- Developmental biology
- Evolutionary biology
- Ecotoxicology

Biology is essential in the drug discovery process, from identifying potential therapeutic targets to developing new treatments. Biological factors play a role in the following ways:

Understanding Disease Mechanisms

Identification of potential drug targets is possible through biology by identifying the molecular mechanisms that cause disease and identifying such targets, for example, in proteins [16], genes, or RNA molecules.

Genomics and Proteomics

Currently, genomics and proteomics [17] advances permit identification of novel targets from the study of gene and protein expression and function in diseased vs. healthy states.

High-throughput Screening

Assays developed in biology are capable of screening large compound libraries to identify compounds that alter the activity of a target.

Structure-Based Drug Design

Since we understand the structure of biological targets (e.g., proteins) using techniques such as X-ray crystallography [18] and cryoEM, we can design molecules that bind specifically to these targets.

Biochemical and Cellular Assays

Ancillary biological assays are used to assess how a potential drug engages with its target, the dispositional consequences, and importantly, to assess whether the drug modulates the disease process as designed.

Systems Biology

The drug effect can be better understood in terms of the impact on cellular pathways and networks, and can give insights into drug off-target effects and toxicity [19].

Pharmacokinetics and Pharmacodynamics

As you might be imagining, you need biological studies to understand the way the drug gets absorbed, distributed, metabolized, and how it is excreted (ADME) and what its effects will be in the body.

Predictive Biomarkers

Biomarkers are subsequently identified by biology to predict a patient's response to a drug to enable personalized medicine approaches [20].

Development of Biologics

The development of biologics, such as monoclonal antibodies, therapeutic proteins and gene therapies, is more important in modern medicine, and biology is integral to that development.

Understanding Resistance

By revealing how diseases, including infectious diseases and cancers, resist drugs, biology helps uncover mechanisms that can guide the development of next-generation therapies.

Stem Cell Research

The contribution of biology to drug discovery lies in the use of stem cells in regenerative medicine to provide new therapeutic options for diseases that are incurable by now.

Contributions of biology are critical for the drug discovery process because biology allows identification, development and optimization of new medicines to enhance human health.

In Contribution with Pharmacology

The execution of the drug research is done by Pharmacology as a control between the discovery and the treatment of patients with new drugs. But it's very useful for characterizing what pharmaceuticals do to biological systems, not just what they do to biological systems. For this reason, pharmacologists study the ADME of medications [21]. Why is that important? It does the least to save the least and has the least side effects. The drug safety profile is also assessed along with pharmacodynamics (the relationship of drug concentrations to treatment outcomes) and pharmacodynamics (toxicology studies are used to assess medication interactions). These elements, together, bring pharmacology to bear for creating safe, individualized, and effective treatments to assure safe novel medications deliver on their promise, impacting patients as little as possible.

In drug discovery, a number of subfields of pharmacology are used for the safety and security of proposed treatments. The primary pharmacological subtypes employed in this procedure are as follows:

- Pharmacodynamics
- Pharmacokinetics
- Toxicology
- Clinical pharmacology
- Molecular pharmacology
- Behavioral pharmacology
- Pharmacoepidemiology
- Pharmacogenomics
- Pharmacometrics

Together, these pharmacological specialities enable a more integral frame to look at potential medications, so that only the safest and most promising medications will advance through the drug development and research process.

Mechanism of Action

Pharmacology is used to specify targets in drug development through the understanding of how possible targets affect [22] disease states and biological processes.

Drug Screening

Assays created by pharmacologists allow them to sort through tremendous libraries of chemicals, picking out those that give the hoped-for effect on biological targets.

Absorption, Distribution, Metabolism, and Excretion

Pharmacology is knowledge about the pharmacological absorption, distribution, metabolization, and excretion of pharmaceuticals in the body. This knowledge is necessary in order to optimize medicine safety as well as efficacy.

Interaction Studies

Pharmacologists need to understand how medications interact with each other and diet in order to understand possible side effects and contraindications.

Formulation Development

Pharmacology has application in the designing of the drug formulation and the drug delivery system for increasing the availability, stability, and patient compliance.

Genetic and Environmental Factors

It supports formulation of individualized treatment plans by supporting in identification of how environmental variables and genetic differences affect a patient's response to the medication.

Study Design and Monitoring

Pharmacologists take part in the planning of clinical trials, in terms of helping to plan correct dosages and even track effectiveness, as well as to assess safety among various patient demographics.

In summary, pharmacology is important for drug development: it supplies the ability to understand how the drug works, how the body processes it, and to what chemicals it could react. The information helps to advance the safety, efficacy and patient-centered development of novel medications [23].

In Contribution with Informatics

As informatics allows the researcher to tackle the massive amount of data generated when discovering new drugs, informatics is a vital component of modern drug discovery.

Cheminformatics and bioinformatics can together be used to predict drug behavior in the body, to discover new therapeutic targets, and refine lead compounds [24]. The effective discovery and improvement of drug candidates is made possible by informatics technologies including virtual screening, predictive toxicity, and molecular modelling. Additionally, the use of AI and machine learning in informatics will observe patterns and project outcomes in ways the conventional approach would not. Using informatics in drug discovery allows for more accurate, efficient, and effective drug discovery that produces safer, stronger, and more potent treatments.

In drug discovery, a variety of informatics techniques are used for evaluating data, finding possible candidates for drugs, creating molecules and speeding up the research depicted in Figure 7.2. The most common forms of informatics utilized are as follows:

- Bioinformatics
- Cheminformatics
- Clinical Informatics
- Pharmacoinformatics

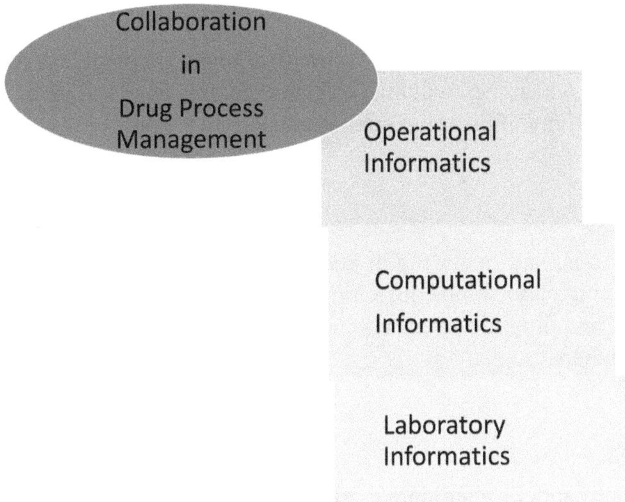

Figure 7.2 Collaboration of informatics in drug discovery.

- Systems Informatics
- Artificial intelligence (AI) and machine learning (ML)
- Health informatics
- Text mining and natural language processing (NLP)
- Data integration and knowledge management

Each of these informatics types is important in each step of the drug development process, from target identification, chemical design, clinical trial management, through to personalized medicine, to key factors in productivity and efficacy of the drug development process.

Informatics, in particular bioinformatics and cheminformatics, enable management, analysis and interpretation of vast quantities of biological and chemical data, which are of vital importance in modern drug discovery. Informatics has made the following significant contributions to drug discovery [25].

Handling Big Data

Informatics helps efficiently store, retrieve and manage large datasets generated by genomics, proteomics, high-throughput screens, and even other such kinds of drug development processes.

Bioinformatics Tools

Using computational models and algorithms, you can analyze genomic and proteomic data to connect genetic variants or patterns of expression with disease and discover possible therapeutic targets.

Cheminformatics

Its computational methods are used to predict chemical compound features, e.g., the affinity with which they will bind to biological targets [26] to maximize the efficacy and selectivity of potential medications.

AI and ML

All of these uses, and many more, are becoming increasingly common AI and machine learning applications, including drug target interactions prediction, drug optimization, and drug discovery automation [27]. They would be overlooked by human researchers.

Data Mining

To find new treatment candidates, learn disease mechanism, and identify potential adverse effects, we apply informatics techniques that mine enormous databases such as scientific literature, patents, and these methods speed up the process of discovery by seeing the trends and making connections from experimental data.

Virtual Screening

Informatics [28] makes possible virtual screening, which is a computational screening of vast libraries of chemicals against a target before any physical testing. This is a technique that cuts down on time and money because it dictates which compounds will be best at succeeding through using the least number of compounds.

Molecular Modeling and Simulation

Molecular modeling software can predict how a medication will interact with a target. Simulations of these interactions reveal the binding affinities, the efficiency of the medication as a whole and possible adverse effects.

Collaborative Platforms

Informatics allows for the creation of collaborative platforms upon which researchers from all around the world can share data, tools, and ideas. These platforms allow drug research to proceed faster, more innovatively, and team-wise.

Basically, informatics has greatly improved data management, predictive modeling, and the incorporation of diverse scientific fields to drug discovery. This makes drug development procedures faster, more efficient, and more economical.

Collaborative Approaches and Team Sciences

Collaborative Approaches

With a plethora of treatments available today, it's no surprise that collaborative approaches to drug discovery are becoming an effective way of speeding new drug development. To overcome the various obstacles of the drug development, these techniques are carried out by means of partnerships between academic institutions, pharmaceutical corporations, biotechnology enterprises and government agencies [29]. Pooling the resources, expertise, and data of the data scientists, they do this. The ways in which drug research could take place using collaboration include a form of consortia, an open innovation framework, or public-private partnerships (PPPs). These partnerships aim to cut costs and raise productivity, increase the odds of spotting and marketing new drugs by sharing risk. Particularly, when traditional, segregated techniques may not suffice, for instance, in rare diseases and global health, this cooperative strategy is especially important. The benefits of collaborative approaches are discussed in Figure 7.3.

Collaborative approaches in drug discovery include collaboration and collaborations across industries, disciplines, and geographic regions for the purpose of speeding up the creation of new medications. Thus, these strategies make the most of the capabilities that different stakeholders (government agencies, academic institutions, pharmaceutical corporations, and research organizations) can bring to the table.

The following are some essential cooperative strategies:

Public-Private Partnerships

PPPs refer to cooperative agreements between the public sector and private sector to fund [30], build, and oversee public services or infrastructure. These collaborations

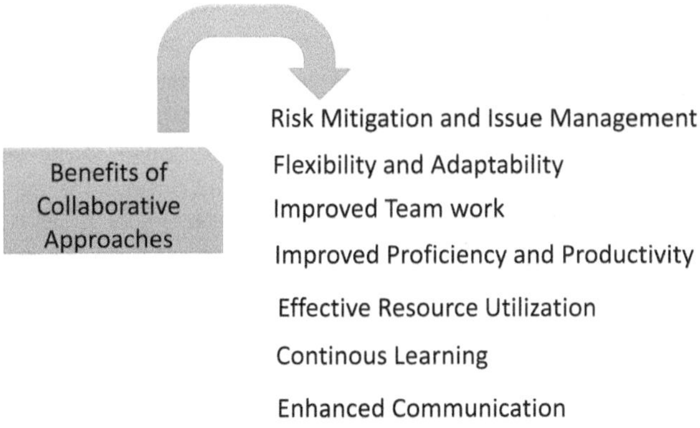

Figure 7.3 Benefits of collaborative approaches.

let the government control and ensure that the private sector is the ones that reap the benefits of these outsourcing ventures. Since the private partner is usually in charge of the initial capital investment as well as design, building, and operation, PPPs—which usually entail long, life contracts—involve risk sharing with the private partner and with the sector. PPPs enjoy a good reputation for performing projects in a more playful and efficient way, but managing them in a careful way to set the balance between private sector interests and public accountability during negotiation may be hard.

Open-Source Drug Discovery

Open-source drug discovery (OSDD) is a novel methodology that incorporates the tenets of open collaboration and transparency into product development in the pharmaceutical sector. The model would encourage participation amongst scientists, researchers, and institutions from around the world to join in drug discovery efforts by placing research findings, data, and resources into the public domain [31]. This collaborative model seeks to empower stakeholders—from academia, to nonprofits, to even citizen scientists—to make their contributions to the discovery and development of new therapies by democratizing the research process. Particularly, in areas where public health challenges and neglected diseases may be less economically viable for traditional pharmaceutical development, OSDD has become remarkably successful. Through group expertise and resources, OSDD utilizes its collaborative approach to speed up drug discovery, develop successful therapies, lower costs, and instill innovation.

Consortia-based Research

Consortium-based research forms a cooperative innovation system that involves a network of different stakeholders, including academic institutions, business partners, governmental organizations, and nonprofits, which is Peace research. Representatives negotiate pooling their resources, knowledge, and data more smoothly. This method enhances inquiries that are largely or completely unanswerable by single associates. The community-centered study approach is a vehicle for sharing information and best practices from different areas when new drugs are being developed, which in turn creates new solutions that are faster and therapeutic innovation is also a subject Civilization sits at the root of the problem, and the development of novel treatments becomes a subject of A. Consortia are said to be innovative documents that may help the conversion of new discoveries into the medical market in record time; thus, public health will be enhanced through the introduction of interdisciplinary collaborative drawing technologies. Moreover, it is a contract with risk-sharing at partners, causing each part to have less financial responsibility, as large-scale ventures can now be performed with the large economic downturn [32].

Crowd-sourcing and Citizen Science

Crowd-sourcing and citizen science are both inventive techniques that involve the masses in scientific research and even problem-solving, significantly affecting areas such as drug development and environmental monitoring. Crowd-sourcing is about pooling knowledge or resources from a very large number of people, mostly through online platforms, to come up with new ideas, solve complex problems or collect data. A variety of this crowd-sourcing is called citizen science, which enables everyday people to engage with scientific research through volunteer time, skills, and beliefs on a variety of projects. Such approaches could dramatically simplify and make whole research pathways speedier in drug discovery, starting from the collection and processing of data all the way to identifying potential drug candidates. Crowd-sourcing and citizen science can improve research quality and stimulate community engagement using multiple perspectives and areas of expertise.

Collaborative Networks and Platforms

Collaborative networks and platforms provide the praiseworthy frameworks for promoting cooperation among researchers, institutions, and organizations in achieving collective scientific ends, especially during drug discovery and development. With information technology, these networks build these connected environments that provide an avenue for stakeholders to share resources and exchange information and data access. Such joint areas make communication better and encourage interdisciplinary relations, which are needed in fighting complex health issues [33]. Examples of such collaborative networks include virtual labs, shared databases, and communication technologies allowing real-time collaboration between participants from all over the world and speeding up the research process. This methodology will collect a variety of inputs and areas of expertise, thereby accelerating the identification of new treatments and the promotion of innovative ideas.

Industry-academia Collaborations

The purpose of industry-academia collaborations is to close the gap between fundamental research and drug discovery and development processes. These collaborations are critical since they are between academic institutions and pharmaceutical or biotechnology companies. By pooling their resources, funding, and experience, industry-individual partnerships turn research findings into actual therapeutic solutions by leveraging the distinct advantages of each sector. Academics provide cutting-edge research and offer innovative methodologies and access to advanced knowledge [34]. Therefore, this fusion is presumed to create new development opportunities, accelerate the pace of scientific discovery, and bring about marketability. Besides, industry-academia partnerships usually foster knowledge transfer and skills development through training programs and internships while offering real-world problems, all of which benefit students and researchers.

Global Health Initiatives

Global health initiatives are concerted attempts to improve health outcomes for populations all over the world by tackling issues related to health that cut across national borders. Governments, nongovernmental organizations (NGOs), international organizations, and the commercial sector frequently work together on these projects, combining resources and knowledge to address urgent problems like infectious diseases, maternity and child health, and access to necessary medications. Global health initiatives seek to improve healthcare systems, execute evidence-based interventions, and guarantee fair access to healthcare services through the establishment of partnerships and the dissemination of knowledge. These programs also highlight the significance of innovation and research in the creation of novel treatments [35] and medical technologies, especially for marginalized groups. Global health initiatives use a collaborative approach to develop long-term solutions that enhance health equity and fortify health systems.

Data-sharing Initiatives

Such collaborative efforts, commonly termed as data sharing initiatives, will break down the silos that usually separate academies, organizational efforts, and businesses so that important datasets may be shared and fast tracked for scientific discovery and innovative thinking. On these initiatives hinge open, useful, and timely applications of research data [36] across a variety of fields, from public health to drug discovery. Data-sharing programs enable research institutions to access and examine enormous amounts of data, and also ease collaboration and improve reporting under reproducibility. Centralized repositories and the establishment of common procedures achieve this. Sharing such data would facilitate drug discovery involving new therapeutics, potency improvements over existing therapies, and a deeper understanding of disease processes.

Drug Repurposing and Repositioning Collaborations

Collaborations between researchers, pharmaceutical companies, and research institutions offer a means for repurposing and repositioning drugs from novel applications to discover commercially available drugs as therapeutics for illnesses. It involves making extensive use of the wealth of historic data and information available on existing drugs, which typically include safety profiles, mechanisms of action, and pharmacokinetics, to speed up the time needed in development and meet unmet medical needs. By bridging disciplines and using patient data, modeling on computers, and new screening technologies, these partnerships will lead to the possible novel indications for any existing medication depicted in Figure 7.4. Thus saving significant time and cost vis-a-vis collaborative drug development. Drug repurposing becomes particularly effective when novel or uncommon diseases emerge, or when there is an urgent need for assessment of effectiveness in a new setting of existing therapy [37].

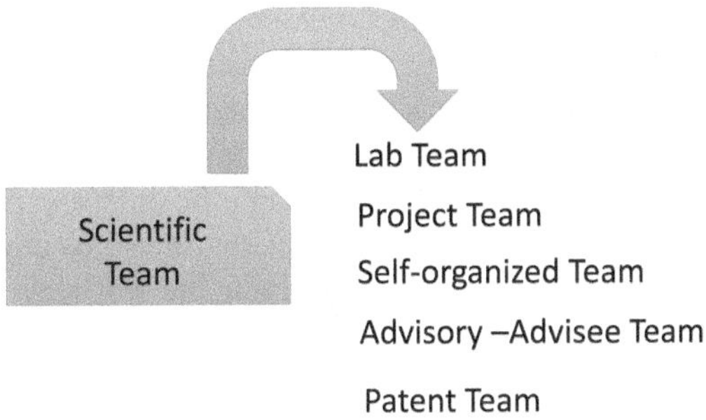

Figure 7.4 Science teams.

Non-Profit Drug Discovery Organizations

Apart from creating new treatment modalities, nonprofit discovery organizations immensely contribute toward the advancement of biomedical research, especially for the neglected populations and diseases. Unlike standard pharmaceutical companies-for-profit projects, nonprofit discovery organizations fill the gaps that would otherwise be left empty in medication research beyond what is deemed market-motivated and put priority on public health needs. To maximize resources, knowledge, and data, nonprofit drug development groups frequently partner with academic institutions, business partners, and governmental entities. They engage in various activities that include but are not limited to the basic research, drug screening, or clinical trials with a focus on cutting-edge models like crowd sourcing, open-source, and drug repurposing adaptation approaches.

Joint Ventures and Alliances

In business perspective, it becomes a strategic partnership among two or more organizations joining their hands in another field and working together to accomplish a specific set of organizational objectives in relation to drug research and discovery activities. Such partnerships offer an opportunity for pooling resourcefulness and faculties in the resolution of complicated issues that ordinarily could not be addressed more brilliantly by one organization working alone [38]. Type of a cooperative venture within the pharmaceuticals is collaborative research, co-generation of novel therapeutic applications, or joint research activities, sharing costs and diversifying risks, for example, could be something like a contract-based formal partnership or an informal one sharing common interests. Alliances come in many shapes.

Integrated Research Centers

Integrated research centers are collaborative entities that bring together interdisciplinary groups of researchers, doctors, and business minds for the creativity and pace of science and drug research development. Among the specializations these integrate are biology, chemistry, engineering, and informatics. Integrated research institutes may speed up research initiatives and offer specific customized solutions depending on given health conditions or around specific medical fields. They generally make available access to high-tech equipment, a shared pool of research resources, and exclusive spaces, thus enhancing efficiency and productivity of research programs. The institutes also encourage partnerships among government, private, and academic organizations, thus bridging the gap between basic research and application.

Using the skills and abilities of professionals who have often received training in diverse domains, team science is a cooperative effort to answer a scientific question. Even while many scientific projects are best handled by traditional single-investigator driven procedures, coordinated teams of investigators with a variety of expertise and experience may be especially useful for taking on challenging scientific and societal issues.

A notable surge in interest in (and funding for) team science can be attributed to the past two decades of heightened emphasis on scientifically addressing complex issues: climate change, the escalation of chronic illnesses and the health ramifications of social stratification. Scientists are increasingly engaging in team-based research initiatives, participating across diverse locations and disciplines [39]. These endeavors encompass both large and small teams, interdisciplinary as well as transdisciplinary groups and initiatives that involve various stakeholders (such as policymakers, scientists, and community members). Team science programs are also garnering financial support from national governments, industry, academic institutions and other sources; however, this funding landscape continues to evolve. Although there are challenges, the commitment to collaborative efforts remains strong because the complexities of today's problems require multifaceted approaches.

Cross-disciplinary science signifies a burgeoning trend in the field of team science, where individuals with varied training and experience (across multiple domains) come together to integrate their viewpoints within a unified research endeavor. One effective way to conduct comprehensive research that tackles a wide array of complex and interlinked variables is, however, through the use of cross-disciplinary team science. This method is considered a promising strategy for expediting scientific innovation and aiding the conversion of discoveries into applicable laws and regulations. Although such collaborations can be difficult, they frequently produce substantial advantages.

In specialized roles, individuals from various professions contribute their distinct knowledge and techniques within the realm of team science. The amalgamation of diverse methods and approaches fosters an interdisciplinary collaboration that can enhance the scope and importance of research. Effective management is essential to organize activities and synthesize results; furthermore, clear communication, mutual respect, and a shared objective among team members are pivotal for successful team science [40]. Scientific challenges are increasingly complex and interconnected, necessitating the collective expertise and insights of a heterogeneous team. Consequently, this collaborative paradigm is gaining significance. However, the effectiveness of such teamwork relies heavily on these foundational elements.

Crucial Elements of Team Science Consist of the Following

Interdisciplinary Collaboration

To effectively address complex challenges and devise innovative solutions, interdisciplinary collaboration unites diverse perspectives and experiences from individuals across various industries. By integrating knowledge from multiple realms—including science, engineering, social sciences and the arts—teams can confront obstacles from different viewpoints, which ultimately leads to more comprehensive and inventive solutions [41]. This approach not only enhances problem-solving abilities; it also fosters a deeper understanding of issues by analyzing them from multiple angles. However, to cultivate a vibrant environment where fresh ideas can thrive and new connections emerge among seemingly disparate fields, effective multidisciplinary collaboration necessitates strong communication skills, mutual respect and a readiness to learn from one another.

Effective Communication

In any given context, effective communication is crucial for fostering understanding and facilitating productive interactions. This process not only involves delivering accurate information but also requires tailoring the message to the specific needs and circumstances of the intended audience. Clarity presenting information in a clear and direct fashion—and active listening, which helps in accurately grasping the words of others and responding thoughtfully, are integral components of this process. Furthermore, non-verbal cues, such as tone of voice and body language, play a significant role in effective communication because they profoundly impact how messages are perceived. People may collaborate more efficiently, build stronger relationships [42] and resolve conflicts more swiftly by emphasizing empathy and transparency. However, it is important to recognize that developing mutual understanding and achieving positive outcomes in both personal and professional realms necessitates a comprehensive understanding of effective communication strategies.

Shared Goals and Vision

Working and collaborating well is due to common aspirations and a common vision, all other efforts unite to this unified goals. A vision that is shared by all members of a team or organization serves as standard to keep everyone moving in the same direction and enables such motivation. Goals that are crystal clear so everyone is focusing on the same things and therefore can conclude with the goals achieved. This alignment cascades well into impact morale and commitment while helping to drive commonality which in turns should lead to efficiency. These common goals get refreshed and reaffirmed periodically, which keeps all the activities in sync. This keeps us all on-point and alert to the shifting conditions. As teams can drive more success and innovation when the contributions of all members are understood and linked back to an overall success.

Role Specialization

Assigning each person specific duties and responsibilities to focus on according to his/her unique assets as an individual in a strategic way where the team can be more efficient and skilled. The result of this narrow division of labor is that everyone pays attention to their strengths, so the work turns out better and problems get solved faster. Specialization, on the other hand, increases productivity, with a simultaneous increase in knowledge and creativity depth at the cost of breadth of specialization. Well-defined roles are required to eliminate redundancy and ambiguity, so that every component of the project is taken care of. Specialist roles must work in harmony via communication and teamwork to ensure that the different elements of the projects configure properly.

Mutual Respect and Trust

In any team or collaborative environment, only a strong, high-performance relationship can be generated when there is respect and trust. When team members genuinely value each other's contributions, input, ideas, and perspectives, an open/collaborative atmosphere is created. Trust, strongly correlated with respect [43] is the idea that there is a safe environment for people to be acknowledged and ideally safe to share their ideas, attempt new things. Tacitly building trust is due to members of cooperative assemblies acting in the best interest of the group at large, and consistent, dependable behavior accompanied by transparent communication. Respect and trust are complementary since mutual respect leads to collaboration, where rapport works in decreasing friction that forms a convergent team working with trust.

Leadership and Coordination

The success of any organization or project relies in turn on having good leadership and coordination. When the team has proper guidance, inspiration and support from its leader, they work in sync and for a common objective. On the other hand, coordination that all parts of the organization align and operate as one. This depends on the flexibility of being able to do situational analysis, resource management and smooth communication. Together coordinated with Leadership provides an enabling environment for creativity [44] to happen, people mobilized to scale the obstacles and goals are hit.

Integration of Expertise

For a team or org to get full and novel solutions, the experts need to come together. By bringing together experts and backgrounds to help with hard problems, organizations can approach issues in many different ways so that no relevant factors are overlooked. Collaboration results in harnessing the different strengths of a team, which enables idea amplification and collectively creates a facilitative space for collective contribution. For a team to truly harness its combined knowledge and accelerate the consistent achievement, openness of communication, respect for one another common vision are integral to a seamless integration.

Flexibility and Adaptability

Today is the world of change, and it requires flexibility and adaptability. Those people and organizations that do adopt these characteristics are able to deal with unexpected obstacles and gain from new opportunities. Adaptation ensures one can adapt quickly to new situations, technology or market conditions, but only flexibility allows one to be willing to change course or to rethink strategies. Resilience built into these attributes enables the company to continue striving and innovating despite the uncertainty. Flexibility and adaptation are developed by organizations and individuals who can remain in an unpredictable situation and keep a competitive edge.

Evaluation and Feedback

For every initiative or organization that has to continuously improve, the evaluation and feedback need to be included and embedded. Regular evaluation would allow a regular view of what is doing well and what needs improvement. Then, it is measured against predetermined goals or benchmarks. Constructive feedback is an opportunity to work with someone on something they're good at doing or how to do something; it will help them get better at or refine how they do whatever it is [45]. Active problem solving and reinforcement of success are used to learn and hold oneself accountable. As part of that, then, they don't just produce the right result, but they provide the right amount of assessment and feedback so you and everyone else can grow personally and professionally.

Case Studies in Interdisciplinary Research

One of the key research areas where interdisciplinary intervention is essential for solving the demanding challenges of creating new therapeutic medicines includes drug discovery. There will be a few case studies that indicate the value involved in applying multidisciplinary methods within the process of discovering drugs.

Imatinib (Gleevec) – A Breakthrough in Cancer Treatment

Disciplines Involved: Molecular Biology, Chemistry, Pharmacology, Clinical Medicine, and Bioinformatics.

Perhaps one of the most striking examples in modern drug discovery is that with imatinib-Gleevec, a classic representation of how crossing boundaries could often lead to revolutionary discovery of medicines. Below, here is an in-depth reflection on some of the numerous disciplines involved in the discovery of Imatinib and the relative contribution of each one in its development

Molecular Biology and Cytogenetics: Understanding the Disease

Key Contribution: The identification of the Philadelphia chromosome and the BCR-ABL fusion gene.

- The Philadelphia chromosome, an abnormally truncated chromosome 22 in individuals with chronic myeloid leukemia, was first identified by researchers in the 1960s. This was one of the landmark findings about the genetics of cancer.
- It was not until the 1980s that researchers in the field of molecular biology discovered that the translocation producing the BCR-ABL fusion gene between chromosomes 9 and 22 gave rise to the Philadelphia chromosome. This gene produces an abnormal tyrosine kinase that is always "on" and signals for cell division, allowing the leukemic cells to develop without control. Understanding that BCR-ABL was the driver of CML established a clear molecular target for drug development.

Medicinal Chemistry: Designing the Inhibitor

Key Contribution: The design and synthesis of Imatinib, inhibiting the BCR-ABL tyrosine kinase, is a very small molecule [46].

- Once BCR-ABL had been identified as the molecular target, the next challenge was to design a molecule that could selectively inhibit this kinase.
- In structure-based drug design, inhibitors were designed to exactly fit into the active site of the target protein based upon its 3D structure. The chemists working at Ciba-Geigy—now Novartis—used.
- As a competitive inhibitor, imatinib was created to attach to the ATP-binding site of BCR-ABL. This stops the kinase from phosphorylating its substrates, which stops the signal for cell proliferation.
- Medicinal chemists had to optimize Imatinib's properties to ensure it was not only effective in inhibiting BCR-ABL but also safe and bioavailable when administered to patients [47].

Pharmacology: Testing the Drug's Efficacy and Safety

Key Contribution: Preclinical testing to evaluate the drug's activity against BCR-ABL and its effects on normal cells.

- Pharmacologists conducted extensive in vitro (cell culture) and in vivo (animal) studies to assess the efficacy of Imatinib.
- These studies confirmed that Imatinib could selectively kill BCR-ABL-positive leukemic cells without harming normal cells, which was crucial for its potential as a targeted therapy.
- Pharmacokinetic studies were also conducted to determine how the drug was absorbed, distributed, metabolized, and excreted in the body, as well as to establish the optimal dosing regimen.

Clinical Medicine: Conducting Clinical Trials

Key Contribution: Conduct safety and efficacy of Imatinib in human subjects using clinical trials.

- Phase I Trials: Human studies with imatinib began in the late 1990s. These were supposed to establish the maximum tolerated dose, along with the safety profile of the drug. It was during this time also that imatinib demonstrated its effectiveness, inducing remission in CML patients for whom other therapeutic avenues had been exhausted [48].
- Phase II and III Trials: Later trials with larger patient populations pitted Imatinib against the current standards of treatment. Indeed, these studies confirmed its greater efficacy and finally gained approval from the regulatory agencies. Imatinib was found to induce complete cytogenetic responses in a very high percentage of patients suffering from CML; that is, the Philadelphia chromosome became undetectable in the blood and bone marrow cells of such patients.
- Clinicians further extended the use of Imatinib to other cancers, including gastrointestinal stromal tumors, where it proved effective through similar molecular mechanisms involving tyrosine kinase activity.

Structural Biology: Understanding the Drug-Target Interaction

Key Contribution: Providing detailed insights into how Imatinib interacts with BCR-ABL at the molecular level.

- Structural biologists used techniques like X-ray crystallography to determine the 3D structure of the BCR-ABL kinase bound to Imatinib.
- This structural information was crucial for understanding why Imatinib was such an effective inhibitor. It also provided insights into how mutations in BCR-ABL could lead to drug resistance, guiding the development of second-generation tyrosine kinase inhibitors like dasatinib and nilotinib.

Bioinformatics and Computational Chemistry: Supporting Drug Design

Key Contribution: Using computational tools to model the interaction between Imatinib and its target, and to predict potential resistance mechanisms.

- Bioinformaticians and computational chemists played a role in modeling the BCR-ABL kinase and simulating how Imatinib binds to it [49–51].
- These models helped in optimizing the drug's design and predicting how mutations might alter the drug's efficacy, which was important for understanding and overcoming resistance.

The invention of imatinib serves as a prime example of the value of multidisciplinary research in drug discovery. Experts from several scientific fields collaborated to overcome difficult obstacles in the project's path, ultimately producing a medication that has improved the lives of numerous CML and other cancer patients. The success of imatinib continues to direct and motivate the creation of novel targeted treatments for a range of illnesses.

Development of Antiretroviral Therapy for HIV/AIDS

Disciplines Involved: Virology, Immunology, Medicinal Chemistry, Pharmacology, Public Health, and Sociology.

A major advancement in medical science, the creation of antiretroviral therapy (ART) for HIV/AIDS is a prime example of the effectiveness of multidisciplinary research. HIV was changed from a deadly disease to a chronic [47], treatable condition by a complicated process that involves the integration of knowledge from virology, immunology, medicinal chemistry, pharmacology, clinical medicine, and public health. Below is a thorough summary of the multidisciplinary initiatives that helped to create ART:

Virology: Understanding the HIV Virus

Key Contribution: Identifying and characterizing the HIV virus, including its life cycle and the mechanisms by which it infects human cells.

- HIV was first identified in the early 1980s as the causative agent of AIDS. Virologists worked to understand the structure and function of the virus, particularly its envelope proteins (gp120 and gp41) and the reverse transcriptase enzyme that allows it to replicate within host cells.
- They discovered that HIV targets CD4+ T cells, a critical component of the immune system, leading to immune system failure in infected individuals.
- This understanding of the virus's life cycle, particularly the key stages of entry, reverse transcription, integration into the host genome, and replication, provided essential targets for drug development.

Immunology: Understanding the Body's Response

Key Contribution: Understanding how HIV evades the immune system and the impact of HIV on the immune system's function.

- Immunologists studied how HIV infection leads to the depletion of CD4+ T cells, resulting in the gradual breakdown of the immune system and making the body susceptible to opportunistic infections and cancers.
- They also explored the body's immune response to HIV, including the production of antibodies and the role of cytotoxic T cells in controlling the infection.
- Insights into immune evasion by HIV, such as its high mutation rate and ability to hide in latent reservoirs, were critical in developing strategies to combat the virus.

Medicinal Chemistry: Designing Antiretroviral Drugs

Key Contribution: Developing small molecules that can inhibit key enzymes and processes in the HIV life cycle.

- Medicinal chemists focused on designing inhibitors for the enzymes critical to HIV replication, including reverse transcriptase, protease, and integrase.
- Reverse Transcriptase Inhibitors (RTIs): The first class of antiretroviral drugs developed. These include nucleoside reverse transcriptase inhibitors (NRTIs) like zidovudine (AZT) and non-nucleoside reverse transcriptase inhibitors (NNRTIs) like nevirapine. NRTIs mimic the natural nucleosides used by the reverse transcriptase enzyme, leading to chain termination during DNA synthesis, while NNRTIs bind directly to the enzyme and inhibit its function.
- Protease Inhibitors (PIs): These drugs, such as saquinavir and ritonavir, inhibit the HIV protease enzyme, which is necessary for the maturation of viral particles. Without protease activity, the virus produces immature, noninfectious particles.
- Integrase Inhibitors: These are a newer class of drugs, including raltegravir, that block the integration of viral DNA into the host genome, a critical step in the viral life cycle.
- Entry Inhibitors: This class of drugs, including maraviroc, prevents HIV from entering host cells by blocking the interaction between the virus and the CD4 receptor or co-receptors like CCR5.

Pharmacology: Optimizing Drug Efficacy and Safety

Key Contribution: Studying the pharmacokinetics (absorption, distribution, metabolism, and excretion) and pharmacodynamics (effects on the body) of antiretroviral drugs.

- Pharmacologists worked to determine the optimal dosing regimens for antiretroviral drugs to maximize their efficacy while minimizing side effects. This included studying drug interactions, as many HIV patients require combination therapy.
- Combination Therapy: To prevent the emergence of drug-resistant strains of HIV, pharmacologists developed highly active antiretroviral therapy, which involves using a combination of drugs that target different stages of the viral life cycle. This multi-drug approach reduces the likelihood of the virus developing resistance.
- Long-Term Effects: Pharmacologists also studied the long-term effects of ART on patients, including potential toxicities, the impact on metabolic processes, and interactions with other medications.

Clinical Medicine: Conducting Clinical Trials

Key Contribution: Testing the safety and efficacy of antiretroviral drugs in human patients and establishing treatment guidelines.

- Clinical Trials: ART drugs underwent rigorous testing through multiple phases of clinical trials. These trials involved evaluating the drugs in terms of their ability to suppress viral load, restore immune function, and reduce HIV-related morbidity and mortality.

- Treatment Guidelines: Based on the results of clinical trials, clinicians developed treatment guidelines for HIV patients. These guidelines evolve as new drugs are developed and as more is learned about the optimal management of HIV infection.
- Adherence: Clinicians also focused on the importance of adherence to ART regimens. Poor adherence can lead to treatment failure and the development of drug-resistant strains of HIV.

Public Health: Implementing ART on a Global Scale

Key Contribution: Ensuring the widespread availability and proper use of ART in diverse populations around the world.

- Access to Treatment: Public health experts worked to make ART widely available, particularly in low- and middle-income countries hardest hit by the HIV epidemic. This involved negotiating with pharmaceutical companies, securing funding, and developing programs to distribute ART.
- Education and Awareness: Public health campaigns were crucial in educating the public and healthcare providers about HIV, the importance of early testing and treatment, and the need for adherence to ART.
- Monitoring and Surveillance: Ongoing monitoring of ART effectiveness and the spread of HIV drug resistance was essential. Public health organizations like the World Health Organization (WHO) and the Centers for Disease Control and Prevention (CDC) have played key roles in this effort.

Sociology and Ethics: Addressing the Human Dimensions

Key Contribution: Understanding the social, ethical, and cultural factors that affect HIV treatment and prevention.

- Sociologists and ethicists explored the social determinants of health that affect HIV transmission and treatment, such as stigma, discrimination, access to healthcare, and socioeconomic status.
- Ethical Considerations: The development and distribution of ART raised numerous ethical questions, such as the right to access life-saving treatment, informed consent in clinical trials, and the implications of drug pricing and patents on global health.
- Behavioral Interventions: Understanding the behavior of individuals and communities in relation to HIV risk and treatment adherence led to the development of interventions that support adherence to ART and reduce the spread of the virus.

The creation of ART for HIV/AIDS is a potent illustration of how interdisciplinary research may result in ground-breaking medical discoveries. Researchers were able to create successful treatments for a disease that was previously considered to be uniformly deadly by combining knowledge from the fields of virology, immunology, chemistry, pharmacology, clinical medicine, public health, and the social sciences. The discovery of treatments for other complicated diseases was facilitated by the success of ART, which not only altered the trajectory of the HIV/AIDS epidemic but also set a precedent.

Development of Statins for Cholesterol Management

Disciplines Involved: Biochemistry, Pharmacology, Clinical Medicine, Public Health, and Chemistry. The creation of statins to lower cholesterol is a shining illustration of how multidisciplinary research may result in a significant advancement in medicine. Statins are a class of medications that decrease blood cholesterol levels [48], which lowers the risk of cardiovascular illnesses like heart attacks and strokes. Many disciplines, including biochemistry, pharmacology, clinical medicine, genetics, and public health, contributed to the understanding of cholesterol's role in heart disease and the subsequent creation of statins. This is a thorough examination of the multidisciplinary initiatives that resulted in the creation of statins:

Biochemistry: Understanding Cholesterol and Lipid Metabolism

Key Contribution: Identifying the role of cholesterol in cardiovascular disease and understanding the biochemical pathways involved in cholesterol synthesis.

- Early in the 20th century, scientists discovered a connection between high blood cholesterol and the onset of atherosclerosis, a disorder marked by the accumulation of plaques high in cholesterol in the arteries.
- By pinpointing the essential enzymes involved in the process, biochemists were able to clarify the liver's cholesterol manufacturing pathway. It was discovered that the rate-limiting step in the synthesis of cholesterol is the enzyme HMG-CoA reductase.
- Knowing this pathway made developing drugs easier because it was possible to efficiently lower cholesterol levels by blocking HMG-CoA reductase.

Pharmacology: Discovering and Developing Statins

Key Contribution: The discovery of statins as potent inhibitors of HMG-CoA reductase and the development of these compounds into safe and effective drugs.

- The first statin, mevastatin, was discovered by Akira Endo in the 1970s from a fungus (Penicillium citrinum). It was found to be a potent inhibitor of HMG-CoA reductase.
- Building on this finding, Merck and other pharmaceutical companies created several statins, including atorvastatin, simvastatin, and lovastatin, the first statin to go on sale.

- In order to increase these molecules' effectiveness, lessen their adverse effects, and enhance their pharmacokinetic qualities—that is, how the body absorbs, distributes, metabolizes, and excretes them pharmacologists attempted to optimize their chemical structures.

Clinical Medicine: Conducting Clinical Trials

Key Contribution: Testing the safety and efficacy of statins in humans and establishing their role in preventing cardiovascular diseases.

- Phase I Trials: Initial trials focused on determining the safety and appropriate dosage of statins in healthy volunteers.
- Phase II and III Trials: Subsequent trials involved larger patient populations with high cholesterol levels or existing cardiovascular disease. These trials demonstrated that statins significantly reduced LDL cholesterol (the "bad" cholesterol) levels and lowered the risk of heart attacks, strokes, and other cardiovascular events.
- Landmark Studies: The Scandinavian Simvastatin Survival Study (4S) and the Heart Protection Study were pivotal in proving the benefits of statins in reducing cardiovascular mortality. These studies provided strong evidence that statins not only lower cholesterol but also significantly reduce the risk of death from heart disease [52–58].

Genetics: Understanding Individual Responses to Statins

Key Contribution: Identifying genetic factors that influence how individuals respond to statins, including both efficacy and risk of side effects.

- Genetic studies have shown that differences in some genes, such SLCO1B1, can impact the body's metabolization and transportation of statins. These differences may affect the statins' efficacy as well as their potential for adverse effects, like myopathy (pain in the muscles).
- Pharmacogenetics: The study of how genetic differences affect individual responses to drugs has led to personalized approaches in statin therapy, where genetic testing can guide the choice and dosage of statins for optimal results and minimal side effects.

Epidemiology and Public Health: Assessing the Impact of Statins

Key Contribution: Evaluating the population-level impact of statin use on public health, particularly in reducing the incidence of cardiovascular diseases.

- Epidemiologists studied the trends in cardiovascular disease incidence and mortality before and after the widespread adoption of statin therapy. These studies showed a significant decline in cardiovascular events, correlating with the increased use of statins.

- Guideline Development: Guidelines for cholesterol management were published by public health groups, including the American Heart Association and the National Cholesterol Education Program (NCEP). These organizations recommend statin medication for persons who have a high risk of cardiovascular disease.
- Health Economics: A cost-effectiveness analysis of statins has also been conducted, and the results indicate that statins are very cost-effective in preventing heart attacks and strokes, especially in high-risk groups, even with the high cost of long-term therapy.

Molecular Biology and Drug Design: Enhancing Statin Efficacy

Key Contribution: Applying molecular biology techniques to design more potent and specific statins, as well as exploring combination therapies.

- Advances in molecular biology allowed for the design of statins that are more selective for HMG-CoA reductase, reducing the likelihood of off-target effects.
- Combination Therapy: In an effort to further cut the risk of cardiovascular events and achieve even higher reductions in cholesterol levels, researchers have also looked into combining statins with other lipid-lowering medications, such as ezetimibe, which lowers cholesterol absorption in the intestines.

Cardiology: Integrating Statins into Cardiovascular Care

Key Contribution: Integrating statins into the broader management of cardiovascular disease, including their use in patients with varying levels of risk.

- When deciding which patients gain the most from statin therapy, cardiologists have been instrumental in identifying the variables that matter most, including age, LDL cholesterol levels, and total cardiovascular risk.
- Risk Stratification: The use of risk calculators (such as the Framingham Risk Score) has been essential in determining who should receive statins, with guidelines recommending statins for those with a certain percentage risk of developing cardiovascular disease over a 10-year period.
- Preventive Cardiology: Statins have become a cornerstone of preventive cardiology, not only for secondary prevention (preventing further events in patients who have already had a heart attack or stroke) but also for primary prevention in high-risk individuals.

Ongoing Research and Future Directions

- Statin Resistance and Intolerance: The goal of ongoing research into the processes underlying statin resistance and intolerance is to create novel treatments or strategies for people who are not able to tolerate or do not respond well to statins.

- Cardiometabolic Benefits: Recent research indicates that statins may offer advantages beyond lowering cholesterol, including the potential to decrease inflammation and stabilize atherosclerotic plaques. These benefits are now being investigated.
- New Therapeutic Targets: Researchers are also looking at new therapeutic targets within the cholesterol metabolism pathway to complement or enhance the effects of statins.

The success of interdisciplinary research is demonstrated by the creation of statins, which are used to control cholesterol. Through the integration of knowledge from several fields such as biochemistry, pharmacology, clinical medicine, genetics, public health, and cardiology, scientists have created a class of medications that has significantly transformed the approaches to illness prevention and treatment. Since they dramatically lower heart disease-related morbidity and mortality and enhance millions of people's quality of life, statins have grown to be among the most often prescribed drugs in the world. The effectiveness of statins continues to impact cardiovascular medical research, with even more advancements possible in the future.

Conclusion

Drug discovery has become more and more dependent on the interdisciplinary convergence of several fields, with each offering its distinct expertise to tackle the complex problems of creating safe and effective treatments. Given the complexity of diseases increasing and the constantly changing field of medical science, an interdisciplinary approach to drug discovery is not just a trend but a requirement.

Fundamentally, multidisciplinary drug discovery research fills the gap between basic science understanding and practical application. The discovery of statins as cholesterol-lowering medications, for example, demonstrates how biochemistry, pharmacology, and clinical medicine can come together to produce a medical revolution. A thorough understanding of biochemistry was necessary to determine the function cholesterol plays in cardiovascular disease. Pharmacologists then used this information to develop medications that effectively target important enzymes involved in the manufacture of cholesterol. The effectiveness of these medications in lowering cardiovascular events was subsequently confirmed by clinical trials, which solidified statins position as a mainstay of preventive medicine.

Additionally, the tale of Imatinib (Gleevec) shows how interdisciplinary cooperation can result in advances in the treatment of illnesses that were formerly thought to be incurable. A medication that could specifically target the genetic abnormalities causing particular malignancies had to be developed, and this required the convergence of molecular biology, genomics, and oncology. This focused therapy emphasized the significance of comprehending disease at a molecular level, which is only possible through interdisciplinary efforts, and it also offered a new paradigm for treatment.

The discovery of ART for HIV/AIDS emphasizes even more the value of multidisciplinary research in solving international health issues. HIV was once thought to be fatal, but with the help of virologists, immunologists, pharmacologists, and physicians, it is now a chronic illness that can be managed. This accomplishment resulted from the synthesis of information from several disciplines rather than just breakthroughs in one area, which sped up the discovery of medications that could stop the virus's replication and boost the immune system.

Beyond these particular instances, the pharmaceutical business as a whole as well as public health are affected more broadly by the multidisciplinary approach to drug discovery. By promoting the exchange of ideas and methods, it stimulates innovation and leads to the identification of new therapeutic targets as well as the creation of more individualized and efficient therapies. Personalized medicine, which reduces the risk of side effects and improves treatment outcomes by customizing medicines to individual genetic profiles, is made possible by advancements in genetics and genomics. Comparably, developments in bioinformatics and computational biology have transformed drug design by making it possible to simulate drug interactions at the molecular level prior to clinical trials, which has saved time and money.

A vital role for public health viewpoints is also played in the multidisciplinary field of medication discovery. Prioritizing research endeavors is based on epidemiology and health economics, guaranteeing that funds are directed toward the most urgent health concerns. These disciplines also aid in comprehending the wider effects of novel medications on societies by evaluating not just their effectiveness but also their affordability and accessibility. By taking a holistic approach, it is ensured that drug discovery initiatives are in line with societal demands, especially when it comes to tackling gaps in global health.

The success of multidisciplinary drug discovery research further emphasizes how crucial it is for experts from many professions to collaborate and communicate with one another. Discipline-specific silos that were previously present have been broken down to produce more thorough and reliable research results. The cooperation of government agencies, business, and academic institutions, for instance, has been essential in quickening the drug development process from fundamental research to clinical trials and regulatory approval.

It is likely that multidisciplinary methods will become even more important in the future for drug discovery. The integration of several scientific fields will be crucial as diseases become more complicated and the demand for tailored therapy increases. With new techniques and approaches that will call for the cooperation of specialists from several domains, emerging fields like systems biology, synthetic biology, and nanotechnology have the potential to further revolutionize drug development.

Finally, in order to effectively address the complexity of contemporary medicine, an interdisciplinary approach to drug discovery is not only beneficial but also necessary. This effective tactic has already produced important medical advancements and keeps stimulating the creation of novel treatments. We can research diseases more thoroughly, create medications that work better, and eventually enhance patient outcomes globally by encouraging interdisciplinary collaboration. It is certain that this collaborative culture will continue to affect drug discovery in the future as experts from all professions collaborate to address the most important health issues of our day.

References

1. Smith J, Brown M, Green S, Harris D. Personalized medicine and precision therapeutics: Emerging approaches and impact on healthcare. J Med Sci. 2022;45(7):122–134.
2. Brown M, Johnson T. The role of genomic sequencing in precision medicine. Genet Med. 2021;23(3):59–71.
3. Harris D, Lee K, Patel R. Targeted therapies in HER2-positive breast cancer. J Cancer Res. 2020;56(9):501–510.
4. Lee K, Park S. EGFR mutation testing in non-small cell lung cancer: Advances in targeted therapies. Lung Cancer Rev. 2023;17(5):103–115.
5. Patel R, Robinson E, Martin L. Biomarker discovery and application in personalized medicine. Biomark Res. 2022;18(4):84–97.
6. White P, Green S. Pharmacogenomics: Improving drug efficacy and reducing side effects. Am J Pharmacol. 2021;42(6):123–132.
7. Zhang W, Johnson M, Robinson E. CRISPR-Cas9 technology in precision medicine: Potential and challenges. J Gene Ther. 2021;34(2):187–199.
8. Johnson M, Harris T. Artificial intelligence in precision medicine: Enhancing diagnostics and treatment. AI Healthc. 2024;5(1):19–31.
9. Kumar V, Singh A. Economic barriers to the widespread adoption of precision medicine. Health Econ Rev. 2020;12(7):77–88.
10. Watson J, Williams R. Ethical considerations in the era of personalized medicine. Med Ethics J. 2023;11(8):223–234.
11. Davis A, Robinson E, Tan Z. The role of companion diagnostics in personalized therapy. J Clin Oncol. 2022;30(6):542–556.
12. Robinson E, Tan Z, Martin L. Pharmacodynamic biomarkers in personalized cancer treatment. Clin Cancer Res. 2021;25(10):1199–1210.
13. Martin L, Kim S, Wong J. Use of surrogate biomarkers in clinical trials: Opportunities and challenges. Transl Med. 2020;18(4):128–139.
14. Kim S, Green T, Singh A. Challenges in biomarker discovery for heterogeneous diseases. J Clin Invest. 2023;39(3):245–256.
15. Tan Z, Liu X. Genetic variability and disease response in precision medicine. Hum Genet Rev. 2021;35(7):302–311.
16. Foster R, Brown M. Biomarker validation and its clinical implications. Biomed Adv. 2020;27(2):101–114.
17. Wong J, Zhao Y. Liquid biopsy as a non-invasive tool in precision oncology. Cancer Ther J. 2022;19(8):74–82.
18. Thompson L, Robinson E, Davis M. Improving patient outcomes with precision therapeutics. Adv Ther. 2021;29(5):213–225.
19. Green T, Tan Z, Brown M. Precision medicine in rare genetic disorders: Tailored approaches. Rare Dis J. 2023;16(4):58–70.
20. Zhang Q, Liu Y. Future directions in precision medicine: New frontiers and technologies. Future Healthc J. 2024;13(3):301–313.
21. Haldeman M, Vieira B, Winer F, Knutsen LJS. Exploration tools for drug discovery and beyond: Applying SciFinder® to interdisciplinary research. Curr Drug Discov Technol. 2005;2(2):69–74.
22. Alber P. Li. An integrated, multidisciplinary approach for drug safety assessment. Adv Pharm Sci. 2004;9(16):687–693.

23. Butler MS. The role of natural product chemistry in drug discovery. J Nat Prod. 2004;67(12):2141–2153.
24. Kolb HC, Sharpless KB. The growing impact of click chemistry on drug discovery. Drug Discov Today. 2003;8(64):1128–1137.
25. Butcher EC, Berg EL, Kunkel EJ. Systems biology in drug discovery. Nat Biotechnol. 2004;22:1253–1259.
26. Surade S, Blundell TL. Structural biology and drug discovery of difficult targets: The limits of ligandability. Cell Chem Biol. 2012;19(1):42–50.
27. Ekins S, Mestres J, Testa B. In silico pharmacology for drug discovery: Applications to target and beyond. Br J Pharmacol. 2009;152(1):21–37.
28. Claus BL. Underwood DJ. Discovery informatics: Its evolving role in drug discovery. Drug Discov Today. 2002;7(18):957–966.
29. Ojima I. Modern natural products chemistry and drug discovery. J Med Chem. 2008;51(9):2587–2588.
30. Jiang X, Hao X, Jing L, Wu G, Kang D, Liu X, et al. Recent applications of click chemistry in drug discovery. Expert Opin Drug Discov. 2019;14(8):779–789.
31. Taylor AP, Robinson RP, Fobian YM, Blakemore DC, Jones LH, Fadeyi O. Modern advances in heterocyclic chemistry in drug discovery. Org Biomol Chem. 2016;14(28):6611–6637.
32. Boyd DB. Computational medicinal chemistry for drug discovery. J Med Chem. 2004;47(25):6433.
33. Tiwari VK, Kumar A, Rajkhowa S. Green chemistry: Opportunity in drug discovery research. Curr Org Chem. 2021;25(20):2257–2259.
34. Scapin G. Structural biology and drug discovery. Curr Pharm Des. 2006;12(17):2087–2097.
35. Jubb H, Higueruelo AP, Winter A, Blundell TL. Structural biology and drug discovery for protein–protein interactions. Trends Pharmacol Sci. 2012;33(5):241–248.
36. Kell DB. Systems biology, metabolic modeling, and metabolomics in drug discovery and development. Drug Discov Today. 2006;11(23-24):1085–1092.
37. Zhu J, Zhang B, Schadt EE. A systems biology approach to drug discovery. Adv Genet. 2008;60:603–635.
38. Anderson DC, Kodukula K. Biomarkers in pharmacology and drug discovery. Biochem Pharmacol. 2014;87(1):172 188.
39. Enna SJ, Williams M. Defining the role of pharmacology in the emerging world of translational research. Drug Discov. 2009;57:1–30.
40. Xia X. Bioinformatics and drug discovery. Curr Top Med Chem. 2017;17(15):1709–1726.
41. Wishart DS. Introduction to cheminformatics. Curr Protoc Bioinformatics. 2016; 53(1):14.1.1–14.1.21.
42. Patel V, Shah M. Artificial intelligence and machine learning in drug discovery and development. Intell Med. 2022;2(3):134–140.
43. Kerasidou A. Trust me, I'm a researcher!: The role of trust in biomedical research. Med Health Care Philos. 2017;20:43–50.
44. Stokols D, Hall KL, Taylor BK, Moser RP. The science of team science: Overview of the field and introduction. Am J Prev Med. 2008;35(2):S77–89.
45. Warburton FE Feedback in development and its evolutionary significance. Am Nat. 1995;89(846).
46. Broder S. The development of antiretroviral therapy and its impact on the HIV-1/AIDS pandemic. Antiviral Res. 2010;85(1):1–18.
47. Grundy SM. Statin trials and goals of cholesterol-lowering therapy. Circulation. 1998;97(15):1436–9.
48. Rasmussen B. The role of pharmaceutical alliances. Cent Strateg Econ Stud. 2002;02:1–19.
49. Atmakuri LR, Peeriga R, Begum S, Vallamkonda B, Baratam A. Novel bioanalytical LC-MS/MS method for determination of metoprolol in human plasma. J Appl Pharm Sci. 2024;14(12):131–138.

50. Peeriga R, Venkata Bangaru GK. Implementation of the POCSO act in schools. In: Child Sexual Abuse: A Public Health Problem in India. Springer publications, Singapore, 2024. p. 391–413. Springer Publications, Singapore.
51. Peeriga R, Yarlagadda LC, Alla NR. Protection of children from sexual exploitation. In: Child Sexual Abuse: A Public Health Problem in India. 2024. p. 191–201. Springer Publications, Singapore.
52. Peeriga R, Shiek Arabath SAM, Manubolu K, Thelappilly BB, Yarlagadda LC. Insilico assessment of phytoconstituents in *myxopyrum smilacifolium* blume against arthritis. Biomed Pharmacol J. 2024;17(1):235–241.
53. Manubolu K, Balagani PK, Gope ER, Peeriga R, Sridevi AR. Unlocking the potential of aquasomes: A comprehensive review on innovative nanocarriers in drug delivery and beyond. Int J Chem Biochem Sci. 2023;24(6):405–410.
54. Manubolu K, Peeriga R, Bonthu MG, Gope ER, Kadirvel D. Evaluation of anti-inflammatory activity of *Millingtonia hortensis* leaf extract. Int J Chem Biochem Sci. 2023;24(6):380–385.
55. Peeriga R, Chandrasekhar KB. Comparative study of anti-inflammatory activity of petroleum ether extract of *myxopyrum smilacifolium* blume and ethanolic leaf extract of *pamburus missionis* swingle. J Pharm Sci Res. 2017;9(6):955–957.
56. Peeriga R, Manubolu K. (2025). Design strategies for waste reduction and enhanced recyclability in pharmaceutical packaging. In: Yingngam, B., Aslam, M.S., Haghi, A.K. (eds) Sustainable Pharmaceutical Product Development and Optimization Processes. Springer, Singapore.
57. Manubolu K, Peeriga R, Chandrasekhar KB. A Short Guide to Clinical Pharmacokinetics. 1st ed. 2024. Springer, Singapore.
58. Manubolu K, Peeriga R (2025). Ecodesign principles. In: Yingngam, B., Aslam, M.S., Haghi, A.K. (eds) Sustainable Pharmaceutical Product Development and Optimization Processes. Springer, Singapore.

8 Personalized Medicine and Precision Therapeutics

Lakshmana Rao Atmakuri, Rajani Vetapalem, Ratna Kumari Yejerla, R. Radha, Udaya Guttikonda, and Angilicam Avinash

Introduction

Precision, or as some might still categorize it, individualized medicine, is the approach to medical treatment that is unique to a certain individual. In contrast to other conventional ways of treatment, which use a single approach for patients diagnosed with a certain disease. Personalized medicine deals with a patient's genetic make-up, environment, lifestyle, as well as the molecular signature of a particular patient to deliver therapy. This method has the intended goals of boosting the results of the treatments, decreasing the impact of the side effects, and taking into account the biological factors in relation to the patient's response to the treatments [1].

Using the results of genetic tests, doctors can understand whether a person has genetic markers that may lead to a particular disease or experience an inadequate reaction to a specific drug. This helps in the diagnosis to a higher level and allows working on individual treatments of diseases, particularly for which they are many-sided, such as cancer, cardiovascular diseases, and autoimmune diseases, where individual differences affect the progression and efficacy of the disease even more [2].

Personalized medicine is not limited to the genetic makeup of a person but also incorporates environmental influencing factors and life decisions that affect one's wellbeing in order to prevent and conquer looming diseases in their totality. Today, the development of technologies in the field of science contributes to the emergence of individualized medicine, which means that treatments are much more efficient; they do not require invasive procedures and are developed for every patient individually. This future is a promise of healthcare that is more accurate, more prophetic, and more focused on the customers—in this case, patients—to enhance their lives [3].

Precision medicine is a new direction in medicine, the core of which is oriented at genetic, molecular and biochemical individual characteristics of the patient. This approach is a typical characteristic of the concept of personalized medicine, designed to focus on the targeted, rather than the general use of drugs. In precision therapeutics, treatment is guided by the patients and the disease genomic profile, biomarkers and other molecular signatures [4].

DOI: 10.4324/9781003564041-8

Precision therapies are mainly aimed at increasing the efficacy of the administered treatment and decreasing the side effects. For instance, in oncology, precision medicines can pinpoint genetic mutation and or molecular profile that fuels cancer, and therefore, therapies such as targeted therapy and immunotherapy are more effective as compared to chemotherapy. Same way, in other diseases like autoimmune diseases, cardiovascular diseases and neurological diseases, precision therapy assists in identifying the best treatment regimen, which may be available from the genetic and molecular individual markers [5].

Genomics and related fields, as well as bioinformatics and biotechnologies, or such technologies as CRISPR (Clustered Regularly Interspaced Short Palindromic Repeats) and gene editing, are pushing the pace of precision medicine progress. It has also facilitated the discovery of novel biomarkers and aims at enhancing drug discovery and definable clinical assessment parameters. In the course of research, precision therapeutics has become identified with the opportunity to revolutionize healthcare by delivering improved, patient-specific, and safer treatment interventions for improved patients' quality of life [6].

Personal medicine and precision therapeutics are two correlated and complementary ideas that, when combined, offer a better, highly specialized treatment strategy. Despite the fact that both are methods of ensuring better treatment outcomes given patient individuality, they are different in their approaches and uses [7].

Overview of Precision Medicine

Precision medicine, also referred to as personalized medicine, is a current model of healthcare delivery where treatments are unique for every patient in consideration of their unique features. The personalization of treatment through a taxonomy of people based on their biological characteristics is the key goal of precision medicine depicted in Figure 8.1 [8].

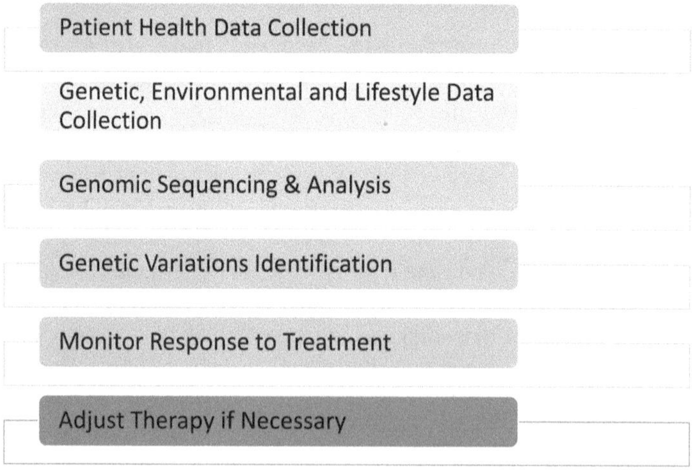
Patient Health Data Collection
Genetic, Environmental and Lifestyle Data Collection
Genomic Sequencing & Analysis
Genetic Variations Identification
Monitor Response to Treatment
Adjust Therapy if Necessary

Figure 8.1 Process of precision medicine.

Principles of Precision Medicine

1 Individualized Treatment: Precision medicine is the approach that implies that every person is different in terms of genes, the environment, and lifestyles that will cause health problems. By doing so, it seeks to differentiate treatment according to these differences [9].
2 Data Driven: It is highly dependent on such data as genetic, molecular, and environmental data for accurate construction of individualized therapies and treatment plans [10].
3 Prevention and Early Detection: In this case, precision medicine uses genetic risks and environmental factors to anticipate, avoid and identify diseases in their initial stages before they become chronically severe [11].

Techniques in Precision Medicine

1 Genomic Sequencing: For instance, approaches like whole-genome sequencing, next-generation sequencing (NGS) reveal genetic markers which may put one at risk of diseases, or how he or she will manage treatment outcomes [12].
2 Biomarker Identification: Precision medicine defines biomarkers as small elements found in the patient's blood, tissues, or any other body fluids that can be used to diagnose a disease or in defining how the body will likely react to particular treatment [13].
3 Gene Editing: With information technology, methods such as CRISPR are employed to edit or repair the genes that bring about diseases, suggesting treatments for genetic diseases [14].
4 Pharmacogenomics: This technique studies how genetic factors determine reaction to drugs; thus, the best medication with few side effects can be prescribed [15].

Advantages of Precision Medicine

1 Improved Treatment Effectiveness: Many of the existing therapies are even more effective due to customization according to the genetic and molecular features of an individual.
2 Fewer Side Effects: Since targeted therapies are drugs that target specific molecular targets, the incidence of side effects is highly reduced when as to conventional medicines. Drugs that are administered for targeted therapies are aptly chosen precisely in the patient's genetic model.
3 Better Disease Prevention and Early Detection: The use of precision medicine makes it possible for the doctor to realize the genetic factors for predisposition, allowing for the development of measures that can prevent diseases or minimize their effects.
4 Personalized Care: This makes it promote a more patient-centric approach where the provider is in a position to provide treatments that are right for them [16].

Disadvantages of Precision Medicine

1 Cost and Accessibility: Genomic sequencing needs state-of-the-art equipment, and personalized care can be expensive, which makes precision medicine an exclusive club and inaccessible to ethnicity, minorities, and impoverished clients.
2 Ethical Concerns: The information based on genes has privacy implications and the possibility of the abuse of the acquired information. The questions concerning consent, security, and genetic discrimination should be solved.
3 Limited Evidence for Certain Treatments: There is no doubt that precision medicine brings a lot of potential for improving the lives of patients, but currently, there are many diseases for which personalized treatments are still not discovered, or not completely substantiated.
4 Complexity: However, the integration of a large amount of genetic, environmental exposure, and lifestyle information makes it challenging for practitioners to practice precision medicine across the healthcare systems [17].

Concepts in Precision Medicine

1 Genetic Variability: Understanding that people are genetically unique, and that genetic variation has several implications for disease susceptibility, disease advancement, and therapeutics, is the basis of precision medicine [18].
2 Biomarker-driven Therapy: The process of diagnosing biomarkers to inform treatment choices, like using certain gene mutations to show that the drugs will work efficiently.
3 Holistic Approach: Precision medicine is also different from gene-targeted medicine; it is a blend of genetic characteristics and predispositions, and environmental and lifestyle factors; disease outcomes stem from a product of gene characteristics and external factors [19].
4 Data Integration: Innovation in data capture, analysis, and artificial intelligence is enhancing the feeding into of multiple patient layers, whether genetic, clinical, behavioral, etc., to support specific ailments.

Precision medicine will only grow in its ability to redefine how we diagnose and treat patients; as technology increases, there are even more opportunities to use these treatments to make medicine better, more tailored and patient-centered.

Biomarker Discovery and Companion Diagnostics

Biomarker identification and companion diagnostic partnerships are essential parts of the maturing field of precision medicine. They facilitate the discovery and validation of diagnostic, prognostic, predictive, and pharmacogenomic biomarkers that are pivotal for disease diagnosis and prognosis, as well as for the selection of therapeutic interventions and evaluation of patient's response thereto. The most salient example of a DxVd is the companion diagnostics, where Dx stands for diagnostics and Vd represents therapeutic drug, which are diagnostic tools that seek to establish the patient's most likely to benefit from any given therapeutic intervention, by an assessment of biomarkers, including genetic and protein-based markers [20].

Biomarker Discovery

Biomarkers are laboratory or imaging tests that signal the presence of a disease, the degree of severity or progression, or alternatively, the impact of a particular treatment. They can exist in the form of blood, tissue or other fluids and are often used to assess disease activity or therapeutic efficacy [21].

Types of Biomarkers: It is illustrated in Table 8.1 and Table 8.2

1 Diagnostic Biomarkers: Applied in diagnosis, in determining whether a specific disease is or is not present in a patient.
   Example: Prostate-specific antigen (PSA) as an indicator of prostate cancer.
2 Prognostic Biomarkers: Describe in an accurate way the probable course of a disease, whether or not a treatment is being administered.
   Example: HER2 in breast cancer as a biomarker with the indication of tumor aggressiveness.
3 Predictive Biomarkers: Predict how a particular patient will perform with respect to a certain treatment regimen.
   Example: Epidermal growth factor receptor (EGFR) mutations in non-small cell lung cancer (NSCLC), which suggest who will benefit from EGFR inhibitors.
4 Pharmacodynamic Biomarkers: Determine the level of biological activity of a treatment.
   Example: DNA in the bloodstream as a biomarker of response to chemotherapy in cancer patients.
5 Surrogate Biomarkers: Provide an alternative to a clinical outcome (such as mortality or changes in disease status) in clinical studies.
   Example: Blood pressure as a surrogate for cardiovascular incidents.

Table 8.1 Types of biomarkers in precision medicine.

Type of biomarker	*Description*	*Example*
Diagnostic biomarkers	Used to detect or confirm the presence of a disease.	Prostate-specific antigen for prostate cancer
Prognostic biomarkers	Predict the likely progression of a disease, regardless of treatment.	HER2 in breast cancer, which predicts tumor aggressiveness.
Predictive biomarkers	Indicate how likely a patient is to respond to a specific treatment.	EGFR mutations in NSCLC predict response to EGFR inhibitors.
Pharmacodynamic biomarkers	Measure the biological effect of a treatment.	Circulating tumor DNA in cancer to measure chemotherapy effectiveness.
Surrogate biomarkers	Substitute for clinical endpoints in clinical trials.	Blood pressure as a surrogate for cardiovascular events.

Table 8.2 Case studies in precision therapeutics.

Therapeutic area	*Disease/ condition*	*Biomarker/genetic mutation*	*Targeted therapy*	*Outcome*
Oncology	HER2-positive Breast Cancer	HER2 overexpression	Trastuzumab	Improved survival, reduced recurrence
Oncology	NSCLC	EGFR mutations (L858R, exon 19 deletions)	Erlotinib, Gefitinib	Increased progression-free survival, fewer side effects

Biomarker Discovery Process

The process of biomarker discovery involves several key steps:

1 Identifying Target Diseases: Identifying diseases or conditions in which biomarkers that will increase in specificity for diagnosing, predicting prognosis or helping in establishing treatment regimens would be useful.
2 Sample Collection and Analysis: Biopsy and blood samples from patients with diseases and healthy volunteers, including blood samples. These are examples of the following sample types: Genomic sequencing, Proteomics, and Metabolomics are technologies utilized to process these samples.
3 Data Integration: Applying genomic data to analyze the genome and its function, detect patterns, and localize biomarkers.
4 Validation: All identified biomarkers have to be further tested using either large clinical trial cohorts or appropriate groups of patients matched to controls in a retrospective manner to confirm their specificity, robustness of the method used for their identification, and their relation to the clinicopathological characteristics of diabetes.

Challenges in Biomarker Discovery

Complexity of Disease: Most target diseases, particularly cancer, are typically heterogeneous and therefore effective biomarkers are difficult to find [22].

Technical Limitations: The prospects of the analytical tissue biomarkers and their detection, particularly in low concentrations or in heterogeneous tissues, are still an ongoing research.

Regulatory Hurdles: There are a lot of regulatory bodies that expect high levels of biomarker certification before they are considered for use in clinical practice, and the process can take a long time.

Cost: To measure biomarkers, researchers oftentimes apply costly technologies that can impede the possibility of applying biomarker-based strategies across different contexts and for various populations.

Companion Diagnostics

Companion diagnostics are defined as tests that give required data for the appropriate usage of a related therapeutic product, often a drug depicted in Figure 8.2. Companion diagnostics usually involve molecular markers such as gene or protein changes that a doctor uses to determine how a particular patient will react to a particular treatment [23].

Role of Companion Diagnostics

1 Guiding Treatment Decisions: Companion diagnostics assist in defining which patients should expect a positive outcome after taking a given medicine. For example, a test can determine if the tumor of a cancer patient has a mutation that can be treated by a given therapy.

  Example: HER2 testing in breast cancer involves determining which patients are likely to benefit from the drug called Trastuzumab.

2 Optimizing Drug Efficacy: Companion diagnostics provide insight into which patients should receive a particular treatment, thereby increasing drug efficacy and decreasing adverse reactions.

3 Personalizing Medicine: Companion diagnostic is an essential in the change from the one-size-fits-all model for treatment to personalized medicine, whereby treatment is adjusted for a specific molecular or genetic characteristic of the patient.

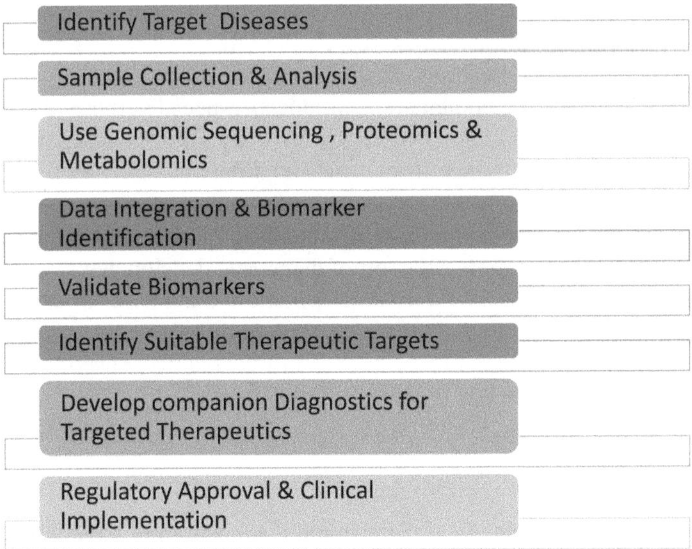

Figure 8.2 Biomarker discovery and companion diagnostics.

4 Regulatory and Approval Process: Most companion diagnostics are co-developed with the drugs and are reviewed and approved by regulatory bodies such as the U.S. FDA, concurrently with the drug. This helps to create a close link between the test and the drug, in a way that they are used in practice and by clients.

Examples of Companion Diagnostics

- EGFR Testing in Lung Cancer: EGFR mutation analysis confirms which patients with NSCLC are likely to benefit from EGFR inhibitors, including Erlotinib.
- KRAS Testing in Colorectal Cancer: Mutations of the KRAS gene in patients with colorectal cancer indicate that a patient will not benefit from the use of EGFR-targeted drugs such as Cetuximab to guide oncologists, their choice of therapy.
- BRCA Testing in Breast and Ovarian Cancer: We know that we have a genetic predisposition to BRCA that may increase susceptibility to breast and ovarian cancer. It has been known that they already planned to use PARP inhibitors like Olaparib.

Challenges and Future Directions

Challenges

- Regulatory Complexity: Companion diagnostics have quite a challenging requirement for obtaining the approval, which needs clinical confirmation and is well-coordinated with the drug's regulatory cycle.
- Cost: The creation of combination products, especially those tied to high-throughput techniques such as NGS, may be costly. Besides, insurance approval and compensation for these tests may also be different.
- Clinical Implementation: Implementation of companion diagnostics as part of the standard patient care requires informing the clinicians, as well as setting up a dossier and systems for the support of diagnostic developments.
- Genetic Heterogeneity: The variety of genetic mutations in diseases such as cancer entails that while biomarkers may be useful for one group of patients, they might not translate to other patients, thus the restricted usefulness of some companion diagnostics.

Future Directions

- Expansion Beyond Oncology: Companion diagnostics are largely practiced in cancer treatment but are steadily moving into oncology-sidelined therapeutic categories like cardiology, neurology, and infectious disease [24].

- Advances in Technology: Technological advancement promotes more detection techniques through liquid biopsy, for example, ctDNA exosomes make companion diagnostics more affordable and detectable.
- Integration with Artificial Intelligence: Molecular and clinical diagnostic data can be utilized to identify new biomarker profiles by the use of advanced AI, support the analysis of the data faster and more efficiently than human analysts [25–29].

Biomarker identification and companion diagnostics are the fundamentals of precision medicine. Biomarkers are used for detection, risk estimation, and assessment of treatment efficacy and safety; companion diagnostics determine which treatments are most efficient and effective for the patient according to the genetic and molecular background data.

Case Studies in Precision Therapeutics

Precision medicines, on the other hand, refer to the packaging of medicine according to patients' characteristics, which include genetics, biomarkers, and disease type in many medical specialties, in particular, oncology, neurology, and rare hereditary diseases. These case studies are based on molecular targets, leading to superior, optimum, and safer therapies. These are presented in detail below across different therapeutic areas to describe how the concept of precision therapeutics works and its effects [27, 30].

Targeted Cancer Therapies: HER2-positive Breast Cancer

Background

Mammal cancer is among the common cancers, which has different subtypes depending on the molecular markers it has. This latter category of factors is exemplified by HER2-positive breast cancer, in which cancer cells have higher-than-normal levels of the HER2 protein.

Precision Therapeutic Approach

HER2-positive breast cancer is particularly treated by means of those drugs that are created to act on the HER2 protein. The best-known treatment is Trastuzumab—a monoclonal antibody that reacts with the HER2 receptors present on the surface of cancer cells and inhibits their further development and calls on the immune system to target the tumor.

Biomarker

HER2 status is determined by IHC or FISH because the presence of the protein is confirmed only by this method. These diagnostic tests determine if a patient's cancer cells overexpress HER2 or qualify for treatments such as Trastuzumab.

Outcome

Other researchers have found that women who have HER2-positive breast cancer, once administered with Trastuzumab, were more likely to live longer than those given standard chemotherapeutic agents. HER2-targeted therapies have produced a perfect model of how to deliver targeted therapies for a chronic disease.

Impact

This case shows how molecular profiling of the cancer cell influences the specific treatment that is chosen, and therefore, good results are achieved with fewer side effects compared to the drug such as chemotherapy.

EGFR Gene Mutations in NSCLC Type

Background

Lung cancer is known as a leading cancer type in most developed countries, and NSCLC is mainly diagnosed in approximately 85% of lung cancer cases. The main treatment for several years of NSCLC is chemotherapy; however, this method has not cured most of the patients with distinct genetic changes.

Precision Therapeutic Approach

For those cancer patients who test positive for EGFR, drugs such as Erlotinib and Gefitinib demonstrate effectiveness in inhibiting EGFR signaling with corresponding increases in survival and quality of life. These therapies help in inhibiting the overexpressed EGFR receptors, which encourage cancer cell division.

Biomarker

EGFR mutations are identified by genetic testing tools PCR or next-generation sequencing NGS. Therapies targeting specific EGFR mutations that are found in NSCLC, including L858R or exon 19 deletions, make it possible to identify targeted therapies

Outcome

Those patients who received EGFR inhibitors had a statistically significant increase in PFS compared to patients receiving traditional chemotherapy if they had EGFR mutation. These therapies usually respond quickly, and the results are very effective.

Impact

This case illustrates the practice of molecular diagnostics/profiling/targeted treatments, which show better efficacy of embracing genetic diagnosis, to enhance the quality of life of patients suffering from cancer.

Cystic Fibrosis: Targeting the CFTR (Cystic Fibrosis Transmembrane Conductance Regulator) Gene

Background

Cystic fibrosis is therefore a genetic ailment resulting from mutations in the CFTR gene, which produces thick, sticky mucus in the respiratory tract and the gastrointestinal system. CF leads to severe respiratory and gastrointestinal manifestations.

Precision Therapeutic Approach

CFTR modulators mark a major advancement in precision medicine in patients with CF, intended for the correction of the defect of the CFTR protein. For example, Ivacaftor corrects specific forms of mutation and enhances the function of the protein. Lumacaftor/Ivacaftor targets genotypes by using CFTR modulators, whereas Tezacaftor/Ivacaftor targets residue 117 His.

Biomarker

Selecting these therapies has to do with the biomarker, and this is the specific CFTR mutation the patient has. Some mutations include G551D or F508del, which make patients eligible for CFTR modulator therapy.

Outcome

CFTR modulators make *P. aeruginosa* more accessible to the immune system, allowing patients with specific CFTR mutations to have better lung function, fewer pulmonary exacerbations, as well as enhanced overall CF-related health. For instance, Ivacaftor understands lung function and improves the quality of life of the patient with GCC with mutation G551D.

Impact

With this case, people can also learn how precision therapeutics can change the world of genetic disorder treatment. Thus, traditional symptomatic management may not address the root of the problem as effectively as the molecular management of the mutated CFTR protein provided by modulators.

Gene Therapy (Luxturna) for the Treatment of Inherited Retinal Diseases

Background

Leber congenital amaurosis (LCA), for example, causes a gradual loss of vision because of mutations within genes that control vision. These conditions have been hard to manage because the peripapillary atrophy of the retina is very hard or impossible to restore with conventional medical procedures.

Precision Therapeutic Approach

In 2017, Luxturna became the first FDA-approved gene therapy for inherited retinal diseases. This viral vector is used to bring in a normal copy of the RPE65 gene to the retinal cells of patients with LCA. The therapy helps to rebuild the function of a protein that is crucial to sight, which in turn helps eyesight in the therapy's subjects.

Biomarker

RPE65 mutation is the only biomarker defining eligibility since its specific variations are present in the patient. This gene therapy has undergone necessary medical examination to determine the patients who are suitable to undergo this gene therapy.

Outcome

People receiving Luxturna treatment also report improvements in their visual ability, as noted during clinical processes. These are helpful outcomes because, in the past, LCA was a condition that caused individuals to lose their sight in early adulthood.

Impact

The case of Luxturna, revealing that gene therapy is a realistic way of targeting and indeed correcting the root of the problems presented by genetic diseases, means that some diseases are no longer untreatable, and patients can have hope.

Immunotherapy in Melanoma: The Case of Pembrolizumab

Background

Melanoma is a malignant skin disorder; for many years, advanced melanoma has been, with few exceptions, a disease which could hardly be treated. Immunotherapy alone has drastically changed the facet of treatment.

Precision Therapeutic Approach

Pembrolizumab is an immune checkpoint inhibitor which attaches to the PD-1 receptor on the T-cell in order to strengthen the immune system's ability to fight against melanoma, which overexpresses PD-L1 on tumor cells; PD-L1 is the protein that helps tumors to avoid being identified by the immune system.

Biomarker

The degree of expression of PD-L1 on tumor cells is the basis for using Pembrolizumab as a biomarker. Detecting the expression of PD-L1 helps clinicians identify those patients who would benefit from immunotherapy treatment.

Outcome

Thus, patients who developed PD-L1-positive tumors receiving Pembrolizumab report durable response, including long-term survivorship. The treatment has helped boost survival among the melanoma patient's especially those in the later stages.

Impact

This case finally supports immunotherapy treatments for melanoma and the validity of biomarkers in choosing the appropriate intervention. This also underlines the rise of precision medication in cancer immunology.

These case studies show that precision therapeutics is changing the face of health care and delivering back to the patient the promise of treatments that are tailored to effectively address the causes of the diseases. They range from cancer to inherited diseases to orphan diseases, and precision therapy is delivering better, miraculous treatment.

Adjustability of Applications of Personalized Medicine and Precision Therapeutics

Personalized medicine, precision therapeutics, and other molecular medicine techniques are rapidly transforming the approach in diagnosis and synthesis of treatment plans, specifically for each patient owing to his or her genetic code, lifestyle, and surroundings. These approaches enhance therapeutic intervention efficacy, reduce side effects, and enhance the overall efficiency of the health systems. Here are some key applications:

Cancer Treatment

- Targeted Therapies: Precision medicine in cancer has changed the way of managing the disease by analyzing unique molecular changes in tumors and then designing treatments based on these findings. For instance, erbB2 overexpressing breast cancer such as HER2-positive breast cancer, drugs such ending Trastuzumab interact only with the excess HER2 proteins present in tumor cells.
- Immunotherapy: Other personalized treatments are immunotherapy, such as checkpoint inhibitors, Pembrolizumab which blocks receptor proteins, for example, PD-L1, on cancer detects in order to boost the immune system of the body to fight against cancer. This type of treatment has worked with melanoma, lung cancer, and other forms of cancer that have special biomarkers.

Cardiovascular Disease

- Genetic Testing for Risk Assessment: Precision medicine is used to identify individuals at high risk for cardiovascular diseases based on genetic markers. For instance, mutations in genes like LDLR and APOB can predispose individuals to familial hypercholesterolemia, prompting early intervention and lifestyle changes.
- Personalized Statin Therapy: Genetic variations can influence how individuals respond to statins. Pharmacogenomic testing allows healthcare providers to personalize statin therapy to optimize effectiveness and minimize side effects, particularly for those at risk of adverse reactions.

Neurology and Psychiatric Disorders

- Alzheimer's Disease: Genetic testing, such as identifying mutations in the APOE gene, helps predict susceptibility to Alzheimer's disease. Personalized approaches, including early interventions and tailored therapies based on genetic risk factors, can slow disease progression and improve patient outcomes.
- Psychiatric Treatment: Pharmacogenomics is used to tailor psychiatric medications to patients based on their genetic profile. For example, genetic testing can determine how a person might respond to antidepressants, antipsychotics, or mood stabilizers, leading to more effective treatments with fewer side effects.

Rare Genetic Disorders

- Gene Therapy: Advances in precision medicine have led to the development of gene therapies for rare genetic disorders. For example, Luxturna, a gene therapy for Leber congenital amaurosis, a genetic cause of blindness, delivers a functional copy of the RPE65 gene to retinal cells, improving vision in patients with specific mutations.
- CFTR Modulators in Cystic Fibrosis: In cystic fibrosis, CFTR modulators such as Ivacaftor and Lumacaftor target specific genetic mutations in the CFTR gene to improve lung function and reduce complications in patients with cystic fibrosis.

Infectious Disease

- Antiviral Therapies: Personalized medicine is applied in the treatment of infectious diseases like HIV and Hepatitis C. Genetic testing helps determine the most effective antiviral drugs based on viral mutations and individual patient characteristics.
- Pharmacogenomic testing: Guide therapy for patients with tuberculosis and other infectious diseases, ensuring optimal drug efficacy and minimizing resistance.

Personalized Pharmacotherapy

- Pharmacogenomics: Precision medicine helps determine how individuals will respond to certain drugs based on their genetic profile.
- Pharmacogenomic testing: Identify genetic variants that affect drug metabolism, such as variations in the CYP450 enzyme family, influencing the choice and dosage of medications. This application is particularly useful in oncology, pain management, and psychiatry, where drug efficacy and side effects can vary widely across individuals.

Autoimmune Diseases

- Rheumatoid Arthritis: Personalized approaches in autoimmune diseases like rheumatoid arthritis (RA) involve testing for specific biomarkers, such as Rheumatoid Factor (RF) and anti-CCP antibodies, to tailor treatment regimens. Biologic drugs, such as TNF inhibitors (e.g., Etanercept), are targeted to specific immune system components, offering more effective control over RA.
- Multiple Sclerosis: Precision therapeutics is also applied in multiple sclerosis (MS), where genetic profiling helps to determine the best disease-modifying treatments. Biologic therapies, such as Ocrelizumab, target specific immune system pathways to reduce MS flare-ups.

Regenerative Medicine

- Stem Cell Therapy: Personalized stem cell treatments are being explored for regenerative medicine applications. By using a patient's own stem cells, therapies can be designed to regenerate damaged tissues, as seen in conditions like spinal cord injuries and heart disease.
- Tissue Engineering: Personalized therapies also include the development of bioengineered tissues and organs, customized to match an individual's specific genetic and biological characteristics, improving the likelihood of successful integration and function.

Conclusion

Personalized medicine and precision therapeutics are revolutionizing healthcare by offering tailored treatments based on an individual's unique genetic, molecular, and environmental profile. These approaches enhance treatment efficacy, reduce adverse effects, and provide hope for patients with conditions that were once difficult or impossible to treat. Central to this transformation are advances in biomarker discovery and companion diagnostics, which enable precise disease prediction and treatment response based on specific genetic mutations and molecular markers. Techniques like genomic sequencing and biomarker profiling lead to more accurate diagnostics and the development of targeted therapies, significantly improving the management of diseases such as cancer, genetic disorders, and chronic conditions. While challenges like high costs and implementation complexity remain, the continuous advancements in genomic research and diagnostic technologies hold the promise of a more individualized, effective, and sustainable future for healthcare. As these approaches evolve, personalized medicine has the potential to reshape healthcare globally, making it more patient-centric, efficient, and impactful.

References

1. Smith J, Brown M, Green S, Harris D. Personalized medicine and precision therapeutics: Emerging approaches and impact on healthcare. J Med Sci. 2022;45(7):122–134.
2. Brown M, Johnson T. The role of genomic sequencing in precision medicine. Genet Med. 2021;23(3):59–71.
3. Harris D, Lee K, Patel R. Targeted therapies in HER2-positive breast cancer. J Cancer Res. 2020;56(9):501–510.
4. Lee K, Park S. EGFR mutation testing in non-small cell lung cancer: Advances in targeted therapies. Lung Cancer Rev. 2023;17(5):103–115.
5. Patel R, Robinson E, Martin L. Biomarker discovery and application in personalized medicine. Biomark Res. 2022;18(4):84–97.
6. White P, Green S. Pharmacogenomics: Improving drug efficacy and reducing Side effects. Am J Pharmacol. 2021;42(6):123–132.
7. Zhang W, Johnson M, Robinson E. CRISPR-Cas9 technology in precision medicine: Potential and challenges. J Gene Ther. 2021;34(2):187–199.
8. Johnson M, Harris T. Artificial intelligence in precision medicine: Enhancing diagnostics and treatment. AI Healthc. 2024;5(1):19–31.
9. Kumar V, Singh A. Economic barriers to the widespread adoption of precision medicine. Health Econ Rev. 2020;12(7):77–88.
10. Watson J, Williams R. Ethical considerations in the era of personalized medicine. Med Ethics J. 2023;11(8):223–234.
11. Davis A, Robinson E, Tan Z. The role of companion diagnostics in personalized therapy. J Clin Oncol. 2022;30(6):542–556.
12. Robinson E, Tan Z, Martin L. Pharmacodynamic biomarkers in personalized cancer treatment. Clin Cancer Res. 2021;25(10):1199–1210.
13. Martin L, Kim S, Wong J. Use of surrogate biomarkers in clinical trials: Opportunities and challenges. Transl Med. 2020;18(4):128–139.
14. Kim S, Green T, Singh A. Challenges in biomarker discovery for heterogeneous diseases. J Clin Invest. 2023;39(3):245–256.
15. Tan Z, Liu X. Genetic variability and disease response in precision medicine. Hum Genet Rev. 2021;35(7):302–311.
16. Foster R, Brown M. Biomarker validation and its clinical implications. Biomed Adv. 2020;27(2):101–114.
17. Wong J, Zhao Y. Liquid biopsy as a non-invasive tool in precision oncology. Cancer Ther J. 2022;19(8):74–82.
18. Thompson L, Robinson E, Davis M. Improving patient outcomes with precision therapeutics. Adv Ther. 2021;29(5):213–225.
19. Green T, Tan Z, Brown M. Precision medicine in rare genetic disorders: Tailored approaches. Rare Dis J. 2023;16(4):58–70.
20. Zhang Q, Liu Y. Future directions in precision medicine: New frontiers and technologies. Future Healthc J. 2024;13(3):301–313.
21. Atmakuri LR, Peeriga R, Begum S, Vallamkonda B, Baratam A. Novel bioanalytical LC-MS/MS method for determination of metoprolol in human plasma. J Appl Pharm Sci. 2024;14(12):131–138.
22. Peeriga R, Venkata Bangaru GK Implementation of the POCSO act in schools. In: Child Sexual Abuse: A Public Health Problem in India. Springer Publications, Singapore 2024. pp. 391–413.

23. Peeriga R, Yarlagadda LC, Alla NR. Protection of children from sexual exploitation. In: Child Sexual Abuse: A Public Health Problem in India. Springer Publications, Singapore. 2024. pp. 191–201.
24. Peeriga R, Shiek Arabath SAM, Manubolu K, Thelappilly BB, Yarlagadda LC. Insilico assessment of phytoconstituents in *myxopyrum smilacifolium* blume against arthritis. Biomed Pharmacol J. 2024;17(1):235–241.
25. Manubolu K, Peeriga R, Bonthu MG, Gope ER, Kadirvel D. Evaluation of anti-inflammatory activity of *Millingtonia hortensis* leaf extract. Int J Chem Biochem Sci. 2023;24(6):380–385.
26. Peeriga R, Chandrasekhar KB. Comparative study of anti-inflammatory activity of petroleum ether extract of *myxopyrum smilacifolium* blume and ethanolic leaf extract of *pamburus missionis* swingle. J Pharm Sci Res. 2017;9(6):955–957.
27. Peeriga R, Manubolu K. (2025). Design strategies for waste reduction and enhanced recyclability in pharmaceutical packaging. In: Yingngam, B., Aslam, M.S., Haghi, A.K. (eds) Sustainable Pharmaceutical Product Development and Optimization Processes. Springer, Singapore.
28. Manubolu K, Peeriga R, Chandrasekhar KB. A Short Guide to Clinical Pharmacokinetics. 1st ed. 2024. Springer. Singapore.
29. Manubolu K, Peeriga R (2025). Ecodesign principles. In: Yingngam, B., Aslam, M.S., Haghi, A.K. (eds) Sustainable Pharmaceutical Product Development and Optimization Processes. Springer, Singapore.
30. Manubolu K, Balagani PK, Gope ER, Peeriga R, Sridevi AR. Unlocking the potential of aquasomes: A comprehensive review on innovative nanocarriers in drug delivery and beyond. Int J Chem Biochem Sci. 2023;24(6):405–410.

9 Emerging Technologies and Their Trends

Talamanchi Balakrishna, Venkateswara Rao Javvaji, Raveesha Peeriga, Sonti Lavanya, Avisa Indira, and Suchitra Monapati

Introduction

CRISPR-Cas9 Technology

Editing is a very precise alteration of the DNA sequences of an organism, hence its genetic makeup. Gene editing uses enzymes, which are a kind of nuclease, to cut open DNA strands at the points where one wishes to make a change to either replace existing DNA with new DNA or remove it and replace it with replacement DNA. This is one of the crucial molecular tools that contributed to developing gene-editing technologies, in which the American scientist Feng Zhang and others have worked. Scientists from the United States and France, led by Emmanuelle Charpentier and colleagues, found it in 2012. Using this tool, researchers precisely deleted and inserted DNA in desired regions owing to its high accuracy with which CRISPR-Cas9 functioned [1].

Clustered regularly interspaced palindromic repeats (CRISPR)/Cas9 is revolutionizing healthcare research by making precise gene regulation in cells and animals easy, fast, and inexpensive. Among its many scientific uses are functional genomic screens, real-time imaging of cellular genomes, and the rapid development of cellular and animal models. It has been established that it can be utilized to rectify defective DNA in mice, enabling their recovery from genetic disorders. It has been conjectured that the same applies to human embryos. Additional prospective clinical uses encompass gene therapy for infectious disorders, including HIV, and the development of autologous patient tissue for cancer and other ailments.

These gene editing technologies are revolutionizing biological research and hold tremendous promise in transforming various industries, including agriculture and medicine. Amidst these technologies, CRISPR-Cas9 stands out with ease of use, accuracy, and adaptability in genome editing. That was initially identified as a component of the bacterial immune system, has been developed into an effective tool that enables researchers to precisely target and alter DNA sequences in living things.

A new technology that is described as CRISPR-Cas9 enables genetic and medical researchers to add, delete, or change DNA sequences in specific regions of the genome.

DOI: 10.4324/9781003564041-9

This is because it's the simplest, most versatile, and most accurate genetic manipulation technique yet.

Microbiome-based Therapeutics

The therapy, which entails the manipulation of microbial communities, seeks to restore balance and health by re-establishing the beneficial populations residing on or within the host, along with the subsequent metabolic networks governed by the microbiome.

The microbiome refers to the species of bacteria and other microorganisms found in the human body, as well as any compounds produced by these microbes. The pleiotropic effects of the human gut microbiome in health and disease can now be studied thanks to technological progress. The substantial role of microorganisms in human health has considerable potential for their application as therapeutic agents in disease treatment. Microbiome therapy offers the potential to address significant issues such as interpersonal variability and stability across various environments, aiming for tailored treatment and showing considerable promise for the management of major health conditions. Investigation of high-resolution data made it possible to design modifiers for microbiome engineering. Because most human diseases are linked with microbial dysbiosis, several approaches are currently employed to re-establish the endogenous microbiota so that the diseases can be managed effectively. There is growing interest in the production and distribution of synthetic microbial consortia for health benefits. Some of the methods for managing diseases due to dysbiosis are fecal microbiota transplantation (FMT) and probiotics that depend on the delivery of exogenous bacteria. Advances in synthetic biology have now allowed the development of cell therapies tailored to target specific cells, tissues, or pathways due to probiotic engineering. Genetic switches [2] would then be activated in altering the pathways linked to the microbiota. It would be able to control a single microbe or an entire microbial consortium to produce specific medicinal compounds or antitoxins. Chemical entities are evolved by the engineering of gut microbiomes.

Integration of Big Data Analytics and Omics Technology

Numerous developments have been made in a number of fields, especially the omics sciences—genomics, proteomics, metabolomics, and so on—with big data analytics and technology working hand in hand, helping to jointly improve our understanding of complex biological systems [3]. The basis of many of the new developments relating to the environmental sciences, agriculture, medicine, and biology continues to emerge. The term "omics" defines the set of high-throughput technologies used in large-scale analysis of biological molecules. This includes the following:

- Genomics: Genomics includes annotation and sequencing in the study of the genome.

- Proteomics: Study of the expression, composition, and roles of proteins in the proteome.
- Metabolomics: Metabolomics is the understanding of metabolic patterns and pathways.
- Transcriptomics: Transcription analysis by RNA transcript was known as transcriptomics, but recently, it has been known as the study of gene expression profile.
- Big Data Analytics involves processing and analysis of huge and complex data stores through the application of complex computing methods. These include
- Data Management: Storing and retrieving large datasets.
- Data Mining: It finds out the hidden patterns and relationships present in the data.
- Machine Learning: This entails algorithms that learn through experience and aid in modeling predictions.
- Statistical Analysis: Techniques for understanding data distributions, relations, and significance.

Emerging Technologies and Trends

Gene editing is a rapidly advancing field of science with numerous emerging technologies and trends expected to outline gene editing's future. Some of the most promising ones are listed below:

No CRISPR/Cas9
No gene editing
No microbiome-based therapies
No integration of data analytics and omics technologies
No epigenome editing
No base editing
No personalized gene editing

CRISPR/Cas9 Technology

- It is a talking point in the scientific community because, at present, it is the simplest, versatile, and accurate technique of genetic modification.
- Two main parts are the CRISPR-associated nuclease (CAS) and the guide RNA sequence (gRNA), which are responsible for directing the CAS nuclease and identifying and cleaving DNA, respectively.
- It was shown to operate in bacterial immunity, digesting the DNA of infecting viruses, known as bacteriophages, so that they could not function.
- It was shortly developed as a genetic engineering tool once the molecular mechanism underlying its ability to cleave DNA was defined.

Importance of CRISPR

- The importance of CRISPR is that nearly any living thing's genetic code can be changed. It is easier, less expensive, and more precise than previous gene editing techniques. It also has some applied uses, such as treatment for inherited diseases and engineered crops resistant to drought.
- The CRISPR may be useful for scientists to correctly manipulate DNA in living things. Genes can be added, removed, and replaced precisely. So, there may be more specialized studies and treatments.

History and Discovery of CRISPR/Cas9

- Genetic illnesses such as sickle cell anemia, muscular dystrophy, and cystic fibrosis may be treated by correcting the genetic mutation through CRISPR. Clinical studies have already started to research these options.
- CRISPR allows the creation of animal models whose genome has very specific changes, which, in turn, sheds light on the hereditary etiology of a variety of diseases, enabling them to be tested with potential therapies under optimal conditions.
- CRISPR is an effective tool for studying the function of genes. Through knockout or modification of such genes, scientists can gain new insights and discoveries by learning about the functions that particular genes play in health and illness. Though it took several years for scientists to understand what CRISPR was and how to use it, it is now widely recognized as an accurate gene editing technology.

Discovery

- Discovery of CRISPR Sequences: Japanese scientist Yoshizumi Ishino and his co-workers discovered the CRISPR sequences first in the genome of *Escherichia coli*, also referred to as *E. coli* for the first time. In such research, they observed that there existed repetitive DNA sequences but did not know what their functions were at this time.
- Drs. Jennifer Doudna of the University of California, Berkeley and Emmanuelle Charpentier of the Max Planck Institute for the Science of Pathogens in Berlin discovered CRISPR in 2012. If their pioneering work from 2012 had been published in the journal Science, Doudna and Charpentier would have become the first women to receive the Nobel Prize for Chemistry. They demonstrated how to use the CRISPR-Cas9 bacterial immune system for gene editing. The two received the Nobel Prize in Chemistry in 2020 for their discovery, which was created over a decade ago and is now employed in labs all around the world [4].
- Virginijus Siksnys, a biochemist at Vilnius University in Lithuania, discovered that CRISPR can modify genes in numerous creatures. George Church, of Harvard Medical School in Boston, Massachusetts, was the first to demonstrate that CRISPR could alter human cells. Feng Zhang of the Broad Institute of MIT and Harvard in Cambridge, Massachusetts, was the first to employ CRISPR on eukaryotic cells to discover novel Cas variations.

History

- CRISPR and Cas Proteins: Philippe Horvath and his team found out that CRISPR sequences are associated with specific proteins, among which Cas (CRISPR-associated) proteins. That proved to be critical in understanding how CRISPR works in bacterial immunity.
- Demonstration of CRISPR Function in Bacteria: Emmanuelle Charpentier and Jennifer Doudna published the first test of its functionality in bacteria, where they demonstrated that the CRISPR/Cas9 system could be targeted to any DNA sequence for modification, a discovery that would form the basis of all future gene editing applications.
- CRISPR/Cas9 as a Gene-Editing Tool: Although this discovery occurred way before Doudna and Charpentier published their paper in 2012, they were the first users of the CRISPR-Cas9 as a gene-editing tool. In 1993, a research scientist, Dr. Francisco Mojica, who was working at the University of Alicante in Spain, reported that repeating palindromic DNA segments were found intermingled with other genetic material pieces within bacterial genomes. These regions were named CRISPR by Dr Mojica, and he further postulated that they constitute one of the mechanisms of defense in bacteria [5]. Research scientists under the guidance of Dr. Philippe Horvath in 2007 carried out an experimental proof of the hypothesis formulated by Mojica.
- This versatile gene editing technique has quickly evolved since its discovery by the scientists, Drs. Doudna and Charpentier. Many applications have been developed on it, such as live imaging, diagnostics, base and prime editing, RNA editing, among them, a human whose DNA has been manipulated.
- It included the collection of cells from SCD patients, in vitro editing, and restoring them into the body. The process is referred to as cell therapy. The first CRISPR clinical trials were initiated in 2019. In 2020, a CRISPR treatment was administered in human patients for the first time after an experiment with SCD cell therapy proved successful. Hereditary blindness is treated through gene therapy, which is a process referred to as this [6].

First Successful Gene Editing in Mammalian Cells

Feng Zhang et al, in the Broad Institute, published the first applications of successful CRISPR/Cas9 technology in mammalian cells in 2013. That was primarily meant to open avenues for deep applications in medicine and biotechnology.

CRISPR Mechanism

- The CRISPR/Cas9 mechanism found its basis on the complex system that bacteria and archaea employ in their fight against viruses and plasmids.
- Components of the CRISPR/Cas9 System:
- CRISPR Array

- In the prokaryotes, the CRISPR array consists of repeated DNA sequences, often referred to as short palindromic repeats, separated by unique DNA sequences often termed "spacers."
- Function: Each spacer sequence is of foreign DNA, like from viruses or plasmids that had previously infected the bacterium. This array can be considered a record of previous infections.

Cas9 Protein: Cas9 is a DNA endonuclease that catalyzes double-strand breaks (DSBs). It combines with guide RNA for its actions to be directed toward specific target sequences.

Function: Cas9 accurately cuts the target DNA.

Guide RNA (gRNA)

- The guide RNA is an artificial short RNA piece guiding Cas9 to its specific DNA target. It has two parts
- CRISPR RNA (crRNA): It contains a sequence that is complementary to the targeted DNA sequence.
- Tracrk RNA (trans-activating CRISPR RNA): It assists in the maturation of the CRISPR array and stabilization of the RNA-Cas9 complex [7]. In reality, crRNA and tracrRNA are frequently bundled into a single guide RNA (sgRNA).
- Function: Guide RNA directs Cas9 to specific location in DNA.

Upon re-infection, the bacteria can recognize the virus and employ Cas9 to eliminate it. Activation of Cas9 requires two components: trans-activating CRISPR RNA (tracrRNA) and CRISPR RNA (crRNA). The tracrRNA serves as a scaffold to associate with the complementary crRNA and choose the viral spacer retained from the initial infection. The two RNAs amalgamate to create a complex known as the guide RNA (gRNA). The gRNA can be viewed as the hands wielding the "scissors," while the Cas9 is analogous to the "scissors" themselves. The protospacer adjacent motif, abbreviated as PAM

During a subsequent infection by the virus, the bacteria can recognize and eliminate it using Cas9. Cas9 activation necessitates the presence of both crRNA and tracrRNA, which are trans-activating CRISPR RNAs. The scaffolding is provided by tracrRNA, and the complementary crRNA is the same as the viral spacer that was conserved from the initial infection. A complex called guide RNA (gRNA) is formed by the two RNAs. If Cas9 were a pair of scissors, the gRNA would be the hand wielding them. Downstream of a target site called PAM, the Cas9 enzyme will find a short nucleotide sequence. Cas9 will begin a DSB if it finds the target specified by the gRNA during its upstream scan after finding the PAM. Viruses are rendered powerless when they experience DSBs since they do not possess DNA repair mechanisms [8].

It raises the question of whether or not it is feasible to cleave at any location in an organism's genome by simply changing the guide RNA sequence and feeding it to Cas9. The molecular mechanism that allows the natural CRISPR-Cas9 system to cleave DNA was explained by Doudna and Charpentier. Their hypothesis is valid and backed by revolutionary data.

The natural gRNA complex was transformed into a chimeric single guide RNA (sgRNA), a simple and inexpensive gene editing method. Researchers may utilize Cas9 to cleave any place in an organism's DNA by giving a unique guide RNA that is reasonably simple to generate, as long as the requisite PAM sequence is present.

To edit genes, CRISPR-Cas9 causes double-stranded DNA breaks, which are then repaired by the cell's own DNA repair mechanism. Along with homology-directed repair (HDR), which involves the introduction of new genes or genetic bits, and non-homologous end joining (NHEJ), which can cause genes to malfunction, DNA repair also includes a third step.

Methods of CRISPR

CRISPR-Cas9

It is the most commonly used and popular CRISPR method. The Cas9 protein acts as a molecular scissors through which DNA is cut at specific locations guided by a complementary RNA sequence, such as the guide RNA or gRNA.

CRISPR-Cas12 (Cpf1)

Another type of endonuclease is utilized in CRISPR technology, known as Cas12. In contrast to Cas9, the staggered cuts produced by Cas12 are sometimes more precise and effective for certain applications.

CRISPR-Cas13

Cas13 is an RNA-targeting CRISPR system. Unlike Cas9 and Cas12, which target DNA, Cas13 can specifically target and degrade RNA.

Base Editing

This is an advanced version of CRISPR that has the capability to convert one DNA base into another directly and does not induce DSBs. It has been achieved through the use of a modified version of CRISPR-Cas9 system, where the ability of a deaminase enzyme is incorporated.

Prime Editing

Described as "search-and-replace" genome editing, prime editing introduces new genetic material to specific DNA regions. The approach combines reverse transcription with a catalytically inhibited Cas9 protein.

Epigenome Editing

This approach modifies histone modifications and other epigenetic markers, including DNA methylation, without any alteration in the DNA sequence by using CRISPR-based technologies.

CRISPRa and CRISPRi (Activation and Interference)

Such strategies involve using customized versions of the CRISPR system-such as CRISPRi, which represses gene expression, and CRISPRa, which activates gene expression-without having to alter the underlying DNA sequence. CRISPRi uses repressor proteins, while CRISPRa utilizes transcriptional activators.

Some of the other approaches are:

- CRISPR gene knockout
- CRISPR Knock-in
- CRISPR screens

Applications of CRISPR Technology

Cell and Gene Therapies

The great promise that CRISPR holds for the revolutionization of medicine is founded on its ability to treat various hereditary illnesses such as cancers, blood problems, eye issues, and neurodegenerative diseases. We had reported a CRISPR cell therapy study in 2019, conducted to treat patients suffering from sickle cell disease. Since healing was required through the restoration of fetal hemoglobin and not the existing copy of adult hemoglobin, it became unnecessary.

One outstanding CRISPR study of the neurological disease transthyretin amyloidosis achieved spectacularly promising results in 2021. As it explains to Shondra Miller at St Jude's in this radio conversation, it is also revolutionizing the treatment of pediatric cancer.

This refers to the development of CAR T cells, which have been applied in immunotherapy to combat cancer by utilizing CRISPR. Importantly, the T Cells are taken out from the patient and engineered to produce chimeric antigen receptors. This may make T cells easier to target the cancer type specific to the patient, thereby killing it. CRISPR could directly correct faulty genes in cells from patients, thereby addressing hereditary disorders.

Diagnostics

CRISPR was applied during the COVID-19 pandemic not only as a potential treatment tool but also as a coronavirus diagnostic tool. Federal officials issued approval of SHERLOCKTM CRISPR SARS-CoV-2 test kit to be used in the laboratory under Emergency Use Authorization. End Listen Here, and in this podcast, you may learn more about SHERLOCK and the more recent STOP Covid diagnostic test. Mammoth Biosciences also engineered DETECTR, a CRISPR-based technology used for COVID-19 testing. Like SHERLOCK and STOP Covid, DETECTR uses the naturally occurring Cas nucleases Cas12 and Cas13 and leverages Cas9's search function for the detection of the virus's genetic material. Listen to this podcast featuring Mammoth Bioscience CEO Trevor Martin for additional information on DETECTR.

Another kind of diagnostics using the search functionality of Cas9 is designed to detect various viral and genetic diseases. Dr. Kiana Aran of Cardea Bio published an article at the beginning of 2021 that combined three Nobel Prize-winning technologies—transistors, graphene, and CRISPR—into a small device capable of identifying dangerous SNPs. SNPs account for half of human disease-causing mutations, thus being a very grand discovery [9].

Agriculture

Experts expect that over the next five to ten years, food sources modified through CRISPR will be available. Gene editing technology has a very bright future in agriculture. This is mainly because it can be used to create crops with a resistance to drought and disease. For example, researchers from the Innovative Genomics Institute and the University of Berkeley joined up with Mars, Inc. in developing a disease-resistant chocolate tree.

This may also be used to enhance the shelf life of other perishable products while saving food and providing more people with healthy, wholesome meals on a budget. To learn more about these applications, read our summary on the use of CRISPR in agriculture.

Crops are being developed with CRISPR so that they become improved in various traits like drought resistance, pest resistance, and nutritional content. Rice and wheat have already been genetically modified to increase yield and stress tolerance.

Livestock genetic editing can result in less susceptible animals falling ill, promoting faster growth, and reducing the environmental effects of these animals in farming [10].

Future of CRISPR

Of course, CRISPR-Cas9 has transformed the field of genome engineering. However, with many promising preclinical research findings and more clinical trials now being authorized, we are only beginning to realize the full potential and the benefits of this great technology in allowing DNA editing for the cure of human diseases.

Also, CRISPR-Cas9 gene editing technology is the main focus of an increasing number of biotech start-ups. A large number of researchers are continuously working on innovative methods to put this technology to use in order to address pressing global issues. This technology has many potential uses, including modifying epigenomes, developing new cell and gene therapies, studying infectious diseases, and protecting endangered species.

The future of CRISPR-Cas9 tool is great in cancer biology, mainly because it is a highly versatile, easy, practical, and effective technology. The process can modify the target cells' genomes in ways previously thought impossible, thereby providing a singular approach toward cancer treatment. The technology would mainly provide the greatest type of cancer treatment in the future because of its adaptability, efficacy, and flexibility. In the near future, it will also impact cancer biology, provided researchers have efficiently developed techniques and tools for delivery of the technology to the intended cell or tissue, as well as guidelines and control measures for any off-target effects of the technology [11].

Gene Editing

Scientists have long been able to precisely modify the genome of a living organism through genome editing, a form of genetic modification that encompasses the addition, removal, or alteration of specific DNA sequences to facilitate a better understanding of gene functions, offer therapeutic benefits for hereditary diseases, or enhance particular traits.

Adding, deleting, modifying, or replacing DNA inside a living thing's genome is known as genome editing, genome engineering, or gene editing. Genome editing differs from previous genetic engineering methods in that it inserts genetic material into specified regions of the host genome rather than randomly. Programmed nuclease genetic manipulations work by first locating genomic loci to target, then repairing DNA DSBs caused by restriction endonucleases like FokI and Cas using methods like HDR or NHEJ [12]. The effectors' DNA-binding domain (DBD) is then bound to these loci. A major step forward has been the development of genome editing tools, which allow for targeted alterations to specific regions of the genome in nearly all eukaryotic organisms. Whether they are bacterial or synthetic, both rely on nucleases. Genome editing has increased our understanding of how genes cause sickness by allowing for the creation of more precise cellular and animal models of disease-causing processes. It has begun to show great potential in a variety of fields, including basic science, biomedical research, and applied biotechnology. Recent advances in programmable nucleases, such as zinc-finger nucleases (ZFNs), transcription activator-like effector nucleases (TALENs), and CRISPR-Cas-associated nucleases, have resulted in gene editing outpacing any comparable trend from conception to clinical application [13]. This study, which focuses on eukaryotic cells and animal models, dives into the most recent breakthroughs in the three major genome editing technologies—TALENs, ZFNs, and CRISPR/Cas9—and their derivative reagents as gene editors for a variety of human illnesses and possible therapeutics. Scientists now understand how certain biological products cause disease thanks to the rapid advancement of genome editing in recent years, which has changed human genome research. In the 1970s, the process of genome editing, which includes modifying DNA or RNA, marked the beginning of a new era in genetic engineering. Over the last ten years, genome editing technologies have had a remarkable surge in development, showcasing their immense importance in various domains such as basic research, applied biotechnology, and biomedical research. Artificial or naturally occurring nucleases are essential to these methods [14].

This will make it easier to modify genomes in vivo or in vitro by delivering the editing equipment to the site right away. The addition, removal, or "knock-in" of genes are some of the high-resolution genomic changes that could result from this. Numbers 3 and 4 The creation of nuclease-induced DSBs is the initial step in targeted DNA alteration. These D SBs enable mammalian cells to perform extremely effective DNA recombination methods.5.6 One promotes targeted integration via HDR, whereas the other disrupts genes via NHEJ [15]. Nuclease-induced DNA DSBs are seen in all cell types and species. Methods for altering the genome and repairing DSBs with existing DNA. Genome editing nucleases create DSBs in strategic locations, which can be repaired using donor templates in a process known as NHEJ or HDR. Indels are produced when NHEJ disrupts gene expression at a specific location. When a pathogenic amplification or insertion occurs on one side of a DNA DSB, therapeutic deletion of intervening areas can result in NHEJ gene repair on the other. A DSB is formed at the specified locus during HDR gene addition or repair with a donor-corrected HDR template. TALEN is an abbreviation for transcriptional activator-like effector nuclease. Zinc finger nuclease is also known as ZFN. The abbreviation CRISPR/Cas9 stands for clustered regularly interspaced short palindromic repeat-associated 9 nuclease. NHEJ and HDR are two labels for the same mechanism.

History

Low editing efficiency hindered the utility of genome editing, which was found in the 1990s. This occurred prior to the widespread usage of nuclease-based gene editing techniques. Nature Methods published an article titled "2011 Method of the Year" that discussed the use of designed nucleases for genome editing. Enzymes like these are frequently categorized into three types: planned meganucleases, TALENs, and ZFNs. Science selected the CRISPR-Cas system Breakthrough of the Year in 2015 [16]. By 2015, four types of modified nucleases had found their way into use: meganucleases, ZFNs, TALENs, and CRISPR/Cas9 systems. There were nine genome editing technologies available by 2017. In this type of editing, the first ever endogenous application of "molecular scissors" or designed nucleases took place. These nucleases cause DNA to split at specific spots called "sites." After that, there are two main ways DNA can be repaired: homologous recombination (HR) or NHEJ. This process causes mutations called "edits." Proposed laws in China will make people pay for any harm that arises from altering the human genome using CRISPR or another genome editing technology, as revealed by Chinese lawyers in May 2019.

The disclosure comes in the wake of assertions that Chinese scientist He Jiankui has successfully produced gene-edited individuals (refer to the Lulu and Nana dispute). Current discussions focus on the stochastic elements of cellular regulatory mechanisms and express a prudent viewpoint regarding the risks and oversights related to CRISPR and related biotechnologies. Pigs exhibiting resistance to the virus responsible for porcine reproductive and respiratory syndrome—a disease that incurs an annual cost of $2.6 billion for pig farmers in the US and Europe—were produced at the University of Edinburgh's Roslin Institute. In a US trial done in February 2020, three cancer patients were claimed to have been safely subjected to CRISPR gene editing. The Japanese government has sanctioned the sale of Sicilian Rouge High GABA tomatoes, recognized for their increased production of an amino acid purported to induce relaxation, in 2020. England, excluding the remainder of the UK, intends to abolish limitations on gene-edited crops and animals this year, aligning regulations with those of the United States and other nations, in contrast to the stringent regulations of the EU. In April, the European Commission published an evaluation indicating "strong indications" that the current regulatory framework is inadequate for gene editing. In 2021, specialists identified a competitor to CRISPR: they determined that the obligatory mobile element–guided activity (OMEGA) proteins of transposons include IscB, IsrB, and TnpB, which are endonucleases directed by small ω RNAs.

Process of Gene Editing

Double Strand Break Repair

Repairing DSBs, a necessary biological function in all living entities, depends on broken DNA strands. Apart from DNA damage by ionizing radiation and endogenous poisons, normal biological mechanisms during DNA replication can also cause DSBs. Many diseases and disorders involve DSBs, which can also lead to aneuploidy, cell death, and mutations should they not be adequately repaired. HR and NHEJ [17, 18] are the two primary ways whereby cells fix DSBs.

Based on ideas of DNA DSB repair, a successful approach for changing genomes is high caliber. Whereas HDR fills in absent DNA sequences at the break site using a homologous sequence as a template, HEJ physically ligates the DNA ends utilizing many enzymes. This allows you to create a vector containing the target genes in a position akin to that of the one just next to the DSB. Consequently, the site of the alteration is the DSB site. Though HR-mediated gene targeting is comparable to HDR-based gene editing, this technique at least three orders of magnitude increases the recombination frequency.

Engineered Nucleases

Cleavage of DNA at specified genomic loci is the backbone of genome editing. Even while classic restriction enzymes have been engineered to cleave DNA more efficiently, they still frequently bind to and cleave at more than one site. To produce site-specific DSBs, three distinct types of nucleases have been created and put into use. This includes the CRISPR/Cas9 system, ZFNs, transcription-activator-like effector nucleases, meganucleases, and others.

Meganucleases

Meganucleases are enzymes belonging to the endonuclease family, first identified in the late 1980s. They can identify and cleave elongated DNA sequences ranging from 14 to 40 base pairs [19]. The most prevalent and renowned meganucleases are proteins from the LAGLIDADG family, named for a conserved amino acid sequence. Meganucleases are normally found in microbial species and are intrinsically highly specific owing to their very long recognition sequences (>14 bp). However, the chances of finding exactly the required meganuclease able to process a selected particular DNA sequence are almost nil. The difficulties this problem presented led to efforts by means of mutagenesis and high-throughput screening approaches that would generate meganuclease variants able to recognize various sequences. Some people have been able to combine various meganucleases to generate hybrid enzymes that can recognize new sequences. Other researchers have endeavored to modify the DNA-interacting residues of the meganuclease to create sequence-specific meganucleases through a technique known as rationally engineered meganucleases. Thirdly, efforts have been undertaken to forecast the specificity of the detected nucleic acid sequence and the efficacy of the modified meganucleases to the utmost precision achievable through computational models. The end product is a big bank holding hundreds of thousands of protein units. Their combination leads to chimeric meganucleases able to recognize the target site to be used in response to all sorts of requirements in research and development: health, energy, agriculture, industry, and basic research, among others. Two meganucleases that can cut the human XPC gene responsible for Xeroderma pigmentosum—an extremely severe monogenic condition characterized by a predisposition to skin cancers and burns whenever the patient's skin comes in contact with UV radiation—are among them. These have been produced at an industrial scale [20]. The advantage of mega nucleases lies in their reduced toxicity to cells compared to approaches like ZFN, attributable to their more precise DNA sequence recognition. Nonetheless, the process of converting each potential sequence into sequence-specific enzymes is both costly and labor-intensive, as it does not leverage the combinatorial advantages offered by ZFNs and TALEN-based fusions.

Zinc Finger Nucleases

ZFNs belong to the class of designed modified proteins. They induce the formation of DSBs at targeted loci in the genome. Consequently, scientists are able to make precise alterations to an organism's DNA sequence through gene deletion, addition of new genetic material, or correction of mutations. Zinc finger motifs are found in many transcription factors. About 8% of human proteins contain the zinc ion, which is very critical to the three-dimensional structure of the protein. The ions help to stabilize the motif at the protein-DNA contact sites, where one should find, in general, the transcription factors. DNA sequence-specific recognition is achieved by the C-terminal end of each finger.

The most common sequences are very short, measuring only three base pairs; but, by joining six to eight zinc fingers with known recognition sites, very specialized proteins can be produced with sequences of about twenty base pairs. Therefore, controlling the amount of a given gene's expression is within the realm of possibility. In animal studies, this approach significantly increased angiogenesis. The catalytic domain of an endonuclease can be coupled with a protein in order to generate a targeted DNA break. Genome engineering can make use of these proteins.

Talen

Some DNA-binding proteins known as TALENs consist of a tandem repeat of 33 or 34 amino acids. A nuclease's DNA-cutting domain fused to TALE domains that could selectively be engineered to bind to a particular DNA sequence can be used to develop artificial restriction enzymes called TALENs. In gene editing applications, the fusion proteins act as easily identifiable "DNA scissors," enabling genome alterations, ranging from insertion to deletion and repair and replacement of sequences, inside live cells [21]. TAL effectors are proteins isolated from plant pathogenic Xanthomonas app. These can attach to DNA and can be engineered to bind any specific sequence for the development of DNA-binding domains. TAL effectors consist of tandem repetitions featuring a highly conserved amino acid sequence of 34 residues per repeat, enabling them to recognize a single nucleotide of DNA at the target site. Until the error-prone process of NHEJ fixes the damage, gene disruptions could occur as a result of small insertions or deletions caused by the nuclease-induced break in DNA at the target region. With the exception of the repeat variable residues (RVDs) at amino acid positions 12 and 13, all repeats are retained. According to the RVDs, the TALE will bind to a certain DNA sequence. The direct one-to-one link between TALE repeats and their associated DNA sequences makes it easier to create repeat arrays for the identification of novel DNA sequences. A trans-activator-like effector nuclease called TALEN can be produced by combining these TALEs with the DNA nuclease catalytic domain of FokI. Successfully, the TALEN constructs produced sequence-specific nucleases that attached to and cut DNA at precise spots. A TALENs target recognition system may be set up using a code that anyone could understand. The binding site of TAL nucleases is very long, lasting more than 30 base pairs, which makes them very specific.

Arcut

Komiyama developed the artificial restriction DNA cutter technology, otherwise known as ARCUT for short. In this method, it identifies the cleavage site in the chromosome by using pcPNA. The cutting is then performed by CE and EDTA-a chemical compound that accomplishes the splicing action once pcPNA identifies the location [22].

- CRISPR
- Nucleobase modification (Base editing) editing

Applications of Gene Editing

Gene editing with tools such as CRISPR-Cas9, TALENs, and ZFNs, has a wide field of applications. It encompasses the following aspects:

- Medicine: It has been used to correct mutations causing genetic disorders cystic fibrosis, sickle cell anemia, muscular dystrophy, among others. For example,

experimentation in clinical trials with CRISPR-Cas9 is being examined to edit the genes of sickle cell patients.
- Scientists are finding ways to modulate immune cells in such a way that they will efficiently target and destroy more cancer cells. This ranges from designing CAR-T cell therapy, which involves how scientists “engineer” T cells bearing specific receptors that can recognize antigens on the surfaces of cancer cells.
- Gene editing promises the possibility of therapy for diseases due to single-gene mutations. It would replace a mutated gene with a functional gene or influence gene expression for the cure of the disease.
- Gene editing may be able to create a therapy for viral infections. For instance, for HIV, a possibility exists to target and disrupt viral DNA or modify the host cell genome to evade infection.

Research

- Functional Genomics: Gene editing allows researchers to knock out or sometimes change the expression of specific genes within model organisms like mice or yeast to see what they do and how they cause disease.
- Disease Models: Accurate genetic models of human diseases enable researchers to understand the underlying biology of diseases and experiment with new therapeutic approaches.
- Cell Biology: Gene editing is used to dissect cellular processes, signal pathways, and molecular mechanisms through mutation of gene expression or function in various cell types.

  - Gene editing in clinical studies
  - Clinical trials of anticancer drugs
  - Clinical trials of antiviral
  - Clinical investigations on hematological disorders
  - Clinical studies for inherited ocular disorders
  - Targeted gene mutation
  - Targeted transgene addition

Creating Chromosome Rearrangement Future of Gene Editing

- This has great promise for revolutionary changes in many disciplines for the future, but there are also disadvantages and ethical dilemmas attached.
- Improvements on the way: We’ll be focusing the most on making these gene editing technologies tighter, fewer off-target effects and more efficient at making the desired change. CRISPR, base editing and prime editing technologies are tougher and will provide greater reliability.
- New epigenome editing and new types of CRISPR/Cas systems, like CRISPR/Cas12 and CRISPR/Cas13 might evolve capabilities to target and function for an increased range of applications
- Improvements will allow simultaneous eds of multiple genes or sites within one genome; thus, more complex genetic manipulations and studies on the interaction between genes are expected to be facilitated.

- Gene editing could be a basis for extremely tailored treatment that is precisely anchored in the genetic makeup of an individual, leading to matched therapies for complex diseases and conditions.
- Gene editing may be used for early interventions, which could prevent genetic diseases even before they come out as symptoms. It can correct genetic risks even before they become problems, so that people can avoid certain suffering related to such disorders.
- More emphasis will be on the efforts of developing universal standards and regulations for safe and ethical use as gene editing technologies advance. Innovation must be weighed out against responsible oversight
- Equity in access to such gene editing technologies is a major factor for considering that the benefits of gene editing are equitably distributed, hence the therapies must be made affordable and accessible to diverse populations
- Debates about the ethical impact of gene editing technologies, especially in humans, will reflect the trajectories that future practice will take. Some of these debates have arisen due to issues involving germ-line modification—a type of modification that seems to produce forward effects generationally, even farther afield, against the possibilities of the technology being prone to abuse and the sensationalistic occurrence of "designer babies."
- AI and ML will be used with ever greater frequency to design and optimize gene editing strategies, predict off-target effects, and conduct massive-scale analysis of genetic data.
- Gene editing combined with synthetic biology can create opportunities in the design of new biological systems and organisms to carry out new functions, which may advance other fields, such as pharmaceutical, environmental management, and bioengineering.

Public awareness and engagement will be an essential component, as widespread use of gene editing is also going to raise many questions for the public. Educating people on the possible benefits, risks, and ethical implications. This would involve considerations of gene editing and help in the fostering of informed discussions and decision-making processes.

In simple words, gene editing is quite promising for the future and can well alter entire fields like health, agriculture, or environmental management. However, ensuring that such technologies are developed and used responsibly and justly calls for serious thought on ethical, social, and regulatory factors [23].

Microbiome-based Therapies

- A very exciting and burgeoning area of medicine is microbiome therapeutics. They encompass a method for changing the microbiome, which is an extremely complex composition of viruses, fungi, bacteria, and others that each human carries with them in and on their body to drive wellness and ideally cure diseases.
- Drug types that are microbiome-based consist of biomarkers—to screen, monitor, stratify patients, and provide therapeutics. Currently, nine types of

therapeutics include: phage therapy, diet alteration, antibiotics, probiotics, synbiotics, prebiotics, FMT, live biotherapeutics and microbiome mimetics.

- Microbiome-based medicines utilize the tremendous power of the microbiome—the vast collection of bacteria that reside in various parts of our body, most prominently in the gut. This manipulates microbial populations into improving or even restoring health.

What Is the Microbiome

Trillions of bacteria, viruses, fungi, and other microorganisms living on and inside humans constitute the human microbiome. These microbes are necessary for digesting food.

Help in the synthesis of essential nutrients along with assisting in breaking down big carbohydrates.

Immune Function

Regulating the immune response and preventing harmful infections.

Metabolism

Effecting absorption of lipids, carbohydrates, and other nutrient types in our body.

Mental Health

Effecting the mood and mental well-being through the gut-brain axis.

How Are Microbiome-based Therapies Used to Treat Patients?

Based on these microbiome treatments they're programmed to treat the gut and other microbes in the body that are based around balancing these problems. To examine an individual's microbiome is to replenish healthy bacteria while reducing pathogenic bacteria, which can control—or at least impact—the immune response, inflammation, and metabolism. This is a new, innovative way in which to tackle diseases, like irritable bowel syndrome (IBS), allergies, and even mental health disorders that are currently being treated with more traditional methods. The aim is to leverage these intricate organism–host physiology relationships to later improve general health and well-being [24].

Several pathologies have been linked to dysbiosis or the imbalance of the microbiome, and even psychological disorders. Therapies based on the microbiome try to fix these imbalances by:

- Rebalanced: To get back a healthy microbial balance, eradicate or reintroduce beneficial bacteria.
- Enhance Function: Enhancing the microbiome capabilities to perform and perform other vital processes, including breakdown of food and others, in addition to maintaining the immune system.

- The treatment is bespoke: tailored treatments to specific individuals based on optimizing outcomes by tailoring treatments to the compositions of the microbiome. Types of microbiome-based therapies

Fecal Microbiota Transplantation

A process called FMT gives a patient's gastrointestinal system the feces of a healthy donor. Restoring the natural balance of gut microbiota is the goal since it can get thrown off by illness, antibiotic use, or other. It is also known as bacteriotherapy. FMT may reinstate the recipient's gut bacterial diversity and the bacterial-derived compounds referred to as the metabolome [25].

How FMT Works

- Donor Screening: Before infusing the stool, a significant screening of donors is done to ensure the safety and usability of the stool by excluding infectious illnesses, medical disorders, and lifestyle concerns. This typically involves blood work, questionnaires, and sometimes other medical assessments.
- Stool Preparation: concentrated preparation of the good bacteria as well as other microbes that are left after the donor feces are processed in a laboratory to remove undigested food fragments and other nonmicrobial elements.
- Administration: The treated stool is administered directly to the patient's gastrointestinal tract. This can be done with one or more of the following;
- Colonoscopy: The stool is directly inserted into the colon.
- Enema: The stool is inserted into the rectum.
- Oral Capsules: The stool material is packaged in capsules and administered orally, though this is less common.

Conditions Treated with FMT

- Clostridium difficile Infection:

  FMT is mostly applied as a treatment to recurrent CDI, an infection most of the times more severe and resistant to conventional antibiotics. FMT has proven very effective at restoring a healthy gut microbiome and resolution of symptoms.
- Inflammatory Bowel Disease:

  Investigations on the utilization of FMT for the treatment of conditions such as Crohn's disease and ulcerative colitis have been undertaken, revealing potential efficacy in reducing inflammation and manifestations of these disorders.

Irritable Bowel Syndrome

Some studies indicate that FMT could reduce the symptoms of IBS, but to determine its effectiveness and proper application would be necessary.

- Metabolic Disorders and Obesity:
  New studies explore the function of FMT in metabolic disorders, including obesity and type 2 diabetes, by exploiting the association of gut microbiota with metabolism.
- Other Conditions:
  Other research is also being done on the use of FMT to treat several other conditions, including some neurological and psychiatric disorders; those are still in the experimental stages.

Probiotics

Probiotics are living microbes that, when introduced to a mammalian host, can improve that host's health. The most common probiotics are Lactobacillus, Bifidobacterium, and Saccharomyces [26]. Live microorganisms referred to as probiotics, which can be bacteria or yeast, may potentially have an improving effect on health if ingested in the right dosage. The microbiome refers to the community of microorganisms that live and adhere to the human body. They have a close relationship with the human body and are actually useful bacteria in their living form, which can potentially impart health if taken in the right dosage. Among the diseases they are currently studied for are IBS, respiratory infections, and other conditions where they are frequently applied to encourage gut health.

Probiotics refer to good bacteria which, when provided in an appropriate amount, are helpful for the host in terms of health benefits. Since they generally help in preserving and restoring the natural balance of gut microbiomes, they are commonly termed good or friendly bacteria.

- Probiotics can be obtained in a variety of food and supplement forms. These include fermented foods such as yoghurt, kefir, and sauerkraut, capsules, pills, and powders.

Mechanism of Action of Probiotics

- Rebalancing the Microbiota: Probiotics may rebalance gut microbiota when it has been disrupted by antibiotics, disease, or an unhealthy diet.
- Competitive exclusion: The means by which probiotics inhibit the setting of pathogenic microbes because they compete with these pathogens for resources and occupation of attachment sites in the gut.
- Immunopotentiation: Probiotics change the immune system, improve the immunity of the body against infections and reduce inflammation
- Producing Beneficial Metabolites: Some probiotics release such products that include short-chain fatty acids (SCFAs) that improve the intestine's health by supplying energy to cells present in the intestine.
- Maintenance or Restoration of the Gut Barrier Function: Probiotics can prevent or preserve the integrity of the lining of the gut, which reduces the permeability of the intestines and leaky gut syndrome. The application of probiotics encourages and controls the balance of the microbiome for overall health. They ought to be applied wisely to benefit at the highest leverage on each individual's needs and in collaboration with healthcare providers [27].

Prebiotics

Prebiotics comprise indigestible fibers and other compounds that enhance the quantity and activity of beneficial gut microorganisms [28]. Prebiotics are substances that nourish and promote the proliferation of beneficial bacteria already existing in the gut, in contrast to probiotics, which consist of live bacteria that are ingested. Prebiotics are drugs that induce the growth or activity of good bacteria in the stomach. Generally, these are forms of fiber that, instead of being degraded in the human digestive system, are fermented by the bacteria that live in the gut.

Common Prebiotics

- Inulin: Vegetables and edible roots of chicory, onions, garlic, and leeks.
- Fructooligosaccharides (FOS): These are present in bananas, onions, and asparagus.
- Galactooligosaccharides (GOS): These are present in legumes and dairy products.
- **Pectin:** This is found in fruits and includes apples and citrus fruits.
- Resistant Starch: This is present in foods such as green bananas and cooked, then cooled potatoes.

Action Mechanism of Prebiotics

- Selective Fermentation: Acetate, propionate, and butyrate are SCFAs that are produced when good gut bacteria ferment prebiotics. Intestinal epithelial cells rely on these SCFAs for energy, and they help keep the gut healthy.
- Increased Microbial Diversity: Prebiotics act as fuel for beneficial bacteria, thus helping to increase the diversity and abundance of these microbes-which is typical with better gut health.
- Modulating Gut pH: The fermentation of prebiotics produces SCFAs that lower the pH of gut environment. This pH environment is favorable to the growth of beneficent bacteria more than to pathogenic microbes.
- Supporting Immune Function: Prebiotics enable enhanced immune function by activating desirable microorganisms, which are involved in the regulation of immunity and prevention of infection. Gut preservation and optimization can only be achieved through the containment of desirable microorganisms. The intake of diets consisting of food sources that are rich in prebiotics assists various components of your health and your overall health [29].

Synbiotics

The interaction of probiotics with prebiotics in a synergistic blend for establishing optimum gut health, leading to general wellness. It is theorized that by combining live beneficial bacteria known as probiotics with nondigestible fibers and compounds which feed them, synbiotics could enhance the functionality of both. Synbiotic blends also allow for the establishment of favorable cross-feeding interactions [30].

Action of Synbiotics

- Synergistic Effect Synbiotics contain prebiotics that feed the probiotics, making the probiotics thrive and remain healthy while accompanied by a healthy flora in the intestine. Ideally, this combination optimizes the effects of the prebiotics and probiotics.
- Improved Survival and Colonization: The functioning of prebiotics is to enhance the ability of probiotics to survive and colonize in the gut. This will actually increase the number of good bacteria entering the intestines and thus start to work.
- Improved Gut Health: Synbiotics contribute to the equilibrium of gut microbiota, which is linked to enhanced health, improved immunological function, and better digestion. They supply advantageous bacteria along with their requirements.
- Synbiotics is a supplementation approach that can improve gut health and general well-being by combining both probiotics and prebiotics. Synbiotics enhance the activity of both the supplemented components while keeping the gut microbiota healthy by feeding beneficial bacteria the required nutrients [31].

Microbiome Modulation

The term "microbiome modulation" describes methods and approaches by which the make-up of activity of a microbiome is changed. The microbiome is composed of a diverse population of bacteria living and thriving within and on human bodies, most specifically within the gut. This was performed through increasing beneficial microbial populations or reducing harmful ones, and the goals were toward improved health outcomes [32].

The Significance of Microbiome Modulation

- Health Impacts: Many aspects of health, including immunity and digestion and, curiously, mental well-being, depend on the well-being of the microbiome. Alterations in the balance of the microbiome are known to be associated with conditions as diverse as IBS, IBD, obesity, diabetes, and psychological disorders [33].
- Personalized Medicine: The microbiome of a particular person can be made unique for specific treatment techniques by altering his/her own microbiome, which may result in more targeted and effective therapeutics. Modulation of the microbiome has a lot of promise because it can eventually make us healthier and aid in treatment with respect to several diseases by changing the composition and functions of microbial communities inside and outside of the body. Methods range from highly complex medical interventions to diet, and ongoing research brings us closer to a grasp of manipulating the microbiome in a safe and efficient manner toward better health. By harnessing the power of our microbial communities, microbiome-based medicines represent a potential opportunity to cure and prevent a wide array of medical maladies. Additional work to be done, these treatments hold a strong potential to be developed into tailored medicine, providing specific treatments for many diseases [34].

Integration of Data Analytics and Omics Technologies

This powerful blend of big data analytics combined with omics technology is proving to revolutionize realms such as proteomics, metabolomics, and genomics. At least as much a philosophical challenge as a practical, everyday processing of omics data calls for the integration of disparate and vast datasets. Biosystems are being researched at a scale never before due to the development of new omics technologies and large-scale consortium efforts resulting in diverse as well as usually enormous data sets. This encourages the research personnel to develop innovative data integration techniques. Development and advancement in emerging technology become highly rewarding through the fusion of data analytics and omics technologies. It fosters innovation in many industries, especially in biotechnology, healthcare, and customized medicine.

High throughput (HT) methods have gained acceptance within the research community over the last ten years, which has facilitated massively parallel examination of the genome, epigenome, transcriptome, and proteome. For computational and quantitative scientists, this has opened new avenues for discovery but posed difficulties in forecasting phenotypic results.

The phrase that denotes datasets produced by technologies that are excessively huge and intricate for ordinary data processing methods is "Big Data." The integration, archiving, sharing, mining, visualization, and transmission of Big Data present issues [35].

This is one of the three principal determinants of phenotype, with genotype essentially indicating genotype-phenotype relationships. Epigenetic factors (DNA methylation, histone modifications, RNA-associated silencing), hereditary factors (DNA sequence), and environmental influences (noninherited) make up the remaining two categories. A study delves into the function of chromatin in correlations between genotype and phenotype. Improving the Gene Ontology Resource to better analyze and understand Alzheimer's disease data is the focus here. Among the many challenges faced by integrative computational biologists and statistical geneticists is the prediction of organisms' genotype-to-phenotype mappings in response to environmental factors. From a collecting perspective, Lewis Frey stated that this establishes a connection between genotypes and phenotypes, which is obvious in Omics data sets. It links encoded genetic information to the macro-scale expression of an organism phenotype.This complicates the identification of the principal molecules responsible for the phenotype from the genotype due to the numerous interactions involved. Frey presents a compelling argument for AI: the amalgamation of genetics and computers that will enable the automation of phenotypes. Numerous issues must be addressed: data proliferation, inaccessibility due to inaccuracies and incomplete heterogeneity, and the existence of data silos [36].

To date, few algorithms utilizing omics data have been implemented in clinical settings and provide sufficient predictive capability.

The majority of health characteristics can be elucidated by clinical and epidemiological data. To enhance algorithmic predictiveness, it must also be well modeled using omics data. This involves the characteristics and diversity of nonomics data, referred to as ascertainment bias, in relation to One data, the existence of interactions, issues with computational model fairness and sub-phenotype existence that prevent One data integration [37]. So far, most of the available data is centered around RNA expression, and the studies that have been conducted have shown minimal dimensionality and have included nonomics data. The three main approaches to modeling are independent, conditional, and integrated modeling. The third choice, joint modeling, which involves analyzing omics and nonomics data together in a supervised and/or unsupervised way, is often the most common. Its assessment of the pattern of correlation between the two types of data makes it a recommended pick. They add more intricacy than conditional or independent models. Essential for the analysis of large omics datasets is Gene Ontology (GO, geneontology.org). Ruth Lovering and colleagues from UCL demonstrated that an improved GO Resource makes it easier to analyze and understand data related to Alzheimer's disease. The UCL biocuration team oversaw this project, which improved the GO database with the help of the Alzheimer's Research UK foundation by adding annotations for gene products associated with dementia and developing new GO terms for the nervous system. Of the 396 prioritized gene products, 276 were related to proteins and complexes classified under neurological Gene Ontology keywords, corresponding to 526 (42.1%) of the 1262 total gene product annotations submitted. More than 70 supplementary GO keywords were created to guarantee the provision of descriptive annotations for gene products linked to Alzheimer's disease.

It can be difficult to assess and understand the large lists of biological phrases connected to proteins that are produced by functional enrichment approaches. With the goal of processing Big Omics data more efficiently, Fiero and colleagues developed NeVOmics, or network-based visualization for Omics. To count the number of substantially enhanced biological terms, this application provides a hypergeometric distribution test. It makes it possible to examine dispersed clusters and link proteins to particular pathway activities [38].

Through the development and widespread use of HT technologies, biostatisticians, geneticists, and biologists have been able to establish a correlation between genotype and phenotype on a scale never before seen. Mass spectrometry for lipid, proteomics, and metabolomics studies and deep sequencing for genomes are all part of these technologies. Topics covered in this issue include methods for integrating Omics data with clinical and biological data, new developments in gene ontology pathways and network algorithms, and integration strategies for Omics systems-level analysis.

Applications

Precision Medicine and Personalized Healthcare

- Tailored Treatments: Merging omics data (such as genetics and proteomics) with sophisticated data analytics, healthcare professionals can comprise individualized treatment programs for each patient based on their exact molecular message. It decreases side effects and increases its therapeutic efficacy [39].

- Disease Prediction and Prevention: The information provided by omics data and predictive analytics facilitates early intervention and preventive actions, first of all, relying on people at risk for some specific disease.

Drug Discovery and Development

- Target Identification: The molecular pathways behind diseases can be fully viewed with the use of omics data. Data analytics can be applied to these very complicated databases and find potential therapeutic targets.
- Accelerating Clinical Trials: The higher the patient classification on clinical trials, the higher the probability of success and shorter and cheaper drug development. It is made possible by the integration of omics data with analytics.
- Biomarker Discovery: This provides advanced analytics over omics data, and now you can find biomarkers to predict treatment response or disease progression, making drug development and monitoring better.

Synthetic Biology and Biotechnology

- Optimizing Biological Systems: Synthetic biology can create more biofuels, more medicines and other vertically integrated bioproducts from engineered metabolic pathways by means of data analytics, omics data.
- Gene Editing: By examining the omics data pre and post modifications, Analytics aids in understanding the effects of gene editing (e.g., CRISPR), and analytics ensures accuracy and reduces off-target effects.

Advanced Diagnostics

- Early Disease Detection: By combining analytics with omics data, advanced diagnostic tools can be developed to detect diseases at early stages, frequently prior to the appearance of symptoms [40].
- Noninvasive Testing: Liquid biopsy and other omics approaches can offer non-invasive means of disease diagnosis and monitoring. There are data analytics that improve the accuracy and reliability of these tests through analysis of the massively complex data.

Agriculture and Food Technology

- Crop Improvement: Together with plant omics data, we will combine analytics to make plants better in terms of drought resistance, higher yield, and more nutritional content.
- Food Safety and Quality: By analysis of food product microbiomes, omics technologies in combination with analytics may be used to monitor food quality, identify the presence of contaminants, and ensure food safety.

Environmental Monitoring and Sustainability

- Ecosystem Analysis: Taken together with metagenomics and other omics approaches, data analytics can provide infrastructure to carry out a deep microbial community study ranging across environments to track biodiversity, monitor ecosystem health.
- Bioremediation: Only with omics data can microbial species that can break down environmental toxins be identified, and analytics may amplify their application in bioremediation projects.

Artificial Intelligence and Machine Learning

- AI-powered Insights: Machine learning algorithms applied to omics data may lead to advances in AI-driven healthcare and research and help predict outcomes that were otherwise completely impossible to understand [41].
- Automation and Scalability: With the addition of AI to omics and analytics, it becomes possible to automate difficult data analysis processes and analyze large-scale data in real time [42–45].

Precision Oncology

- Cancer Genomics: Examining genomic changes in tumors can pinpoint which mutations lead to cancer, big data analytics. We construct the customized therapies that do much less harm and are much more successful than the traditional therapies based off of this information [46–48].
- Therapeutic Resistance: By understanding omics data, we can teach ourselves why some tumors survive therapy, and possibly how to treat that resistance.

Synthetic Biology and Bioengineering

- Metabolic Engineering: The integration of omics data allows big data analytics to be used to design and optimize microbial strains for the production of biofuels, medicines, etc.
- Gene Editing: Big data analytics can be used to identify important genes or pathways from which creatures can be created with desired features through gene editing [49–53].

Conclusion

Biotechnology, biology, and healthcare are transforming thanks to the convergence of cutting-edge technologies like CRISPR, gene editing, microbiome-based medicines, and omics technologies. The field of precision medicine is entering a new era driven by these breakthroughs, wherein individuals' specific genetic, microbiological, and molecular profiles may be used to tailor treatments and interventions.

Together, CRISPR, gene editing, microbiome-based medicine, and omics technologies are driving a paradigm change in biology and medicine. As well as helping us understand life at the molecular level, these advances are boosting the door to incredible medical procedures and hopefully the long-term answer to the world's problems. The further development of these technologies could enable them to transform healthcare, agriculture and environmental management by moving individualized and precise approaches to center stage in medical care and other research.

Due to the convergence of modern advancements such as CRISPR, gene editing, microbiome-based therapies, and omics technology, precision medicine, the tailoring of treatments to individual patients, is about to arrive. Together, these technologies are powerful possibilities for substantial changes in biomedical research and healthcare. With gene editing and CRISPR, scientists can edit genetic sequences with previously unheard-of precision, so they can zero in on the causes of diseases. The implications for diseases that were thought to be incurable are this. Meanwhile, research into the use of microbiome-based therapeutics should spur the development of treatments for a plethora of health conditions that take advantage of this sophisticated symbiosis of gut microbiota and overall health, and offer a means to enhance well-being and bring balance.

The combined application of these domains in conjunction with the knowledge gained from omics technologies (for example, gene, proteomic, and metabolomic information) gives better insights into the biology and disease systems, opening the door to discovery of novel disease biomarkers that will facilitate rapid diagnosis as well as targeted treatment. As these technologies progress, we will eventually be better able to predict treatment responses and, in turn, improve patient outcomes. Moreover, it will also speed up drug discovery and development. And a fair amount of ethical baggage, but along with appropriate use and fair access, these potent instruments need to be properly handled.

However, these obstacles need to be overcome and interdisciplinary collaboration supported to fully realize all of these transformative technologies: CRISPR, gene editing, microbiome therapy, and omics. Together, this will help bridge to a future where everyone attends to treatments and disease management of personal considerations.

References

1. Ishino Y, Shinagawa H, Makino K, Amemura M, Nakata A. Nucleotide sequence of the iap gene, responsible for alkaline phosphatase isozyme conversion in *Escherichia coli*, and identification of the gene product. J Bacteriol. 1987;169(12):5429–5433.
2. Jinek M, East A, Cheng A, Lin S, Ma E, Doudna J. RNA-programmed genome editing in human cells. eLife. 2013;2:e00471.
3. Jinek M, Doudna J, Charpentier E, Chylinski K. Methods and compositions for RNA-directed target DNA modification and for RNA-directed modulation of transcription. US patent US20130177983A1. 2013 Jul 11.
4. Gasiunas G, Barrangou R, Horvath P, Siksnys V. Cas9-crRNA ribonucleoprotein complex mediates specific DNA cleavage for adaptive immunity in bacteria. Proc Natl Acad Sci U S A. 2012;109(39):E2579–E2586.
5. Mojica FJM, Juez G, Rodriguez-Valera F. Transcription at different salinities of *haloferax mediterranei* sequences adjacent to partially modified *PstI* sites. Mol Microbiol. 1993;9(3):613–621.

6. Shao M, Xu T, Chen C. The big bang of genome editing technology: Development and application of the CRISPR/Cas9 system in disease animal models. Sci Press Zool Res. 2016;37(2):1–11.
7. Mei Y, Wang Y, Chen H, Sun ZS, Ju XD. Recent progress in CRISPR/Cas9 technology. J Genet Genomics. 2016;43(2):63–75.
8. Kaur R, Gupta S, Chauhan A, Mishra V, Sharma MK, Singh J. Harnessing the power of clustered regularly interspaced short palindromic repeats (CRISPR)-based microfluidics for next-generation molecular diagnostics. Mol Biol Rep. 2024;51(1):896.
9. Mishra S, Nayak S, Tuteja N, Poosapati S, Swain DM, Sahoo RK. CRISPR/Cas-mediated genome engineering in plants: Application and prospectives. Plants (Basel). 2024;13(14):1884.
10. Liu C, Zhang L, Liu H, Cheng K. Delivery strategies of the CRISPR-Cas9 gene-editing system for therapeutic applications. J Control Release. 2017;266:17–26.
11. Cohen-Tannoudji M, Robine S, Choulika A, Pinto D, El Marjou F, Babinet C, et al. I-sceI-induced gene replacement at a natural locus in embryonic stem cells. Mol Cell Biol. 1998;18(3):1444–1448.
12. Nature Methods Editorial. Method of the Year 2011. Nat Methods. 2012;9(1):1.
13. Esvelt KM, Wang HH. Genome-scale engineering for systems and synthetic biology. Mol Syst Biol. 2014;9(1):641.
14. Tan W, Carlson DF, Walton MW, Fahrenkrug SC, Hackett PB. Precision editing of large animal genomes. Adv Genet. 2012;80: 37–97.
15. Puchta H, Fauser F. Gene Targeting in plants: 25 years later. Int J Dev Biol. 2013;57(6–8):629–637.
16. Boglioli E, Richard M. Rewriting the Book of Life: a New Era in Precision Genome Editing. *Boston Consulting Group*. 2015.
17. Church GG. The future of genetic codes and BRAIN codes. Philos Trans A Math Phys Eng Sci. 2017;375(2099):20160361
18. Cyranoski D. China Set to introduce Gene-editing regulation following CRISPR-baby furore. Nature. 2019.
19. Cheong KH, Koh JM, Jones MC. Black swans of CRISPR: Stochasticity and complexity of genetic regulation. BioEssays. 2019;41(6):1900032.
20. Stokstad E. U.K. set to loosen rules for gene-edited crops and animals. Science. 2021;372(6541):908–909.
21. US trial shows 3 cancer patients had their genomes altered safely by CRISPR. *ScienceAlert* [Internet]. 2020 [cited 2025 May 15]
22. Altae-Tran H, Kannan S, Demircioglu FE, Oshiro R, Nety SP, McKay LJ, et al. The widespread IS200/IS605 transposon family encodes diverse programmable RNA-guided endonucleases. Science. 2021;374(6563):57–65.
23. New programmable gene editing proteins found outside of CRISPR systems [Internet]. Cambridge (MA): Broad Institute; 2021 Jun 28
24. Jasin M. Genetic manipulation of genomes with rare-cutting endonucleases. Trends Genet. 1996;12(6):224–228.
25. Stoddard BL. Homing endonuclease structure and function. Q Rev Biophys. 2006;38(1):49.
26. De Souza N. Primer: Genome editing with engineered nucleases. Nat Methods. 2012;9(1):27.
27. Smith J, Grizot S, Arnould S, Duclert A, Epinat JC, Chames P, et al. A combinatorial approach to create artificial homing endonucleases cleaving chosen sequences. Nucleic Acids Res. 2006;34(22):e149.
28. Seligman LM. Mutations altering the cleavage specificity of a homing endonuclease. Nucleic Acids Res. 2002;30(17):3870–3879.
29. Chevalier BS, Kortemme T, Chadsey MS, Baker D, Monnat RJ, Stoddard BL. Design, activity, and structure of a highly specific artificial endonuclease. Mol Cell. 2002;10(4):895–905.

30. Arnould S, Chames P, Perez C, Lacroix E, Duclert A, Epinat JC, et al. Engineering of large numbers of highly specific homing endonucleases that induce recombination on novel DNA targets. J Mol Biol. 2006;355(3):443–458.
31. Redondo P, Prieto J, Muñoz IG, Alibés A, Stricher F, Serrano L, et al. Molecular basis of xeroderma pigmentosum group c DNA recognition by engineered meganucleases. Nature. 2008;456(7218):107–111.
32. Rebar EJ, Huang Y, Hickey R, Nath AK, Meoli D, Nath S, et al. Induction of angiogenesis in a mouse model using engineered transcription factors. Nat Med. 2002;8(12):1427–1432.
33. Gaj T, Gersbach CA, Barbas CF. ZFN, TALEN, and CRISPR/Cas-based methods for genome engineering. Trends Biotechnol. 2013;31(7):397–405.
34. Khan SH. Genome-editing technologies: Concept, pros, and cons of various genome-editing techniques and bioethical concerns for clinical application. Mol Ther Nucleic Acids. 2019;16:326–334.
35. Waller KMJ, Leong RW, Paramsothy S. An update on faecal microbiota transplantation for the treatment of gastrointestinal diseases. J Gastroenterol Hepatol. 2022;37:246–255.
36. Brown JRM, Flemer B, Joyce SA, Zulquernain A, Sheehan D, Shanahan F, et al. Changes in microbiota composition, bile, and fatty acid metabolism, in successful faecal microbiota transplantation for *clostridioides difficile* infection. BMC Gastroenterol. 2018;18(1):131.
37. George Kerry R, Patra JK, Gouda S, Park Y, Shin HS, Das G. Benefaction of probiotics for human health: A review. J Food Drug Anal. 2018;26(3):927–939.
38. Sanders ME, Merenstein DJ, Reid G, Gibson GR, Rastall RA. Probiotics and prebiotics in intestinal health and disease: From biology to the clinic. Nat Rev Gastroenterol Hepatol. 2019;16:605–616.
39. Pandey KR, Naik SR, Vakil BV. Probiotics, prebiotics and synbiotics—a review. J Food Sci Technol. 2015;52(12):7577–7587.
40. Hoek MJA, Merks RMH. Emergence of microbial diversity due to cross-feeding interactions in a spatial model of gut microbial metabolism. BMC Syst Biol. 2017;11(1):56.
41. Lopez de Maturana E, Alonso L, Alarcón P, Martín-Antoniano IA, Pineda S, Piorno L, Malats N, Díez-Villanueva A, Tornero-Esteban P, Carretero-Iglesia L, Dopazo J. Challenges in the integration of omics and non-omics data. Genes. 2019;10, 238.
42. Kramarz B, Roncaglia P, Meldal BHM, Huntley RP, Martin MJ, Orchard S, Poux S, O'Donovan C, Lovering RC. Improving the gene ontology resource. Genes. 2018;9(593).
43. Zuniga-Leon E, Carrasco-Navarro U, Fierro F. NeVOmics. Genes. 2018;9(569).
44. Atmakuri LR, Peeriga R, Begum S, Vallamkonda B, Baratam A. Novel bioanalytical LC-MS/MS method for determination of metoprolol in human plasma. J Appl Pharm Sci. 2024;14(12):131–138.
45. Peeriga R, Venkata Bangaru GK. Implementation of the POCSO act in schools. In: Child Sexual Abuse: A Public Health Problem in India. Springer publications, Singapore, 2024. p. 391–413.
46. Peeriga R, Yarlagadda LC, Alla NR. Protection of children from sexual exploitation. In: Child Sexual Abuse: A Public Health Problem in India. 2024. p. 191–201.
47. Peeriga R, Shiek Arabath SAM, Manubolu K, Thelappilly BB, Yarlagadda LC. Insilico assessment of phytoconstituents in *myxopyrum smilacifolium* blume against arthritis. Biomed Pharmacol J. 2024;17(1):235–241.
48. Manubolu K, Balagani PK, Gope ER, Peeriga R, Sridevi AR. Unlocking the potential of aquasomes: A comprehensive review on innovative nanocarriers in drug delivery and beyond. Int J Chem Biochem Sci. 2023;24(6):405–410.
49. Manubolu K, Peeriga R, Bonthu MG, Gope ER, Kadirvel D. Evaluation of anti-inflammatory activity of *Millingtonia hortensis* leaf extract. Int J Chem Biochem Sci. 2023;24(6):380–385.

50. Peeriga R, Chandrasekhar KB. Comparative study of anti-inflammatory activity of petroleum ether extract of *myxopyrum smilacifolium* blume and ethanolic leaf extract of *pamburus missionis* swingle. J Pharm Sci Res. 2017;9(6):955–957.
51. Peeriga R, Manubolu K. (2025). Design strategies for waste reduction and enhanced recyclability in pharmaceutical packaging. In: Yingngam, B., Aslam, M.S., Haghi, A.K. (eds) Sustainable Pharmaceutical Product Development and Optimization Processes. Springer, Singapore.
52. Manubolu K, Peeriga R, Chandrasekhar KB. A Short Guide to Clinical Pharmacokinetics. 1st ed. 2024. Springer. Singapore.
53. Manubolu K, Peeriga R (2025). Ecodesign principles. In: Yingngam, B., Aslam, M.S., Haghi, A.K. (eds) Sustainable Pharmaceutical Product Development and Optimization Processes. Springer, Singapore.

10 Regulatory Considerations and Ethical Issues

Talamanchi Balakrishna, Cheruku Jigeesha Naga Durga Sai Paidi Pranitha, Raveesha Peeriga, Venkateswara Rao Javvaji, Avisa Indira, and Yadlapalli Vamsi Abhiram

Introduction

Biomaterials have now become an important component in many fields, ranging from tissue engineering to biomedical engineering. But when it comes to biomaterials' implementation in clinical practice, there must be a high level of compliance with these regulations and ethical concerns. The framework governing biomaterials is vast and is specific to the region in which they are implemented. Many important agencies oversee the approval of biomaterials for medical use, including China's National Medical Products Administration, Europe's European Medicines Agency, and America's Food and Drug Administration. Due to these factors, the regulatory approval processes always follow elaborate preclinical and clinical evaluation and post-marketing safety [1, 2].

These are all ethical issues regarding biomaterials creation, application, and disposal. There are many situations where ethical quandaries could be raised, from human subject research to protocols for obtaining informed consent to fair access to biomaterials-based treatments. In addition, the acquisition of biomaterials (such as tissues or cells) raises ethical questions related to the donor's permission, confidentiality and commercialization. Societal implications of global health justice and environmental sustainability extend beyond any particular individuals: biomaterials themselves. We seek to reduce resource depletion and environmental impact, and biodegradability and remont are becoming more and more important in biomaterials. If we incorporate ethical and regulatory compliance in our development and use of biomaterials, they can be harnessed to be capable of their revolutionary potential and retain health and societal value for humans and nature as a steward of.

In order to operate within this sector, it is imperative to be subject to a comprehensive regulatory framework that supervises the legal operations of numerous significant organizations. The Central Drugs Standard Control Organization (CDSCO) [3] is a considerable entity in the context of national regulatory supervision of pharmaceuticals and medical apparatus. The primary responsibility for ensuring the efficacy, safety, and quality of publicly available pharmaceuticals is vested in CDSCO, a division of the Ministry of Health and Family Welfare [4]. It is crucial to recognize that CDSCO is merely one

DOI: 10.4324/9781003564041-10

of numerous regulatory agencies when examining the regulatory landscape as a whole. Examples of such organizations include the National Pharmaceutical Pricing Authority (NPPA) and the Indian Council of Medical Research (ICMR) [5, 6]. To achieve this goal, these organizations ought to work together and provide assistance to one another in order to maintain a robust regulatory environment [7].

In the context of drug development, efficacy is the capacity of a medicinal product to yield a favorable outcome under carefully monitored circumstances, usually ascertained through clinical trials. It includes the medication's ability to fulfil its intended therapeutic result, varying from the removal of symptoms to the healing of the illness. The idea of efficacy encompasses more than just a binary definition of effectiveness; rather, it's a comprehensive knowledge of the medication's effects, taking into account variables including dosage, patient features, and length of treatment. Assuring maximum effectiveness is not only essential to the health of the patient but also a basic ethical factor in medical growth [8].

Food and Drug Administration

The Food and Drug Administration (FDA), a branch of the US Department of Health and Human Services, controls foods, drugs, cosmetics, medical equipment, and a great variety of other health-related products. Safety of the public is the responsibility of the FDA. Much of it began in the early 1900s, around the time the Pure Food and Medication Act of 1906 was created in response to popular outcry over the typically poor working conditions in the food and pharmaceutical sectors. Upton Sinclair's novel The Jungle elevated this topic to the front stage. Still, the first statute that greatly expanded agency authority was the Federal Food, Drug, and Cosmetic Act (F D and C Act) of 1938. This law formed the main legislative structure of the FDA. A drug is under continual observation even after it has been launched and promoted. This allows it to keep an eye on the product and respond before it ever finds mass consumption. To find any side effects, extensive clinical studies, post-market monitoring, and testing both before and after the product launches in the market are needed. The United States Department of Agriculture is always under an obligation to guarantee the safety of meat and poultry. Apart from medications, the FDA oversees ensuring that medical equipment, cosmetics, biologics (including vaccinations), radiation-emitting goods, and even the national food supply are safe to consume. The Food and Drug Administration (FDA) continues to be very important in the fight against tobacco use, even if the Family Smoking Prevention and Tobacco Control Act was passed in 2009. There are several different specialist centers under the FDA division of structure. Among such facilities are the CFSAN, CBER, and CDER, which stand for Drug and Biologics Evaluation and Research facilities. Every one of these sites supervises several different product categories. The approval process is absolutely fundamental to the work of the FDA. This approach consists of a careful review of data from clinical trials to evaluate new drugs, medical devices, and biologics. The FDA only grants clearance to those products that demonstrate a favorable balance between the risks and benefits [9–11].

Once these products go to market, the FDA has the authority to issue recalls or safety alerts if problems should arise with these products. And they're MedWatch's safety keeping eye. Another important role for the FDA is that they help enforce the rules businesses must follow, seize dangerous items, and order recalls [12]. The FDA has also been in the middle of public health emergencies such as the COVID pandemic, granting Emergency Use Authorizations for vaccines and treatments for the purpose of slashing the time to market. The agency must also address ongoing pandemic-grade public health issues such as the opioid epidemic and the vaping threat, and do so while simultaneously balancing resource limitations and innovation. The rules and guidelines imposed by the FDA really make a lot of difference in that many other countries follow the same framework or an FDA model. Furthermore, the FDA is helping to foster scientific and health innovation through its Fast Track and Priority Review programs, designed to speed the FDA's approval of new drugs for serious diseases and medical conditions where no adequate therapy exists. As the FDA and the United States, it is still essential that its expansive gaze, contentious as it has been, and probably will be in the future, be augmented with value for public health. It evolves in being adaptable to a never-ending technological wiring of the hitches.

The Regulatory Authority of the FDA

The regulatory authority of the FDA is drawn from a number of important laws:

- In 1938, Congress passed the Federal Food, Drug, and Cosmetic Act (FDCA), which gave the US FDA broad regulatory powers over food, medicine, and personal care products.
- The Public Health Service Act establishes the authority of the Food and Drug Administration to regulate medical devices and sets standards for the control of immunizations and other biological agents.
- The power to regulate tobacco products was awarded to the FDA by the Family Smoking Prevention and Tobacco Control Act of 2009 (FSPAC).
- These acts have vested the FDA with the responsibility to review facilities, impose sanctions upon things that violate the law, as well as to set up rules and standards that the industry must follow.

Overview of FDA Guidelines

A number of product categories are regulated by the FDA. The purpose of these regulations is to ensure products' effectiveness, safety, proper labeling and post-market surveillance. The rules vary based on the kind of product:

Guidelines for Food Safety

Modernization of Food Safety Act

With more than 70 years of lasting, the Modernization of Food Safety Act (FSMA) is the biggest reform law of food safety. Among its notable characteristics are:

Preventive Controls: In order to minimize the risk of foodborne illness, food manufacturing producers have to have in place preventive controls and maintain records.

Inspection and Compliance: As the FDA ensures adherence to the FSMA guidelines, facilities are not only checked but also inspected regularly, through and forth.

Import Safety: Import Safety: Import/exporter's guarantor requires importers to verify that foreign suppliers comply with US safety standards [13].

Good Manufacturing Practices

The basic hygienic and processing requirements of food producers are described in good manufacturing practices (GMPs).

Facilities and Equipment Sanitation

Appropriate handling, storage, and labeling of food products [14]

Labeling and Managing Allergens Food labels should be truthful in listing ingredients and nutritional facts, and labeling for allergies. Statements such as "organic," "non-GMO", or "gluten-free" are all bound by legislation and require specific compliance.

Medication Guideline

Procedure for New Drug Applications

All new drugs need to be processed through the new drug applications (NDA) process to be sold in the US. The application consists of Clinical Trial Data: Clinical trials based on proof of the drug's efficacy and safety.

Manufacturing Information: Specifics regarding the facilities and methods of manufacturing.

Labeling: The right way to annotate a drug for safe application.

Regulations for Over-the-counter (OTC) Drugs

Through monographs that outline: Through monographs that outline:

Excipients, formulations, and doses—the FDA governs over-the-counter drugs.

Commencement of mandatory labeling with directions for use and potential adverse effects.

Risk Assessment and Mitigation Techniques

A risk assessment and mitigation techniques (REMS) program involving extra safety precautions is available for certain drugs that pose significant safety concerns. These may involve monitoring requirements, distribution regulations or triage training for healthcare professionals.

Guidelines for Biologics

Application for Biologics License (BLA)

Blood products, gene treatments, and vaccines are all biologics and must undergo a BLA submission in order to make sure that they're potent, safe, and pure.

There has to be:

Clinical Data: Data collected from clinical research, which shows the biologic is safe and effective.

Manufacturing Specifics: There must be strict regulatory criteria followed by the processes.

Post Market Surveillance: We continually see more safety issues with biologics, and follow (observed and watch) biologics for negative reactions [15].

Immunizations and Blood Products

On behalf of the Food and Drug Administration, the Centre for Biologics Evaluation and Research (CBER) reviews supplementary vaccinations. After a medicine hits the market, it must undergo post-market surveillance to ensure patient safety and track any adverse effects.

Guidelines for Medical Devices

Classification of Devices

Based on the risk they present to patients, medical gadgets are divided into three categories:

Bandages and other low-risk devices fall under Class I

Class I: They need very little in the way of regulatory oversight.

Class II: X-ray machines and other moderately risky gadgets. These call for stricter monitoring and might need 510(k) submissions for premarket clearance.

Class III: Devices that pose a high danger, like pacemakers. Premarket approval (PMA) and comprehensive clinical testing are necessary for these.

Human Factors Engineering

Medical equipment need to be developed with human factors engineering (HFE) in mind to reduce the possibility of user mistakes. The ease of use and safety of the gadgets in practical situations are guaranteed by human factors engineering.

Guidelines for Cosmetics

Safety and Labeling

Cosmetics must follow specific safety and labeling criteria even though they are not subject to premarket approval:

All components must be listed on labels, and goods cannot make deceptive or false claims (such as "FDA approved" when none has been reviewed by the FDA).

Ingredients used in cosmetics must be safe to use. The FDA is able to take a product off the market if it harms consumers.

Reporting Adverse Events

It is mandatory for manufacturers to disclose significant adverse occurrences linked to the usage of cosmetics. Direct reports of these instances to the FDA are also accepted from consumers and medical professionals.

Guidelines for Tobacco Products

Applications for Premarket Tobacco Products (PMTA)

Things become much simpler after 2007—if it's a new tobacco product that's offered, it must undergo a PMTA review. The maker must prove the product's suitability for safeguarding the public's health.

Marketing Limitations and Labeling

The FDA sets stringent regulations for restricting young access to tobacco product marketing. It includes restrictions on labels with graphic warnings and advertising.

Authorization for Emergency Use (EUA)

During public health emergencies, the FDA may authorize for Emergency Use of an unapproved medical product or an unapproved use of an approved medical product. This ensures that in the event of substitution nonavailability, we have the available products promptly and urgently, for example, a vaccine or therapy against a new disease.

Post-market Monitoring and Compliance

After a product hits the market, the FDA has good ways of monitoring things and an eye on things. This comprises:

- Systems for reporting adverse events (AERS): This system publishes manufacturer, medical expert, and consumer-reported adverse events for medicines and biologics.

- Recalls and Enforcement Actions: Under law, the FDA can recall products that are not ready or put the public at threat of its health by stopping production, confiscating goods, or warn to public.
- Inspections: GMPs compliance is guaranteed by routine inspections of manufacturing facilities and GMPs.

European Medicines Agency

The European Medicines Agency (EMA) regulates a wide range of pharmaceuticals for both humans and animals. Its primary responsibilities include developing technical guidelines, coordinating nationwide referrals, and evaluating and monitoring medications that are centrally authorized. Pharmaceutical sponsors can also receive scientific guidance from the agency. Its duties encompass a broad spectrum of pharmaceuticals, such as herbal remedies, biologics, and sophisticated treatments. About 4,500 professionals from more than 40 National Competent Authorities (NCAs) in EU member states provide help to the EMA in its operations. Because of its decentralized structure, the EMA may use a wealth of experience while still having administrative control from its management board.

The agency is divided into many sections, such as the Directorate, Patient Health Protection, Veterinary Medicines, and Human Medicines Development and Evaluation.

In addition to approving the budget and choosing the executive director, the Management Board is in charge of the administrative responsibilities of the Emergency Management Agency. The board is comprised of delegates from each of the 27 member states of the European The European Union, along with lawmakers and commissioners from the EU, and groups that advocate for people's health (including vets, patients, and farmers).

Seven specialized committees make up the EMA, which is in charge of supervising the agency's scientific activity. This group of committees includes the following: CHMP, CVMP, COMP, HMPC, PDCO, CAT, PRAC, and the Committee for Medicinal Products for Veterinary Use and Orphan Medicinal Products.

It is vital to have each of these committees in order to conduct the review of specific categories of medications. It is the responsibility of the COMP, for instance, to designate medications for unusual conditions as orphan drugs, but the CHMP is in charge of appraising human medical products. The Pharmaceutical Risk Assessment Committee (PRAC) was established in 2012 with the intention of utilizing pharmacovigilance in order to assess the safety of medications. The EMA's participation in the unified marketing authorization process is a top priority. Pharmaceutical businesses can now apply to the EMA once and receive a marketing license applicable in all EU member states, Iceland, Liechtenstein, and Norway with only one application.

Certain types of medications, such as those produced from biotechnology, sophisticated therapies, and treatments for illnesses including HIV/AIDS, cancer, and neurological disorders, require this centralized approach. Additionally, items that offer substantial medicinal, scientific or advances in technology. The European Union can more swiftly and effectively make innovative medicines available thanks to the centralization of marketing authority. The history of the EMA has been marked by a number of significant crossroads. Until the agency was formally founded in 1995, the countries that make up the EU engaged in negotiations for a period of seven years. The body for Veterinary Medicinal Products and the Committee for Proprietary Medicinal Products were both replaced by this body, despite the fact that both committees were reconstituted as significant scientific advisory organizations. Beginning in March 2019, the EMA relocated from its previous home in London to Amsterdam. The Brexit, or British exit from the European Union, is the catalyst for this transfer. After a long and difficult selection process involving many EU member states, Amsterdam was chosen as the new host city in November 2017. Throughout its history, the EMA has played a significant role in numerous significant projects. The 2012 World Health Assembly accepted the Global Vaccine Action Plan as one of these initiatives. The group has a number of global collaborations going on as part of its operations. There are a number of collaborations in this area, such as IPRP, CEPI, and the ICH (International Council for Harmonization of Technical Requirements for Pharmaceuticals for Human Use).

The EMA was instrumental in 2020 in the effort to speed up the approval and development of COVID-19 vaccines and medications as a component of the European Union's (EU) reaction to the pandemic. It was a part of the public-private partnership known as the Accelerating COVID-19 Therapeutic Interventions and Therapies (ACTIV) program, which aims to speed up research and development of pharmaceutical products and vaccines by setting priorities and coordinating several initiatives [16]. In spite of this, the EMA's dedication to evaluating, supervising, and authorizing pharmaceutical products for public and animal health purposes has made it the European cornerstone in protecting public and animal health. Ensuring that patients in the European Union have access to safe, effective, and high-quality medications requires the agency depends on its scientific committees, international collaborations, and centralized marketing authorization system. As a result of its commitment to the fight against COVID-19, the EMA has demonstrated its significance in both the ordinary regulatory role and the response to global health crises.

Guidelines for Quality

Good Manufacturing Practices

The GMP principles set forth by the EMA guarantee the consistent production and control of pharmaceutical products in accordance with quality requirements. From the distribution of the final product to the raw materials, they cover every facet of production. GMP adherence is a requirement for all EU pharmaceutical producers [17].

Biosimilars and Biologics

Because they are derived from live organisms, biological drugs are inherently unpredictable due to their chemical composition. The EMA has established specific standards that address the quality, safety, and efficacy of biologics and biosimilars. Biosimilars are modifications to commercially existing biological drugs that do not significantly modify the outcomes of treatment.

Methods of Analysis

In the context of quality control, accurate analytical data is a very important issue. The EMA offers guidelines for the validation of analytical techniques used to test raw materials, intermediates and finished products.

Safety Instructions

Studies on Nonclinical Safety

Before it begins human clinical trials, drugs need to undergo considerable non-clinical (preclinical) safety testing. The EMA [18] provides comprehensive instructions on how to conduct these investigations; investigations that look at a substance's toxicological profile, including its potential mutagenic, carcinogenic and reproductive effects.

Information on Clinical Safety

However, as explained by the EMA, getting solid clinical safety data across different phases of clinical trials is very important. In addition, guidelines apply to the reporting and monitoring of adverse events in order to ensure prior to market approval, that the drug's risk profile is fully known.

Plans for Risk Management (RMPs)

An RMP is needed by pharmaceutical businesses to monitor and diminish product-related risks from one point to the next within the product lifecycle. Pharmacovigilance initiatives, post-authorization safety studies, and risk minimization strategies will be part of these plans.

Efficacy Criteria

Research Studies

Guidelines for planning and carrying out are provided by EMA. The recommendations pertain to patient selection, trial design, ethical issues, and statistical methods for the statistical collection of credible efficacy data.

Drug Development for Pediatric

EMAs guidance emphasizes the importance of conducting pediatric-specific clinical studies to ensure that drugs intended for pediatric use are safe and show efficacy. The stage of the development of medicinal products in the EU requires a mandatory Pediatric Investigation Plan (PIP).

Pharmacovigilance

Reporting Adverse Drug Reactions

Any adverse drug reactions (ADRs) experienced during the course of a drug's lifetime must be reported by pharmaceutical companies and healthcare professionals. The purpose of the EMA's ADR reporting rules is to guarantee that all pharmaceuticals are continuously monitored for safety [19].

Periodic Safety Update Reports

Periodic safety update reports (PSURs) are essential for keeping the safety profile of pharmaceuticals on the market current. Manufacturers are required by the EMA to produce PSURs on a regular basis. These reports provide an overview of all safety data gathered.

Signal Recognition

Guidelines for "signal detection," or the process of spotting early indicators of problems with medication safety, are provided by the EMA. Numerous data sources, like clinical trials, unplanned reporting, and scholarly publications, are used to generate these signals.

Rare Diseases and Orphan Medications

Beneficiaries of orphan medications include those who suffer from uncommon illnesses with the benefit of exclusive market access. The EMA dictates on its website the orphan drug application for orphan drug designation.

Post-authorization Protocols

Modifications to the Marketing Authorization

The EMA details procedures for handling post-authorization modifications of drug composition, labeling or manufacturing processes. Holders of marketing authorizations are obliged to observe some regulations to preserve the integrity of their products.

Advanced Therapies

Advanced Therapy Medicinal Products (ATMPs), such as gene treatments and tissue-engineered products, are "because of their intricacy and their unique nature," regulated in a particular way. The EMA provides a regulatory framework to help bring these new cutting-edge treatments to the market [20].

Evaluations of Environmental Risks

The EMA requires pharmaceutical companies to assess the possible environmental risks their medicines may pose. They assess the possible effects that drug residues can have on ecosystems, in particular in aquatic systems.

All pharmaceutical companies wishing to do business in the European Union are bound to comply with the EMA guidelines. The result is an in-depth regulatory framework guaranteeing quality, safety, and efficacy of medicinal products in the EU. The guidelines apply to the entire drug lifecycle, from the development to post-marketing surveillance, especially for advanced therapies, orphan drugs and environmental risks.

Ethical Considerations in Drug Discovery

That is a hard and important process of finding, creating and approving new therapeutic agents. For saving human subjects and protecting the integrity of science, this procedure must be performed according to strict ethical guidelines. History has given us lessons from drug discovery ethics; morality's precepts, the framework of law, what could go wrong in human research, etc.

Historical Background

Malpractice in Health Research

Medical research is considered a very long-established branch of history, and such unethical practices have seriously injured the public's confidence in this field. In the United States, in 1932, 1972, this case in point of the Tuskegee Syphilis Study, African American males were utilized and used in a study without their knowledge, and treated unconscionably. This is about WWII testing with the same sort of disdain for human personhood and dignity as Nazi physicians. On the other hand, human participant studies also seem obvious [21] and require ethical supervision.

Creation of Ethical Standards

Given these breaches, some ethical standards were created:

- The Nuremberg Code (1947) lays out the basic rules for ethical research and requires informed consent.
- The World Medical Association created the Declaration of Helsinki in 1964, which is a comprehensive set of moral guidelines for medical research involving human subjects with an emphasis on participant welfare and informed consent.
- The three principles of beneficence, justice and respect for people are outlined in The Belmont Report (1979) and still apply today.
- These standards set expectations and obligations for researchers and are the cornerstone of ethical behavior in drug discovery.

Fundamental Ethical Concepts

Individual Respect

Respect for people, which means valuing their freedom and dignity, is an important principle in the development of new medicines.

Informed Consent: Participants in research should understand what this research involves, including its aims, methods, potential risks and benefits, and the option to stop at any time. With a clear and easy-to-understand visual system, they should be able to make clear, informed choices without stress.

Vulnerable Populations: People with cognitive impairments, inmates, and children are among the vulnerable groups that need special attention. Researchers are responsible for making sure that these subjects' rights are upheld and that they are not mistreated [22].

Help

Researchers have a duty to minimize harm and maximize potential benefits, which is known as beneficence.

Risk-Benefit Analysis: Prior to starting a study, researchers must perform extensive risk-benefit analyses. In order to properly analyze the expected advantages of the research, it is necessary to look closely at any possible social, psychological, and bodily hazards [23].

Safety and Monitoring: To quickly detect negative effects, experiments must be subjected to constant monitoring. The trial should be stopped to protect participants if, at any point, the dangers exceed the benefits [24].

Justice

Equity theory emphasizes fairness in the selection of research participants and the allocation of good and bad.

Fair Recruitment: Diverse recruitment methods that represent the communities affected by the research are an important goal for researchers. This prevents the exploitation of certain groups and ensures that all groups benefit from the research.

Reducing Health Disparities: It is important to include disadvantaged groups in clinical trials because their exclusion can lead to differences in treatment outcomes and access to health care.

Normative Structures

Institutional Review Boards (IRBs)

An Institutional review board, or IRB, reviews research proposals to ensure compliance with ethical standards. Their responsibilities include:

Examining Protocols: IRBs review research policies to ensure that they are ethical and protect the rights of participants [25].

Informed permission: They oversee the process of obtaining informed consent and ensure that participants are adequately informed about the study [26].

Risk Assessment: The IRB is responsible for determining whether the benefits of the study outweigh the risks [27].

Good Clinical Practice

The International Committee for Harmonization (ICH) guidelines for GCP provide the basis forethical and scientific conduct of clinical trials.

Quality assurance: From design to reporting, GCP emphasizes the importance of maintaining high standards throughout the course.

Accountability: Researchers must ensure that all research procedures are documented so that all procedures can be reviewed and audited.

International Law

The importance of adhering to international law cannot be overstated when considering the fact that pharmaceutical research frequently involves multinational collaboration.

There is a possibility that protections are less stringent in nations with low and moderate incomes, and the World Health Organization (WHO) offers guidelines for research misconduct.

In order to guarantee that clinical trials adhere to both scientific and ethical standards, it is the responsibility of the EMA to regulate and enforce legislation across the entirety of Europe.

Obstacles in the Discovery of Legal Drugs

Populations at Risk

Good judgment is important when conducting research with vulnerable populations.

Informed Consent for Minors: In addition to the consent of the child, obtaining parental consent is also critical to obtaining the consent of the child. Researchers must exercise caution in the ethical arena and put the best interests of the child first.

Studies with People with Cognitive Impairments: Alternative methods should be used in research involving people with intellectual disabilities to ensure that participants are willing and knowledgeable.

Variety in the Field of Study

A key ethical question relates to the lack of diversity in clinical trials.

The Implications of Using Homogeneous Samples Are as Follows

Research findings obtained from homogenous groups may not be generalizable to larger and more heterogeneous populations. Health disparities can perpetuate inefficient treatment.

Inclusive Recruitment Strategies

Interrogating a diversity of cultures and environments by being immersed in and providing a space where mutual trust can form, all by utilizing culturally sensitive recruitment strategies, will make research more diverse.

Financial Payments

Although payment in cash for participating in scientific trials is standard, it leads to ethical problems.

Risks of Coercion: Scientists have to ensure that money doesn't push people who shouldn't be pushed to act in spite of what is good for them, what is in the best interest of their own survival.

Regulatory Oversight: To minimize coercive effects, concrete guidelines on the form and amount of recompense should be defined.

Particular Ethical Problems

Placebo Use

There are certain ethical questions related to the application of placebos in clinical studies.

Ethical Justification: The use of placebos, according to the Declaration of Helsinki, is not allowed if there are no significant risks and no other alternative treatment. Placebo use cannot be unethical and scientifically admissible to be used by researchers.

Potential Hazard: Patients in placebo groups may have more extreme symptoms or a greater duration of treatment, which would be worrying from the patients' standpoint [28].

Research on Stem Cells

There are many ethical issues in stem cell research, especially when it comes to the source of the stem cells. The utilization of embryonic stem cells gives rise to ethical concerns regarding the ethical standing of embryos. Countries have very different regulations, which makes research more difficult.

Ethical Substitutes: Developments in induced pluripotent stem cells (iPSCs) offer substitutes that could alleviate some of the moral issues surrounding embryonic stem cells.

Transparency of Data: Ethical integrity in research requires maintaining transparency.

Publication Bias: It is common for good results to be published more frequently than negative ones, which distorts opinions about the effectiveness of drugs.

Clinical Trial Registries: These open databases support accountability and openness by guaranteeing that all research, no matter how they turn out, is recorded and available to the public.

Important Clinical Trial Ethical Issues

Clinical trial researchers have a core concern for striking a balance between scientific advancement and patient safety. The public will be presented with a possibly life-saving procedure if all goes as planned. Nevertheless, the therapy will be rejected if the search for a novel treatment jeopardizes patient safety in any way during the trials. Yes, there is a lot on the line, which is why ethical issues are so important. When conducting trials, researchers need to take into account the following five crucial ethical issues:

Phase I: To assess a new medication or treatment's safety, establish a safe dosage range, and pinpoint any side effects, researchers test it initially on a small number of participants [29].

Phase II: A broader population is administered the medication or treatment to assess its efficacy and further assess its safety [30].

Phase III: The medication or therapy is administered to sizable cohorts in order to verify efficacy, track adverse events, contrast it with standard treatments, and gather data necessary for the medication or therapy to be used safely [31].

Phase IV: Research is conducted on the effects of the medication in different demographics and evaluates potential long-term side effects after the treatment or medication has been commercialized [32].

Laws and Standards Regarding Drugs

Drug Guidelines

The United States uses the following set of drug standards: Pharmacopoeia of the States (USP). Our country's Pharmacopoeia, with the National Formulary, a reliable resource (USP-NF). Regarding medication standards (dosage, forms, medicinal ingredients, excipients, supplements, biologics, and compounded preparations), they are released once a year. Experts in microbiology, chemistry, pharmaceutics, nursing, and pharmacology all make contributions. Medications have rigorous requirements for therapeutic use, patient safety, quality, purity, strength, and packaging safety in order to be listed in the USP-NF. As well as the dosage manner. The initials "USP" are included in the official name of drugs that achieve these requirements, signifying their widespread acceptance as superior products. In 1951, the International Pharmacopoeia was initially released. It provides a foundation for the World Health Organization's (WHO) requirements on the potency and make-up of medications for use all over the planet [33].

Drug discovery, the process of discovery, generates a variety of complex ethical issues that need to be taken into consideration in order to protect subjects and the integrity of the research. Compliance with ethics and the ability to cope with new challenges will be an iterative process, as the drug development environment changes. It is critical that there is collaboration among stakeholders, such as the public, regulatory authorities and investigators, to establish ethical guidelines to protect human dignity and advance scientific understanding.

Future Directions and Challenges

The Role of Bioethics in Drug Development Going Forward

The pharmaceutical sector is one of several that have had to change as a result of scientific and technical advances. Pharma companies are looking for ways to modernize the drug development process to keep up with the rapid pace of change caused by the rise of new technologies such as artificial intelligence (AI) and the resulting complex ethical and regulatory challenges. Pharmaceutical researchers may soon be dealing with an altogether new set of bioethical challenges, such as the following:

Both Machine Learning and AI

Software with AI is already being used to automate a number of drug development processes, including evaluating therapeutic compounds and keeping an eye on product quality. The technology of AI and machine learning is developing quickly, and as we become increasingly reliant on it, a number of ethical issues arise.

While automating certain procedures with AI can save both time and money, there's a chance that algorithmic decision-making void of human judgment won't detect research bias, and if mistakes are made, there won't be any personal accountability. Regulators will place a high premium on resolving these moral conundrums as AI grows in significance for Pharmaceutical companies.

Environmental Morality

Pharmaceutical companies are only one of many businesses and governments throughout the world that have made reducing climate change a primary concern. Pharmaceutical corporations currently go to great lengths to ensure that their products comply with environmental laws, and given the ever-changing ethical landscape around global health, they will also be striving to adopt sustainable production practices. Ensuring an equitable allocation of remedies for global health emergencies will become increasingly important as medicine becomes more globally interconnected.

Information Security

Data sharing versus individual privacy is something clinical researchers are often struggling with. Since computer systems are increasingly being used to store vast amounts of sensitive data, this moral dilemma is only going to be more difficult to resolve. Data security issue is raised by the data collected using wearables and electronic health records, and regulators will be watching very carefully in the future.

In clinical trial processes, ethical problems should be given utmost importance to ensure the patients' privacy, the integrity of scientific research and patient safety. Informed consent should be obtained, subjects should be selected carefully, risk-benefit analysis has to be performed, patients' information should be protected, post-interventional follow-up care has to be performed.

Advances in the drug development world will lead to new bioethical problems related to data security, environmental sustainability, and moral use of AI. The pharmaceutical industry can continue to roll out improved medical therapies while maintaining public safety and trust by placing ethics at the heart of drug development.

Difficulties in the Discovery of Drugs

Time-consuming and Expensive Procedures

Drug discovery is notoriously expensive and time-consuming. Development times typically exceed 10 years, and costs are often in excess of $billions. Very high attrition rates drive up the cost burden and delay the introduction of new therapies, in particular in advanced clinical studies. However, the complexity of biological systems, stringent regulations and high rates of failure due to unexpected toxicity or lack of efficacy are all factors that are involved [33–35].

Challenges Related to Regulations

The surroundings of regulation for drug discovery are one of the most challenging issues to tackle. Regulatory agencies demand a high level of evidence of both safety and efficacy, and permission can be a lengthy process and very expensive. Approval process becomes more challenging due to the necessity to meet evolving, different regulatory requirements in multiple regions [36–38]. The increasing complexity of regulation also increases the responsibility to perform extensive testing and documentation, making it necessary, further lengthen development timelines.

Validation of the Target and Biological Complexity

Since biological systems are inherently complex, it remains a significant challenge to effectively validate pharmacological targets [39, 40]. Because of an insufficient understanding of disease processes and of off-target effects, a large number of potential targets do not make it to successful drugs. The multifactorial nature of human biology, driven by both genetic diversity and environmental factors, adds further complexity to the assessment of treatment effect [41].

Adaptation and Resistance

Establishment of resistance to medication (e.g., in the case of cancer and infectious diseases is a significant challenge. Pathogens and cancer cells' fast adaptation to therapeutic forces makes the use of current therapies ineffective. Long-term treatment efficacy is tied to the emergence of resistance-busting approaches, including combination treatments and novel pharmacological targets [42–48].

Social and Ethical Aspects

Concerns about ethics and society are brought up by developments in drug discovery, particularly in fields like gene editing and customized medicine. It is important to carefully consider issues pertaining to genetic privacy, equal access to cutting-edge medicines, and the possibility of unforeseen repercussions from genetic interventions. Properly advancing drug discovery technology requires recognizing societal implications and upholding ethical standards [49–53].

Conclusion

In the future, it is anticipated that AI will play a role in the rapid acceleration and simplification of the pharmaceutical development process. AI has the ability to revolutionize drug development by utilizing robots and models of genetic targets, medications, organs, diseases and their evolution, pharmacokinetics, safety, and efficacy. This could lead to a major data and capital-intensive industry. The use of AI has the ability to streamline and reduce the expense of drug discovery and development while simultaneously increasing its speed and efficiency. Unlike the expectation that selecting a single lead chemical would ensure the creation of a cure that is both safe and effective, AI is already being utilized in the process of discovering potential medicines against the Ebola virus. This is similar to the process that is used in the drug development cycle.

References

1. Gupta P, Kumar A. Regulation of pharmaceuticals in India: Challenges and prospects. Indian J Health Res. 2018;34(2):123–130.
2. Sharma R, Mehta S, Singh A. The role of CDSCO in India's pharmaceutical landscape. J Regul Aff. 2017;25(1):50–58.
3. Choudhury N, Agarwal P, Rao K. Regulatory challenges in drug pricing and research ethics in India. Indian J Pharm Policy. 2020;19(4):200–210.
4. Reddy B, Aparasu R. Pricing and research policies in India pharmaceuticals: An overview. Int J Health Policy Manag. 2019;8(3):155–162.
5. Bhambulkar K, Patil M. Coordination of regulatory agencies in India's pharmaceutical sector. J Public Health Policy. 2020;22(1):100–108.
6. Nayak CB, Singh A, Kumar P. Ethical dimensions of efficacy in drug development: A review. J Med Ethics. 2018;44(1):90–98.
7. Carpenter D. Reputation and Power: Organizational Image and Pharmaceutical Regulation at the FDA. Princeton University Press; 2010.

8. Swann JP. FDA and the practice of pharmacy: Prescription drug regulation before the food, drug and cosmetic act of 1938. Pharm Hist. 1990;32(1):21–36.
9. Angell M. The Truth About the Drug Companies: How They Deceive Us and What to Do About It. New York: Random House; 2004.
10. Hilts PJ. Protecting America's Health: The FDA, Business, and One Hundred Years of Regulation. Alfred A. Knopf; 2003.
11. Carpenter D. Is health politics different? The political economy of the FDA. Annu Rev Polit Sci. 2014;17(1):77–96.
12. Daemmrich A. Pharmacopolitics: Drug Regulation in the United States and Germany. University of North Carolina Press; 2004.
13. U.S. Food and Drug Administration. Federal Food, Drug, and Cosmetic Act. 1938. Available from: https://www.fda.gov/regulatory-information/laws-enforced-fda/federal-food-drug-and-cosmetic-act-fdc-act
14. U.S. Food and Drug Administration. Current Good Manufacturing Practice (CGMP) Regulations. 2023. Available from: https://www.fda.gov/drugs/pharmaceutical-quality-resources/drug-manufacturing
15. U.S. Food and Drug Administration. Biologics License Application (BLA). 2023. Available from: https://www.fda.gov/vaccines-blood-biologics/biologics-licensing-applications
16. European Medicines Agency. Guideline on non-clinical safety studies for the conduct of human clinical trials and marketing authorization for pharmaceuticals (ICH M3(R2)). 2018. Available from: https://www.ema.europa.eu/en/documents/scientific-guideline/ich-guideline-non-clinical-safety-studies-conduct-human-clinical-trials-marketing-authorisation_en.pdf
17. European Medicines Agency. Guideline on the quality, non-clinical and clinical aspects of gene therapy medicinal products. 2019. Available from: https://www.ema.europa.eu/en/documents/scientific-guideline/guideline-quality-non-clinical-clinical-aspects-gene-therapy-medicinal-products_en.pdf
18. Katz J. The Nuremberg code and the Nuremberg trial: A reappraisal. JAMA. 1996;276(20):1662–1666.
19. Sugarman J, McCrory DC, Powell D, Krasny A, Adams B, Ball E, et al. Empirical research on informed consent: An annotated bibliography. Hastings Cent Rep. 1998;28(6):S1–42.
20. Emanuel EJ, Wendler D, Grady C. What makes clinical research ethical? JAMA. 2000;283(20):2701–2711.
21. Lindegger G, Milford C, Slack C, Quayle M, Xaba X, Vardas E. Beyond the checklist: Assessing understanding for HIV vaccine trial participation in South Africa. J Acquir Immune Defic Syndr. 2006;43(5):560–566.
22. Lemmens T. The role of institutional review boards in the regulation of research. Bioethics. 2009;23(3):139–148.
23. Fisher CB. Ethics in Research With Children and Adolescents: A Casebook. New York: John Wiley & Sons; 2004.
24. Benson P, Gutterman EM, Grady C, Hull SC, Joffe S, McGraw D, Miller FG, Wendler D.. The IRB: A guide for investigators. Ethics Behav. 2006;16(2):149–157.
25. Hurst SA, Liddell K. Ethics and the use of placebo in clinical trials. Br J Clin Pharmacol. 2009;68(2):133–134.
26. Friedman LM, Furberg C, DeMets DL. Fundamentals of Clinical Trials. 5th ed. Springer; 2015.
27. Kuehn BM. Ethical issues in clinical trials. JAMA. 2011;306(24):2725–2726.
28. Califf RM, Sugarman J, Sargent J. The role of clinical trials in improving health care. N Engl J Med. 2014;371(22):2058–2060.
29. United States Pharmacopeia (USP). *United States Pharmacopeia and National Formulary (USP-NF)*. 2023. Available from: https://www.uspnf.com/
30. Ekins S, Rees S, Williams A, Williams G. The role of automation in high-throughput screening. Drug Discov Today. 2019;24(1):203–210.

31. DiMasi JA, Grabowski HG, Hansen RW. Innovation in the pharmaceutical industry: New estimates of R&D costs. J Health Econ. 2016;47:20–33.
32. Paul SM, Mytelka DS, Dunwiddie CT, Persinger CC, Munos BH, Lindborg SR, Schacht AL. How to improve R&D productivity: The pharmaceutical industry's grand challenge. Nat Rev Drug Discov. 2010;9(3):203–214.
33. Gupta A. Navigating regulatory requirements in drug discovery. Regul Aff J. 2020;12(2):89–102.
34. U.S. Food and Drug Administration. FDA approves first gene therapy for cancer. 2017 Sep 1. Available from: https://www.fda.gov/news-events/press-announcements/fda-approves-first-gene-therapy-cancer
35. Relling MV, Evans WE. Pharmacogenomics in the clinic. Nat Rev Genet. 2015; 16(4):252–260.
36. Bologa CG, Muresan S, Shoichet BK. Polypharmacology: The design or identification of multiple ligands or single targets that modulate multiple targets. Nat Rev Drug Discov. 2014;13(11):790–807.
37. June CH, O'Connor RS, Kawalekar OU, Ghassemi S, Milone MC, Grupp SA, Weissman IL. CAR t cell therapy: The first year in review. J Clin Oncol. 2018;36(17):1744–1753.
38. Sanchez-Rivera FJ, Jacks T. Use of CRISPR/Cas9 for cancer research and therapy. J Clin Oncol. 2015;33(5):567–574.
39. European Medicines Agency. EudraLex - Volume 4: EU guidelines for good manufacturing practice for medicinal products for human and veterinary use. 2023. Available from: https://health.ec.europa.eu/system/files/2023-03/eudralex_vol4_en_0.pdf
40. Jiang Q, Reichert JM. Bispecific antibodies: A mechanistic review of their structure and function. MAbs. 2017;9(3):386–396.
41. Pardi N, Hogan MJ, Porter FW, Weissman D. mRNA vaccines—a new era in vaccinology. Nat Rev Drug Discov. 2018;17(4):261–279.
42. Torchilin VP. Multifunctional, stimuli-sensitive nanoparticulate systems for drug delivery. Nat Rev Drug Discov. 2014;13(11):813–827.
43. Kuo TT, Kim HE, Ohno-Machado L. Blockchain distributed ledger technologies for biomedical and health care applications. J Am Med Inform Assoc. 2017; 24(6):1211–1220.
44. Atmakuri LR, Peeriga R, Begum S, Vallamkonda B, Baratam A. Novel bioanalytical LC-MS/MS method for determination of metoprolol in human plasma. J Appl Pharm Sci. 2024;14(12):131–138.
45. Peeriga R, Bangaru V GK. Implementation of the POCSO act in schools. In: Child Sexual Abuse: A Public Health Problem in India. Springer publications, Singapore. 2024. p. 391–413.
46. Peeriga R, Yarlagadda LC, Alla NR. Protection of children from sexual exploitation. In: Child Sexual Abuse: A Public Health Problem in India. Springer publications, Singapore.2024. p. 191–201.
47. Peeriga R, Shiek Arabath SAM, Manubolu K, Thelappilly BB, Yarlagadda LC. Insilico assessment of phytoconstituents in *myxopyrum smilacifolium* blume against arthritis. Biomed Pharmacol J. 2024;17(1):235–241.
48. Manubolu K, Balagani PK, Gope ER, Peeriga R, Sridevi AR. Unlocking the potential of aquasomes: A comprehensive review on innovative nanocarriers in drug delivery and beyond. Int J Chem Biochem Sci. 2023;24(6):405–410.
49. Manubolu K, Peeriga R, Bonthu MG, Gope ER, Kadirvel D. Evaluation of anti-inflammatory activity of *Millingtonia hortensis* leaf extract. Int J Chem Biochem Sci. 2023;24(6):380–385.
50. Peeriga R, Chandrasekhar KB. Comparative study of anti-inflammatory activity of petroleum ether extract of *myxopyrum smilacifolium* blume and ethanolic leaf extract of *pamburus missionis* swingle. J Pharm Sci Res. 2017;9(6):955–957.

51. Peeriga R, Manubolu K. (2025). Design strategies for waste reduction and enhanced recyclability in pharmaceutical packaging. In: Yingngam, B., Aslam, M.S., Haghi, A.K. (eds) Sustainable Pharmaceutical Product Development and Optimization Processes. Springer, Singapore.
52. Manubolu K, Peeriga R, Chandrasekhar KB. A short guide to clinical pharmacokinetics. 1st ed. 2024. Springer, Singapore.
53. Manubolu K, Peeriga R. (2025). Ecodesign principles. In: Yingngam, B., Aslam, M.S., Haghi, A.K. (eds) Sustainable Pharmaceutical Product Development and Optimization Processes. Springer, Singapore.

11 Conclusion and Future Prospects on Drug Discovery

Talamanchi Balakrishna, Raveesha Peeriga, Krishnaveni Manubolu, K. N. V. Chenchu Lakshmi, Miriyala Preethika, Nimmagadda Sai Sruthi, and Afsar Shaik

Introduction

A new drug discovery field has come of age, with dramatic progress and the exposure of difficult challenges befitting a new age. Drug discovery historically has been an expensive, combative process that depends on random hits and a long and expensive search and variation process. Early methods were empirical and involved testing of compounds with no predictability, where occasionally success would be had, but with sometimes discrepant results and little predictive accuracy. Although foundational, the traditional approach was inadequate for ensuring the efficient and effective development of drugs, laying the foundation for more advanced approaches [1, 2].

Unfortunately, HTS technology came along much later and has turned the field upside down by allowing researchers to quickly assay thousands of compounds with greater precision in recent years. As they did, these advancements have sped up the initial stages of drug discovery and helped to identify promising candidates at a greater efficiency than prior [3]. Advances in these technologies, coupled with the development of advanced computational models and bioinformatics tools, have improved the prediction of drug interactions, lead compound optimization and the streamlining of the drug development process.

The second is the integration of genomic and proteomic data to define the landscape of targets for new drug discovery. Certain genetically mapped diseases have since led us to understand the mechanisms by which certain diseases operate from the mapping of the human genome and learning of genetic variants associated with various diseases [4]. Using this genomic knowledge, targeted therapies have been developed that seek to address spliceable molecular pathways thought to contribute to disease, and these therapies have been more personalized and more effective. Such developments in systems biology and molecular modeling have also enabled a greater understanding of complex biological systems, to better inform the identification of drug targets.

These are exciting times, and promising, but the path from drug discovery to market remains treacherous. A big barrier is the high cost of research and development—and estimates suggest it can take over $2.6 billion to develop a new drug. Adding to this, the regulatory requirements are extremely stiff, and the attrition

DOI: 10.4324/9781003564041-11

rate in clinical trials is very high. Problems with safety, efficacy, or unforeseen side effects account for many of the reasons why so many promising compounds don't make it past initial testing. Also, drug resistance is mounting, and treatments are needed that individualize to genetic profiles, making the drug development process even more complex

Some new trends and technologies in the future could really solve these problems and dramatically change drug discovery. Increased application of AI and machine learning (ML) in drug discovery and their offer of new visions of looking at big data, guessing how drugs will be active, and creating compounds gives the industry hope for growth and further development. Improved nanotechnology and drug delivery enhance the ability of treatment to be much more targeted and efficient. Such advancement may help in lowering the rate of side effects and even raise results for patients [5, 6]. Furthermore, personalizing medicine and making plans in an individualized way may shift the approach through which treatments are developed and administered, so that options for patients can become better and more fitting.

This chapter intends to trace an explicit image of drug discovery in its current times. It will, therefore, focus on some recent important discoveries and explain their implications in the field and look forward into trends and technology changes that are likely to influence future development. This analysis examines the success and the problems it currently faces to offer information regarding the future of drug discovery. It looks forward to demonstrating how it can meet medical needs and enhance health around the globe.

Summary of Key Findings

Overview of Results: The "Overview of Results" section summarizes the most important findings and insights arising from research or analysis in drug discovery. Recent studies have been marked by several significant achievements and trends that have altered the face of this field. Technologies of HTS make researchers search for potential candidates more speedily and effectively, and decrease the time and costs related to the early stages of drug discovery significantly. Besides, breakthroughs in genomics and proteomics have discovered new drug targets as well as provided targeted treatments that are designed for a specific genetic profile. The new drug delivery systems studied, such as nanoparticles and liposomes, have shown promise to enhance effectiveness while reducing the side effects of treatments. With all these advancements, problems are still there. Those issues involve a high dropout rate among people in clinical trials and the problem of not turning early research results into real therapeutic drugs [7]. Both emphasize progress in improving the efficiency of drug discovery and more importantly need to handle issues remaining to hasten the development of new and viable drugs.

Patterns and Trends: The drug discovery field is undergoing significant change in several key aspects and trends. AI's algorithms predict drug interactions sometimes even before a computer finally decides which is the best compound. In this way, they also make HTS technologies skillfully, which is a big step toward an efficient way to test compounds. Genomics and pharmacogenomics are the primary reasons why personalized medicine is becoming more and more common nowadays. This method positively affects research that is focused on the genetic condition of every person. Biologicals, monoclonal antibodies, and advanced treatments that include gene and cell therapies are the options for patients who are on the rise. Regenerative medicine, about stem cell research and biomechanical effectiveness, brings hope to address diseases which were earlier untreatable. The main issue here is global health—it is the low-cost availability of the medicines and the collaboration on high levels between countries in its improvement, especially in low- and middle-income ones [8, 9].

Universal practice has already started using omics technology (proteomics, genomics, and metabolomics). This allows them to understand the health problems of diseases and to detect the existence of the drugs' targets. The era of targeted treatments and personalized medicines is currently and consistently increasing with the evolution of the interlocked molecular considerations or genetic changes that are predominantly pursued through therapeutic intervention. Using digital health tools and big data analysis improves real-time patient data in drug discovery and Eumenes large sets of data. There is more and more teamwork and open science within research and development. Open data projects and public-private partnerships (PPPs) are helping much to accelerate innovation and remove the existing problem of wasting time and resources from repeated research. Regulation is changing through agile plans and the increased use of real-world evidence (RWE), which accelerates drug development. Finally, sustainability is also essential, with new research emphasizing green chemistry in the drug production process. These new technologies and phenomena follow each other closely, driving the drug discovery process and finally leading to better health for the patient and reducing global health concerns.

Significant Data Insights

Lexical, syntactical, and grammatical errors are disallowed. In pharmacology, the importance of compiling data insights is necessary for driving clinical biotechnology development and improving patient responses. Such omic data would be, for example, delicate genomic sequencing or proteome, meaning in-depth understanding of disease mechanisms, such as characterizing genetic mutations and variations and revealing protein interactions and metabolic pathways. HTS initially yield many vital insights into the efficacy and specificity of series derived from large libraries tasked with identifying potentially ideal drug candidates [10]. Clinical trial data that expresses how efficacious the drug is and how safe the electronic health records and patient registries are in providing information advisory to drug development and other regulatory approvals decisions. Pharmacokinetic and pharmacodynamic data basically help all parties concerned with characterizing a drug regarding its absorption and metabolic activities and its relieving effect on the targets in order to optimize effective dosing and identify a wide range of adverse reactions. Biomarker discovery enables tracking of disease progression as well as treatment response, leading to individualized patient therapy. Digital health tools, e.g., wearables and mobile apps, track health indicators in near real-time, increasing the understanding of drug effectiveness and compliance. Computer modeling and simulation provide a platform for an attempt to unify all data at its center in attempt to explain drug interaction and guide drug design. Finally, through collaborative data-sharing/open data initiatives, research has been accelerated; knowledge pooled together forms the basis for furthering innovation. Therefore, these collections of data insights are at the fore-ground in sublimating drug development processes and targeting complicated health issues [11, 12].

Key Matrix and Statics

Drug discovery key metrics and statistics are critical to understanding the success and efficiency of the entire drug development process. Metrics such as hit rate and lead optimization success indicate the effectiveness of mixture-based HTS and the transition of drug candidates from early-stage discovery to optimized leads. Success rates for clinical trials are key statistics offering the percentage of drug candidates advancing through the many phases of the clinical development process to finally gain regulatory approval [13]. The time-to-market metric records how long the whole drug-development process takes, from discovery to availability on the market, indicating the overall speed of the development process. Return on investments, determining how much money goes from the overall development processes, providing analysis on how much money will be made or lost versus how much was spent. Clinical trial safety and efficacy statistics provide deep insights into the performance of the drug, its side effects, and therapeutic outcomes, all of which are central to any approval from a regulatory authority and to the acceptance of this new drug in the market. Biomarker validation shows the rates of how reliable they might be in disease diagnosis and treatment monitoring. Finally, patient compliance rates and drug effectiveness data describe how patients comply when prescribed therapy and how effective the drug is outside a clinical environment [14]. These statistics and metrics are important for directing decision-making on the proper and optimized development of strategies to ensure a successful launch of new therapies into the market.

Comparative Analysis

In drug discovery comparative analysis is the process of comparing and contrasting different aspects of drugs, approaches, and technologies for the purpose of learning what is worse or better. During the process, several drug compounds are contrasted regarding their efficacy and the safety profile, as well as the mode of action. For instance, the effectiveness of a treatment might be determined by the effectiveness of a new drug in the treatment compared with an established standard of care, and the safety profile might be determined by the incidence and severity of adverse events during clinical trials. Moreover, the methodological analysis itself may also ultimately become methodological methods that provide a mechanism by which HTS methods versus other methods might be used to compare HTS methods to alternative methods in the course of screening to determine the validity and accuracy of HTS screens in discovering drug candidates. Technologies based on AI and ML vs. conventional drug discovery approaches for their influence on time, cost, and power to predict. Cost-effectiveness is also one of the significant issues where the cost of development of various drug candidates is compared with their predicted return in the market, therapeutic value and utility. Through comparative analysis, investigators and developers can rationally select the most likely candidate drug molecules and/or approaches, and iteratively adapt the development process in order to improve the prospect that therapeutic responses will be successful. By means of a systematic screening, this selection can not only facilitate drug screening, but also enhance resource utilization and, hence, expedite the development of successful novel therapeutics.

Unexpected Findings

Particularly, surprising results have dramatically changed the horizon of drug discovery, which have, in many cases, paved the way to significant breakthrough developments. Serendipitous findings, e.g., penicillin and sildenafil, have changed the treatment strategy by showing novel uses outside of their originally intended use. Historically considered to be pure literals, off-target events have been shown to have novel therapeutic benefits, as evidenced by the transition from a sedative to an anti-cancer drug of thalidomide. In addition, clinical trial failures have also driven drug repositioning, as, for example, the case of raloxifene, which evolved from a less attractive breast cancer drug to an osteoporosis treatment [15]. Unanticipated serendipitous discoveries have led to the search for biomarkers, e.g., HER2 in breast cancer, which are currently brought to the forefront by the application of targeted therapies. Sometimes these surprising results can be used to uncover new mechanisms of action (e.g., the discovery of immune checkpoint inhibitors as anticancer treatments).

Drug discovery in the future will be aided by the acceptance, and more importantly, systematic derivation of paradoxical findings. Drug repurposing and repositioning are anticipated to provide timely and cost-effective therapeutics, especially in the context of novel emerging diseases. Personalization of treatment and AI-driven analysis of these will also contribute toward the detection and exploitation of these in a more targeted and effective manner, resulting in more precise therapies. Open sharing and data collaboration among research teams and the pharma industry will be of great importance to speed up the frequency of innovations. Given the ongoing progress of drug development, ethical considerations have to be addressed, particularly when repurposing a drug to a new indication. For the most part, serendipitous discoveries will continue to be an impetus to drug discovery innovation and medical evolution in the future [16].

Highlights of Success and Failures

In the drug discovery process, successes and failures are equally important to the development of this field. Successes can be recognized in discoveries that resulted in important drug approvals and life-saving treatments. The drug repurposing (i.e., failure to be successful at first use) has also turned out as an extraordinary success, showing the industry's capability to transform. Coordinated effort between pharmaceutical companies, academic centers and the authorities has provided a drug development boost, whereas the introduction of AI and personalized medicine has led to more focused and successful therapy for patients [17]. But the route to success is normally littered with failures. Clinically driven trials are often abandoned prematurely because of toxicity issues or lack of efficacy, and thus require revisited strategies. Off-target effects may result in unexpected properties, stopping the progress, but also sometimes replacing them with new therapeutic applications. Both economic and regulatory hurdles frequently result in significant delays or the failure of potentially successful initiatives. Also, inability to keep up with the innovation can leave companies behind in competing in a rapidly changing science and technology landscape. These advances and setbacks provide examples of the intricate and sometimes mysterious process of drug development.

Implications of Findings

Success and failure are equally important at the drug discovery stage to influence the future of the field. There is a success that can be identified in successful drug approvals that led to lifesaving drugs [18]. Drug repurposing, which has previously been as futile as the intended drug use, has also proven to be an enormous success, as it has revealed the capacity of the industry to turn and innovate. Collaborative efforts of the pharmaceutical and academic research centers and authorities have favored drug development. At the same time, utilization of AI and personalized medicine, in unprecedented times, has continuously offered patients more targeted and effective treatment strategies. Yet the road to achievement is not riding on a paved highway in smooth and predictable directions, but with bumps, potholes, and mistakes. In many clinical trials, trials are stopped due to safety or efficacy concerns, which makes us reconsider strategies. Off-target effects can cause unwanted side effects that may stymy progress further. In other situations, however, the unintended therapeutic effects can lead to new applications. Economic (and regulatory) constraints can lead to such large delays, or to abandoning promising projects. Also, a failure to keep pace with innovation can trap an organization in a race to catch up with a rapidly shifting body of scientific knowledge, with no prospect of being able to successfully survive when innovation is ahead of its ability to react. These successes and failures represented the inherent complexity and sometimes random behavior of drug discovery [19].

Potential Impact on Stake Holders

The potential impact of pharmaceutical development advancements on stakeholders is profound and multilayered, with consequences for a wide variety of individuals and organizations across the health system. Patients' health can be best benefitted from the development of more precise prognostic and predictive treatments that can lead to important advances in treatment response and quality of life [20]. The examples of novel and innovative approaches, such as the customization of medicine and novel drug delivery systems, pave the way for the development of treatment unique for the individual needs, accompanied by reduced toxicity and increased therapeutic efficiency. This could lead to improved management of chronic diseases and even progress to a cure for what has long been considered a fatal disease.

Healthcare Providers

Experience may lead to alterations in how they diagnose and care for patients. Drug discovery is advancing with novel tools and drugs, which will provide them with more precise and effective interventions. Furthermore, clinical trial design and RWE innovations will facilitate informed treatment decision-making among providers based on the evolving evidence.

Pharmaceutical Companies

Stand to gain from the financial success of a successful drug development and from the strategic success of keeping a leadership role in technology and science innovations. As reported by this study, such enterprises will benefit from an acceleration in the efficiency of drug discovery workflow, further leading to a reduction in time-to-market and cost for the commercialization of new treatments. Furthermore, successful innovation not only strengthens their market share but also encourages expansion through the introduction of novel therapies [21].

Regulatory agencies will be involved with both to comply with the latest technologies and methodologies, and also to approve new drugs, based on the parameters of safety and efficiency. This transformed landscape of drug development requires ongoing evolution of the regulatory framework and processes, providing a delicate balance between stimulating innovation by fostering social change and providing robust regulatory oversight to protect public health.

Researchers and teaching/research institutions will be provided with the opportunity to spearhead the development of new scientific areas and major findings in them. More funding, higher resources and R&D and greater collaboration will encourage innovation and platform the advancement and development of new methods of research and instruments.

For instance, policymakers and public health officials will now need to grapple with the underlying implications of these innovations, including access and cost. It will also be vitally important for novel therapies that the outcomes of drug discovery are equally applicable to a variety of populations and are responsive to global health inequalities.

Drug discovery technologies in general hold the promise for highly beneficial outcomes for a number of stakeholders, thereby enhancing patient outcomes, healthcare delivery, and economic outcomes for the pharmaceutical industry [22].

Challenges and Limitations

Drug discovery is rife with challenges and constraints that can have a large effect on the evolution of novel therapeutics. A significant obstacle is the high cost of research and development. The discovery and development of a new drug is a very expensive effort, typically spanning more than a decade and billions of dollars. This financial outlay is made worse by clinical trial dropout rates, which include a large proportion of agents that do not show the anticipated efficacy/safety, resulting in costly failures.

Regulatory requirements present another significant challenge. The burden and inconvenience of dealing with regulatory agencies can inhibit the introduction of new drugs so it is costly to develop. The demand for gross documentation and good testing and adherence to safety standards can take time and resources [23].

Scientific limitations also pose substantial obstacles. Drug anticipation of human drug response based on preclinical animal studies has a fundamental bias, as the animal model is rarely a reliable predictor of human biology. Such discrepancies can lead to spurious results in clinical trials, in which drugs fail to work as they should or in which drugs have side effects never seen at the previous stages of the development continuum.

Moreover, the complexity of therapeutic intervention for certain diseases raises the additional difficulty [24]. For diseases, including cancer, which are highly heterogeneous and adaptive, action beyond the adequate level of understanding of disease mechanisms needs to involve novel mechanisms with which to overcome resistance and disease heterogeneity among patients.

Antibiotic resistance is a persistent problem that is problematic for the discovery of new antimicrobial drugs. Along with the rapid increase in resistance against current medications, there is a pressing need for novel agents, but the development of these agents is a long and arduous road, involving high cost and resistance formation [25]. Personalized medicine presents both an opportunity and a challenge. With all the possible advantages of using patient genotypes to tailor treatment, the outcomes will likely have to be accompanied by a high level of technical skill, massive data processing, and high cost/complexity of implementation.

In the final analysis, the equitable access to advanced technologies and data remains far from being achieved among the community of researchers. Limited access to high technology and a lack of data sharing with others can also limit progress, particularly in the case of modesty institutions and researchers with limited resources.

These challenges and restrictions point to the difficulty involved in drug discovery, and give are reason for ongoing innovation, collaboration, and funding so that the field can be further developed and barriers to the creation of novel and effective treatments can be broken through.

Opportunities for Innovation

There are numerous areas of opportunity for innovation in drug discovery, which can be harnessed to overcome current deficiencies and bring new therapeutics to the market. AI together with ML could be a safe path, in such a way that the development process of the drugs can be expedited by understanding large quantities of data that will suggest potential drug candidates, estimate the efficacy, and also modify clinical trial design. By utilizing AI-driven applications, it will be possible to obtain also deeper understanding of the pathophysiology of those complex diseases, which, in turn, will contribute to the identification of novel therapeutic targets [26].

Personalized medicine: Offers another significant opportunity for innovation. In the paradigm of personalized therapies using individual genetic profiles, researchers can then design more effective and tailored therapies (with lessened adverse effects) and improved patient outcomes. Genomics and biomarker development are at the core of this approach, leading to more focused and specific diagnostic and therapeutic efforts.

Biotechnology advancements: CRISPR-mediated gene editing technology provides a promising application to new therapeutics. These agents can be used to modulate genes involved in diseases, offering a disease-modifying treatment for genetic disease and further applied to develop more targeted disease treatments, for example, cancer.

Collaboration and open innovation: Key to unlocking new opportunities. Interactions among academia, the pharmaceutical industry and technology promise to construct knowledge and resource sharing networks, and thus to bring new solutions to light and accelerate drug discovery. Cooperative action may also be used to help access sophisticated technologies and skills that would otherwise be unavailable through independent organization efforts. Furthermore, the design of the drug delivery system may benefit the effectiveness and safety of the therapy. Advancements in delivery devices, including nanotech, are promising to improve targeting of pharmaceuticals, reduce off-target events, and improve patient adherence.

Drug repurposing using available formulary drugs of known drugs is a potential and cost-effective approach to drug discovery. Researchers can find new indications for drugs that are already on the market and accelerate the development of those drugs to market faster and with less risk, compared to the development of entirely new drugs. These innovation corridors have the capacity to change drug discovery in a more targeted, streamlined, and efficient way. Adoption of such developments will be essential for addressing current limitations and pushing the field toward next-generation, novel, and ultimate therapeutic interventions.

Future Research Directions

The future research directions in drug discovery are also promising, with certain important directions going to strongly influence the research and development of future drugs. An important line of inquiry is the investigation of new drug targets, in particular those associated with previously unknown, undiscovered biological processes and disease etiologies. Systems biology methodologies will further our efforts to understand the complexity of biological systems, enabling the discovery of novel therapeutic targets and approaches to modulate whole pathways. Further, studies of the human microbiome offer the potential for identifying the role of microbial communities in drug metabolism and pharmacokinetic and pharmacodynamic effects and could contribute to the development of personalized therapies [27].

Resistance overcoming is also one of the most important, and the future research is to design strategies which can break resistance mechanisms by new drug design and combination therapy. The growing application of AI and ML will also continue to transform the field to the benefit of predictive modeling, virtual screening, and drug formulation optimization. Novel screening technologies will allow for high-throughput, accurate screening of compounds and will therefore accelerate drug discovery.

It also examines clinical practice of orphan and rare diseases, thus applying the positive aspects of gene therapy and individualized medicine to meet expressed medical needs. Trial decision-making could be enhanced with the help of various strategic trends and concepts, for example, trial adaptivity and RWE, which make trials work and relevant. Moreover, global health equity will also be required for the achievement of such worthwhile objectives; it will guarantee accessibility of new technologies and processes to everyone all over the world.

Last, the construction of ethical and regulatory settings will be required to address such problems as new technologies bring forward; to protect patients' privacy; and to ensure appropriate utilization of new therapeutic options. In the following research areas, the drug development will go on with perfection: a New frontier in innovative medicine and patient care outcomes. Future directions were depicted in Figure 11.1.

Recommendations for Practitioners

To researchers working in drug discovery, a number of suggestions are made to improve both impact and respond to new challenges. However, the creation of new technologies (specifically, AI and ML) is highly urgent. Such agents have the potential to optimize the drug discovery pipeline, spanning the selection of drug targets to the optimization of clinical trial design. Practitioners are, however, always going to require staying abreast of the latest technological advances and considering how to integrate these new tools with how they practice in order to enhance efficiency and mastery [28]. Second, more robust links between academic, pharmaceutical, and technology/venture capital organizations can encourage innovation

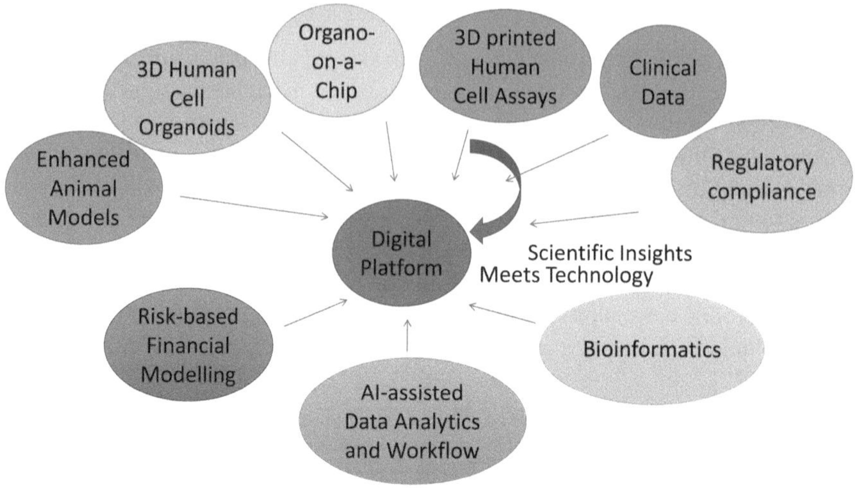

Figure 11.1 Directions of future research.

and facilitate engagement with state-of-the-art resources and competencies. It may be possible for collaboration to permeate with knowledge transfer, speed up the flow of research and lead to a richer set of solutions to these challenges.

Third, clinicians should embrace personalized medicine strategies by taking advantage of genomic and biomarker discovery breakthroughs to develop treatments against individual patient profiles. Not only does this methodology help improve therapeutic efficacy, but it also reduces the rate of toxicity. Fourth, adaptive and flexible clinical trial designs should be employed. Real evidence and adaptive methodology can be used to make clinical trials more practical and useful in the effort to get quicker, more accurate results.

Furthermore, practitioners should consider global health equity considerations relating to the availability and cost of novel therapeutics. If the new treatment is beneficial to a heterogeneous population and accessible to all people within the health system, then the full potential of this new treatment will be achieved. Next, awareness of changes in regulation and implications of ethics is most critical. For the practitioners, it is a continual process of learning, a process of engaging with and adapting to the evolution in the regulatory and ethical landscape to maintain currency and retain public trust. If applied by practitioners, the following recommendations open the way to meaningfully address the problems in drug development, encourage innovation, and participate in the creation of new strategies that will ultimately lead to better patient care and scientific advancement.

Long-term Vision and Goals

A common vision about drug discovery exists, which is aiming to modify the field by innovation, with the aid of a combination of efforts and commitment for improving global health. The main goals are the development of the process of drug development toward greater effective, efficient and accessible drug development procedures for neglected medical problems and increasing the patient's satisfaction.

Advancing Personalized Medicine

A key goal of personalizing medicine is developing therapies tailored to a patient's genetic, environmental and a lifestyle determinant combined. Genomics and biomarker discovery applied with data analytics allow for very targeted therapies in combination with improved efficacy and decreased side effects, this is possible. From the perspective of evolutionary change in the theory and practice of treatment development and delivery, the term "personalized medicine" concerns a process of treatment customized to each patient's clinical features of the treatment. This is motivated by the integration of such information as genetic, genomic and phenotypic to patient individualizing therapeutic agents tuned to a patient's biological distinct profile. This personalized approach goes beyond the standard environmental, genetic and lifestyle factors responsible for disease risk and drug response, in line with the general one-fits-all medical model.

Genomics and Biomarkers

They play an important role in the advancement of personalized medicine. Through mapping of the human genome and finding the genetic variations that lead to diseases, researchers will be able to pinpoint the disease biomarkers that can predict who will respond to these types of drugs. This allows designs of personalized therapies which are more specific to patients with a specific genetic profile. For example, in oncology, personalized medicine is used to select targeted therapies focusing on patients' tumor genetic mutations so that a more effective and toxic treatment is given.

Pharmacogenomics

Research on the role of genes in treatment response of a specific patient is also of paramount importance, i.e., based on knowledge of drug metabolism and efficacy, through understanding drug metabolism and response from the genes, personalized medicine will coincide to predict drug toxicity and dose schedule. In addition to this approach enhances the safety and efficacy of pharmaceuticals, the empirical (trial-and-error) approach for finding the ideal treatment is also minimized.

Recent Advances in Data Analytics and AI

The recent breakthroughs in Data Analytics and AI are changing personalized medicine, leveraging complex datasets including genetic data and electronic health records, and patient-reported outcomes. AI algorithms can be used to identify patterns and correlations that are missed by traditional methods, leading to more precise predictions and personalized intervention plans. In addition, in order to delineate the specificity and release of therapeutics more, personalized drug delivery systems are also an aim to be achieved. Technological improvements with nanoparticle and smart drug delivery systems realize drug delivery to the target site more specifically, and the therapeutic effect of drugs can be increased, and their side effects can be minimized.

Ethical and Privacy Problems

Ethical and privacy issues are no less serious to the discipline of personalized medicine. As genetic and personal health data lie at the heart of making treatment decisions, it is fundamental that the security and privacy of that health data is maintained. Lay practitioners are confronted with the current ethical challenge as they try to deliver the benefits of personalized medicine to underserved groups.

Enhancing Drug Discovery Technologies

Future envisioning is broad, spanning the use of emerging technologies, such as AI, ML, and the upgrading of screening technology. An aim of these technologies is to accelerate the translation of promising pharmaceuticals from target identification through to preclinical trial optimization, in so doing to save time and money. Continuing to develop novel technologies in the area of drug discovery is also crucial for accelerating the development of novel therapeutics in order to streamline the drug discovery landscape and optimize the cost and efficiency of drug discovery itself. At the vanguard of this progress are several technological advances that are transforming conventional approaches for drug discovery, development and assessment.

AI and ML

Transforming drug discovery through the ability to make sense of big data and to find patterns that traditional methods fail to discover. AI algorithms can speed up the drug target identification workflow, predict the binding characteristics of chemicals and their targets, and advance drug design. ML models hold the promise of mining complex biological data to extract a novel information pool of disease processes and drug targets, and putative novel therapeutic drugs.

HTS and Advanced Screening Technologies

Offer researchers the capacity to rapidly screen thousands of compounds toward each biological target. Advances in microfluidics and automation have dramatically increased the throughput and reproducibility of such screening experiments, carrying out the "lead finding" of potential drug candidates in a reasonable time. This increase is represented by the decrease in the drug discovery time and money in the early stages.

Genomic and Proteomic Technologies

This chapter summarizes main lessons on the underlying mechanisms of diseases and the pharmacology aspects of drugs and their targets. Tools, including gene editing (CRISPR), next-generation sequencing (NGS) and mass spectrometry allow researchers to screen, image and analyze gene expression at unprecedented scales. These technologies are used for the identification of new drug targets and elucidation of the underlying molecular mechanisms of the action of drugs in cellular function [29].

Structural Biology and Computational Chemistry

Represent the state-of-the-art tools used in three-dimensional structural analysis of biological macromolecules and interactions between macromolecules and drugs. Structural data on drug-target interactions is obtained from applications including X-ray crystallography, cryo-electron microscopy, and molecular docking simulations and is used to create targeted therapeutics with enhanced potency and specificity.

Lab-on-a-chip (LOC) and organ-on-a-chip (OOC) technologies are developing platforms mimicking the physiologically meaningful microenvironment of the human organs at microchip scale. These approaches enable better predictions of drug action and toxicity based on a biologically relevant model of the human system as opposed to standard cell culture or animal models [30]. RWE and big data analytics are both coming with the aim of being incorporated into the drug discovery pipelines. Based on the analysis of longitudinal datasets of EHR, patient registries, as well as register data, researchers can play various roles in the understanding of efficacy in the real-life settings of the immunotherapy drugs, but also in their recognition of adverse events and in optimizing the design of clinical trials.

Nanotechnology is also used for drug development with a view to the development of new drug delivery systems. Nanoparticles and nanocarriers can be designed such that nanomedical agents are selectively directed to a predefined tissue/cell, solubilize the drug, release the drug, and thereby simultaneously enhance the efficacy and safety of the therapy. In general, drug discovery technology development is a field with great potential to generate major innovation in the field at substantially greater speed, accuracy, and substantially reduced cost of discovery. Through these advances, the translational process can be expedited to harness the power of novel therapies in a broader array of medical indications with greater effectiveness and safety.

Promoting Global Health Equity

Another important aim is to make new therapy widely accessible and affordable globally. This includes reducing care access disparities, lowering the cost of drug development, and using strategies to ensure access to life-saving therapies to marginalized communities. To facilitate benefits to populations globally and regardless of their socio-economic status, the goal of global health equity promotion is central to drug discovery. This undertaking requires the mitigation of healthcare and medication access inequities that are often found between high- and low- to middle-income states.

Access to Medicines

Despite the advances in novel therapies, substantial barriers exist for a large number of populations in low-income countries in accessing these therapies due to the cost of therapy, scarcity of therapy, and a weak healthcare infrastructure. Efforts to achieve global health equity require action to lower the cost of novel drugs by means of (i) price negotiations, (ii) generic drug manufacture, and (iii) PPPs that will lower the cost and availability of medicines.

Capacity Building

The Healthcare system is also of great value for achieving health equity. Improvement of healthcare infrastructure, healthcare professional training and diagnostic/therapeutic resources in the underserved population will have a beneficial impact on providing new therapeutic options to patients and ultimately on improving clinical status. Actions can be supported through collaborative work between organizations on an international level, governments and NGOs, who can all make available resources, knowledge and financial assistance.

Equitable Distribution of Research Benefits

Make sure that the fruits of drug development are not enjoyed only by the global elite. This encompasses research into diseases that have the greatest public health burden for the vulnerable population (e.g., neglected tropical diseases), as well as the development of new therapies that are produced with this vulnerable population in mind. Research and development (R&D) promoting global health priorities can be used to exploit these neglected fields and reduce health inequalities.

Regulatory and Policy Frameworks

It plays a crucial role in promoting health equity. Governments and international organizations need to develop and execute medicines and healthcare resource policies with fair distribution in mind. This will involve establishing regulatory frameworks that will enable affordable drugs to be approved and distributed, and will encourage research on diseases that afflict developing countries.

Community Engagement and Participation

Health applications are created to be used by populations with different members. To assure culturally sensitive, efficaçy, and acceptable solutions, the participaţion of local communities in the planning and implementation of health interventions has been shown to be the optimal approach. Patient advocacy groups and community-based organizations provide valuable information to help us understand the needs and issues of particular community groups.

Addressing Health Inequities

The latter also calls for a social determinant of health at a wider scale, education, economic stability and housing. If the long-standing origins of these factors are addressed, the health and well-being of populations may be improved, with greater impact and reach of new therapies.

Globally, action to reduce health inequity extends far beyond any one action and involves a range of approaches including drug affordability measures, health system strengthening, fair participation of communities in drug research and development and community engagement in health interventions. If these hurdles are overcome, the drug discovery community has a role to play in establishing a more equitable and fair global health care system that can improve clinical outcomes for populations [31].

Fostering Innovation Through Collaboration

There is a need to establish a strong network of partnerships among academic, pharmaceutical, and technology organizations, and with regulatory bodies. This vision encompasses the development of a collaborative ecosystem that promotes innovation, supports knowledge exchange, and enables translation of research into real-world therapeutics. Collaborative innovation is one of the critical factors that can drive drug discovery and the development of novel therapeutics for tackling the complex medical challenges. The interface between heterogeneous stakeholders—academic institutions, pharmaceutical companies, biotechnology companies, regulatory bodies and NGOs—forms a synergistic space that fosters accelerated research and innovation.

Cross-sector Partnerships

This is central to the collaboration. However, academic researchers can work together with industry scientists so that their expertise can be utilized to close the gap between basic research findings and practical applications. It is at academic institutions where the most advanced research and the germ of the lowest level of understanding emerge from as historically, pharmaceutical and biotechnology companies are at the front of the translation of technology, resources, and industrial application into scale-up and commercialization of new discoveries. This is a chance to build better, faster drug development pipelines while accelerating discovery to market.

Public-private Collaborations

It also plays an important role in addressing their basic concerns in global health. Government agencies, non-profits, and the private sector can collaborate together to address such challenging problems as rare diseases, neglected tropical diseases, and pandemic preparation. Every time this kind of collaboration has existed, the pooling of funding, resources, and expertise is the motivation behind these large-scale research projects and innovative solutions thought to be very difficult or impossible to carry out separately.

International Collaborations

In the drug discovery process, it is vitally important. International collaborations lead to the sharing and production of knowledge, data, and resources to enable the research of health issues of various populations globally. Collaborative research may create novel therapeutics between strikingly dissimilar genetic and environmental backgrounds with greater impact.

Innovation Hubs and Consortia

Offers a place for collaborative research and development. All of these hubs do what they are called, they're bringing the researchers, the companies, the institutions together where they work on specific challenges or are interested areas of interest. They often enable participants to share their ideas, speed technology development and access shared facilities and resources. Examples include consortia formed by PPPs directed toward certain diseases or therapeutic areas where a combination of different expertise and funding is used to drive the innovation.

Collaborative Networks and Data Sharing

Modern drug discovery now relies increasingly on them. By sharing data, resources, and research findings through networks, it should also support improved transparency, reduce duplication of effort, and help achieve progress more quickly. By combining others' work and indeed sharing it, researchers are finding that they are able to do so in open access databases and collaborative research platforms more effectively, and faster, to make more discoveries.

Patient and Community Involvement

The research process can also bring about innovation. Together, we're engaging patients and communities in research to ensure that new treatments work as prescribed for real-world patients and their preferences. For example, it could be of help to see what the patient groups perceive to be the disease burden, their experiences with treatment, and possibly lead to research questioning of interest in a patient-centered drug discovery paradigm [32].

Collaborating to promote innovation generally means combining the understanding, body of work, and viewpoints of different stakeholders to achieve significantly more productive and useful drug discovery. Despite this, silos reign in the field and breaking them down along with a building a collaborative culture will accelerate development of new therapies and address some of the most pressing health problems of the time.

Addressing Emerging Health Challenges

It also involves long-term vision in being ahead of emerging health challenges—antibiotic resistance, rare diseases, and complex chronic conditions. That also includes research on new treatments, new ways to stop these threats from evolving. New and evolving responses to drug discovery have been produced in response to new and evolving threats to global health, and they have strengthened drug discovery's toolbox to identify new diseases and new challenges based on changes in disease patterns, environment, and progress in medical sciences [33]. It's no surprise that researchers and healthcare providers in the face of change—specifically in global health research and practice—are navigating their way through never-ending needs to research and adapt to the challenges.

Antibiotic Resistance

That's a growing concern, since bacteria are developing resistance to existing antibiotics and many treatments are failing. The drug discovery, therefore, is directed to the development of new antibiotics and to alternative therapies that might bypass resistant strains. What we call research actually consists of looking for new drug targets, finding new classes of antibiotics, new ways to do things like bacteriophage therapy and combination therapy to reanimate the stereo powers of old drugs.

Emerging Infectious Diseases

Novel viruses and pathogens are a threat to public health. Two recent examples: They are present in perfect timing for COVID-19 pandemic when one needs a fast response or preparedness. To do this, surveillance systems must get better at very early detection of new pathogens, vaccine production sped up and international cooperation based especially on countries sharing information and resources, especially when they come from countries that share information and resources. To be able to produce treatments and preventors for emerging infectious diseases, drug discovery must be agile and responsive.

More effective treatments for chronic diseases and complex Conditions including cancer, cardiovascular disease, and neurologic disorders require ongoing research. To identify new drug targets in these diseases and to develop therapies that target the underlying causes, more understanding about the molecular and genetic basis of these diseases is currently needed. Having its focus on the targeted therapies and personalized medicine, along with new drug delivery systems to improve outcomes for patients who suffer from chronic and complex disease conditions, drug discovery efforts are highlighting its use.

Neglected Tropical Diseases

It affects millions of people in low-resource settings and usually gets less attention and less funding compared to other diseases. New treatments for NTDs have to be developed, and current treatments improved through adequate research. Given the challenges of finding treatments for NTDs, the selection of drugs for the reduction of the burden of disease in the affected community is critical, and efforts should be made to find innovative and affordable treatments, along with improving diagnostic approaches and treatment strategies.

Environmental and lifestyle factors like pollution, climate change, and bad lifestyle choices are all naturally going to play a big role in the development of health challenges. In research of drug discovery and intervention of related diseases, these factors have to be bridged on. The environmental changes are changes that cause health problems, say, how environmental changes cause health effects of environmental pollutants, as well as the development of drugs to prevent or mitigate such effects.

Global Health Inequities

In bit to amplify the impact on emerging health challenges. It may also be the case that some differences in health access, resources and infrastructure can obstruct an effective response to new threats to health. To do that, we need research and development strategies that are sensitized to the underserved population, and efforts to put therapies within the reach and the pocket of as many people as possible.

At its own levels, an emerging health problem must be addressed with a proactive and integrative approach through cutting-edge research and an underlying international coalescence and global health equity. Drug discovery is out in front of evolving threats and can support new research and new technologies to better prepare and respond to future health challenges.

Improving Drug Delivery and Formulation

Aiding in new drug-delivery systems, which aim to improve the precision, efficiency and safety of therapies is aim one. Also included are advances in nanoparticle-based delivery, sustained release formulations, and smart drug delivery systems. Improvement in drug delivery and formulation is a key requirement for advancing therapeutic efficacy and safety in drug discovery. The question this area of research is about is how best to give, absorb and use drugs in the body to maximize their effectiveness and minimize or eliminate side effects [34].

Innovative Drug Delivery Systems

Boasts a leading track record of improving the delivery of medications to their intended targets. However, many of the traditional methods of delivery suffer from low bioavailability, poor tissue penetration, and undesirable side effects. There are advanced delivery systems that form solutions, such as nanoparticles, liposomes, micelles, for drug encapsulation in carriers offering drug protection from degradation, increasing drug solubility and facilitating the drug delivery to the specific tissue or cells [35]. Here, nanoparticle-based delivery systems can provide drug-delivery precision to tumor cells, where the tissue damage is minimized and effective therapeutic efficacy of cancer treatments is enhanced.

Controlled and Sustained Release Formulations

It is a means of achieving maximum drug levels in the body so that the patient would be more compliant regarding compliance in the body, and so that the frequency of the drug dose would be minimized. Formulations based on these technologies have included polymer matrices, hydrogels and degradable materials for the slow release of drugs. This should enable chronic disease management by facilitating stable medication use to lower the number of doses administered daily and minimize fluctuations in drug levels.

Targeted Drug Delivery

However, a lot of it is about getting the drugs into the disease site, in particular, a greater therapeutic effect, and fewer systemic side effects. In order to achieve this precision, we employ techniques including antibody drug conjugates, ligand-receptor interactions, and targeted nanoparticles. This is demonstrated by designing drug delivery systems that allow greater drug delivery at tumor sites with lower amounts delivered to healthy tissues through selective binding to cancer cells.

Improving Oral Bioavailability

This is a huge problem since very few drugs are effective via the oral route. Bioavailability of oral medications has been improved by advances in formulation technologies (tablets based on solubility enhancers, permeation enhancers, advanced tablet technologies, etc. Moreover, it can also deliver drugs to specific locations over the body across biological barriers, i.e., blood-brain barrier [36]. Treatments for central nervous system diseases or other diseases in which highly specific targeting is to be achieved can be delivered in this manner.

Nanotechnology

Revolutionizing drug delivery through the ability to engineer highly specific drug carriers and delivery systems. Nanocarriers are capable of penetrating the biological barriers, i.e., the blood-brain barrier, and release drugs at targeted sites in the body. The same technology works on the treatment for central nervous system disorders and other patients who need precise targeting.

Personalized Drug Formulations

There is a benefit to give care according to each patient's characteristics, in terms of genetic and metabolic and physiological profiles. Personalized medicine is a strategy in which the compositions of medications are specific to the specific requirement(s) that an individual may be experiencing: to that against which he/she is receiving one drug, or even to that against which he/she will be susceptible in terms of the metabolism of that drug. Conventionally, the current strategy may be optimized to achieve the desired therapeutic benefit with minimal adverse effects.

Addressing Drug Stability and Storage

In order to extend their shelf life and be effective over time, better formulation techniques are used to improve the stability of drugs. The process is basically creating formulations or packaging that will shield the drugs from the environmental factors, such as moisture, light, or temperature excursions.

In general, drug delivery and formulation is in need of improvement, with the aim of increasing the effectiveness and safety of treatments. Advances in new strategies and emerging technologies allow researchers to formulate drug delivery systems with therapeutic advantages, enhance patient adherence to treatment and decrease adverse reactions to optimize health outcomes.

Emphasizing Sustainability and Ethical Practices

The paramount importance of environmentally sustainable and ethically responsible drug discovery procedures cannot be overstated. Vision encompasses decreasing pollution of drug production, ethical research and corporate responsibility in the making process. Pressure to achieve ethics and sustainability in drug discovery has an impact on the capability to bring to market medical breakthroughs that offer a positive impact, such as the environment and the people, all at the same time, while maintaining a value on ethical standards of conduct in research and development. The method aligns with the growing demand to reconcile scientific advances with informed environmentalism and moral concerns [37].

Sustainable Research Practices

Reduces the environmental impact of the drug discovery process mainly. It encompasses the elimination of waste creation, utilizing ecofriendly solvents and reagents, and serving to improve laboratory power intake. Applying green chemistry principles can be used in the development of greener processes and the decrease of the ecological footprint of drug production. For example, if we consider synthetic routes that are more efficient or facilitate solvent recovery, then we can make this research more sustainable.

Ethical Considerations in Clinical Trials

It has also been applied to improve research rigor and respect for research subjects. This, therefore, involves the processes of obtaining informed consent, maintaining participant confidentiality and privacy, and conducting research with participant safety and welfare at center. Since ethical behavior also involves the designing of clinical trials, to obtain scientifically meaningful outcomes and minimal risk to the study participants, cultivating a sense of responsibility is essential. Adhering to ethical codes and legal statutes builds public confidence in clinical trials.

Access to Medicines and Affordability

These are just some of the major factors of driving equity and social responsiveness in drug development. Activities aimed at delivering new therapies to the marginalized in a convenient, affordable and inexpensive manner are necessary for addressing global disparities in health. This might involve techniques such as price-gradations, license sharing, and partnerships with nonprofit organizations for drug provision in resource-limited settings [38]. There is a growing awareness among corporations of a trade-off between financial return and improving access to life-saving treatments.

Ethical Sourcing of Materials

That is, the raw materials used to manufacture drugs must be sourced ethically. This includes an embargo on the application of such compounds as synthesized using manipulation of ethics, and on the provision of equitable and transparent supply chains. Companies are mandated to follow ethical principles and laws through the supply chain, i.e., the avoidance of conflict minerals and the reaching of fair labor standards [39].

Reducing Animal Testing

It is an important ethical consideration in drug discovery. Research is also still being carried out in an effort to identify alternative methods to animal testing, such as in vitro assays, computational models and organ-on-a-chip technology, to reduce the use of animals, while also achieving informative and reliable data. This trend in no way contradicts ethical recommendations, but it contributes to the progress of scientific research by producing increasingly human-related data [40].

Corporate Social Responsibility (CSR) activities are the manifestation of a corporate engagement in ethics and sustainability. Pharmaceutical companies are becoming increasingly active in CSR activities, which are perceived to be social and environmentally related issues being addressed as health education promotion, disaster relief, and environmental sustainability. Such programs also help to sustain the image of the organization as well as the broader goal of improving global health.

Stakeholder Engagement: A particularly relevant topic for the background of drug discovery agents in general, e.g., patients, clinicians, regulators, the public, etc. Engaging stakeholders in discourse and decision-making processes helps to guarantee that drug development is in line with social values and responds to real-life needs and issues.

Sustainable and ethical behaviors during drug discovery can be realized through the incorporation of three elements (environmental, social, and ethical) in every step of the R&D cycle. By adhering to these principles, the pharmaceutical community is able to promote medical science to the highest levels of scientific advancement and use medical research to benefit society, all while having low environmental impacts

Enhancing Patient Involvement and RWE

Integration of the patient voice and RWE into drug development pipelines is necessary in order to ensure that treatments match real-world patient needs and experience. The aim is to engage patients more directly in research and draw on real-world data in order to guide therapeutic approaches.

These multi-decade-long goals are only achievable through the combined action of all the stakeholders in the drug space value chain. Concentrating on these priorities, the field can make an impactful contribution to healthcare, to better manage patients' outcomes, and to answer some of the global medical challenges facing the future.

Implications for Healthcare Innovation

By allowing the application of more effective precision treatments targeted to disease mechanisms, precision drugs and biologics contribute to better patient outcomes and the elimination of "trial and error" treatments.

Personalized Medicine

From the perspective of patients' individual genetic profiles, tailored treatments can be used to reduce unnecessary side effects and maximize treatment efficiency, therefore leading to better control of chronic and complicated diseases.

Enhancement of drug development process, by optimization of drug design, prediction of drug interactions and analysis of massive data, AI and ML can be used to expedite the drug discovery and development process. This has, in turn, resulted in lower costs and faster time to market for pharmaceuticals, thanks to the ability through HTS to accelerate drug development and shorten time-to-market for pharmaceutical drugs, thanks to the ability for early identification of candidate drug chemicals.

Advanced Screening Methods

Diagnostic assays and therapeutic interventions are optimized by more and more precise and informative tests made possible by technologies like organ-on-a-chip devices and CRISPR screens [41].

Better Toxicity Predictions

Adverse effects are fewer in the novel drugs due to drug metabolism and toxicity risk profiles being improved because of the development of more powerful modeling methods to predict drug metabolism and toxicity. Integration of multi-omics data is currently receiving more and more attention for toxicity prediction. By integration of genomics, proteomics, metabolomics, and transcriptomic data, investigators can also better understand drug action in biological systems. Multi-omics approaches allow the identification of candidate toxicity markers and toxicity pathways, ensuring a high degree of integration of the cellular response across biological organization. Subtle toxic effects can also be detected, which are not obvious by means of single-omics analyses [37].

Development of Advanced in Vitro Models

Enhancements of toxicity predictions based on more accurate and interpretable biological context. Progress in fields including human-induced pluripotent stem cell (iPSC)-derived tissues and organs (e.g., being used to construct physiological models as representative of humans as possible. These complex in vitro models are able to better represent drug mechanisms of action on human tissues, so that toxicity testing becomes more reliable and animal testing is reduced.

Application of Systems Toxicology

Pertaining to the use of computational models to interpret the intricate relationships between drugs and biological systems. Systems toxicology integrates data from various sources (HTS and omics technologies) to construct integrated models for drug-induced toxicity. These models reproduce the effect of drugs on cellular networks and pathways, which can be used in research to better predict frank adverse effects.

Novel Toxicity Pathways covers the discovery and analysis of hitherto unknown mechanisms of drug-induced toxicity. There are researchers currently investigating new mechanisms and molecular targets that may be involved in the occurrence of ADRs. By discovery of these emerging pathways, researchers are able to formulate more targeted strategies to develop toxicity prediction and protection, ultimately, safer drug candidates [42].

Enhanced computational toxicological tools provide an increased capacity for prediction in drug safety evaluation. Algorithms and software tools are also in the making for the analysis of intricate data sets and predictions of early toxic effects.

These tools have also been constructed on the basis of advanced statistical models and ML methods, such that they aim to enhance the prediction accuracy of toxicity and to integrate information from a variety of sources, such as chemical structure and biological associations.

Drug discovery based on early-stage safety profiling involves identifying drug candidates for early in vivo toxicity. If safety assessments are integrated into the early stages of the drug development process, it is possible to detect and prevent the emergence of potential toxicity and thereby avoid its advancement to later stages in the development process. Beginner-level safety profiling may help to identify promising drug candidates early that would reduce the likelihood of attrition in the late stage.

Enhanced Drug Metabolism Studies aim to elucidate the metabolism and processing of drugs in the body. Drug metabolism pathways research is used to discover possible toxic metabolites and drug interactions. Through detailed investigation of these processes, researchers are able to predict and avoid drug toxicity resulting from drug metabolism, and ultimately, safer drug formulations are produced.

Predictive Toxicology Databases are tools of great utility for the safety evaluation of drugs. Databases aggregating data about drug toxicity, chemical structures and biological interactions are accessible to researchers, allowing them to retrieve historical data and make predictions of potential side effects based on related compounds. These databases assist drug development decision-making and also aid in the early identification of potential safety concerns.

Through the use of these state-of-the-art techniques and technologies, investigators will be able to increase the reliability of toxicity predictions, optimize drug safety profiles, and speed the introduction of safe therapeutic interventions [43–47].

Prospects for Developing Novel Therapeutic Domains in Regenerative Medicine

In the application of stem cells and tissue engineering, previously intractable diseases, such as certain cancers and neurological disorders, could potentially be treated. In its willingness to address the root genetic basis of hereditary diseases directly, gene therapy brings with it the promise of cures and a new paradigm of treatment for these diseases.

Medication Repurposing and Cost-effectiveness Medication Repurposing

By reassessing current medications for novel applications, it is possible to yield new medicines quickly and affordably without having to invest heavily in the costly process of creating new medications.

Cut Development Expenses

Spend on drug development can be minimized by the efficient use of resources, enabled by the AI-powered intelligence of drugs and the power of high-throughput technology.

Accelerated Drug Availability

Faster drug discovery and research processes can lead to novel therapies being introduced sooner, thereby improving access to and delivery of healthcare to patients.

Through merging the breakthroughs in drug development and digital health tools (wearable and mobile health apps), personalized cure and real-time delivery of healthcare are achievable.

Data-driven Insights

Big data and analytics are used to come up with insights that have public health and personal medicine relevance on a larger scale in drug development.

Faster Drug Approval Regulatory Streamlining

AI and advanced discovery approaches can speed up the drug approval process, enabling patients to receive effective therapies more rapidly.

Advances in drug discovery, including the development of new technologies in drug delivery, support the development of better drug delivery systems in order to improve patient adherence and bioavailability. Technological progress provides a light at the end of the tunnel for the creation of therapeutics for rare and orphan diseases, satisfying unmet medical needs.

AI and prediction models can assist in managing and reducing possible interactions in patients who take numerous drugs. By integrating it, RWE from patient data, post-market surveillance, and drug development can be advanced, because verification that therapies are effective in populations other than those involved in the drug development study is ensured.

Enhanced Patient Arrangement Customized Interventions

The ability to classify patients with the help of advanced genetic and biomarker analysis has been applied in order to provide more precise and targeted treatment plans [48, 49]. Developments in immunotherapy cancer treatment: Improved drug discovery tools are pushing immune-therapies to the forefront, providing new hope for cancer patients in the form of more potent, immune-system-based treatments. Novelty facilitates the development of combination therapies that can enhance therapeutic efficacy and reduce resistance to medication, particularly in chronic diseases.

Drug discovery knowledge can help reduce the number of illnesses by informing vaccine and preventive medicine development.

AI technologies also provide an aid to identify new uses of drugs that are already approved, thereby speeding up and simplifying to overcome the process of repurposing. Using modern drug discovery technology, clinical trial designs are becoming more flexible and adaptable, thereby facilitating better patient recruitment and trial outcomes.

Extending Therapeutic Horizons

Novel therapeutic targets:

Recent drug discovery studies have identified novel therapeutic targets and relieved the symptoms of previously intractable diseases [40, 50]. These examples demonstrate that advances in pharmaceutical development have a systemic impact on all the elements of providing care, from enhancing treatment effectiveness to fostering innovation and efficiency throughout the system.

Future Directions in Drug Discovery

Quantum Computing

As an application for the simulation of molecular interactions at a level of detail not previously available while at resolutions not previously accessible. Quantum computers have the potential to provide answers that classical computers cannot, such as a precise prediction of the dynamics of very large biomolecules and of biomolecular-drug-target interactions. This technology can also be applied to accelerate the rate of candidate drug discovery by shortening the cycle in one step of the process, or by changing the mode of candidate drugs binding to their biological targets.

Synthetic Biology

It is increasingly relevant in drug discovery; however, it can also be used to develop and engineer custom biological systems and organisms with targeted characteristics. Synthetic biology methods, e.g., modification of microbes or cell lines, can be applied toward the generation of new compounds and the implementation of high-throughput drug screening. In this context, it is possible to study orphan drugs and create novel biosynthetic routes [51].

Organs-on-chips

Technology will have a role to play in advancing drug discovery by providing more representative human physiological and pathological models [6]. These microfluidic devices recapitulate the structure and function of human organs, and therefore, it is feasible to apply drug substances to an in situ study within a more physiologically relevant biological environment. Organs-on-chips can reproduce drug absorption, metabolism and toxicity and can also be used to study drug effects in vivo.

Epigenetic Targeting

An important contribution will arise when the impacts of modulation of DNA and histones on gene expression and drug response are investigated by researchers. Epigenetic regulators have been successfully manipulated to alter otherwise disease processes from outside causative genetic lesions if the latter is considered. This strategy opens up new directions of study to be explored for the cure of diseases such as cancer, a disease with extensive epigenetic alterations.

Advanced Biomolecular Imaging

The methods will be advantageous for drug discovery via minute-scale, high-resolution, molecular-scale, real-time movies of drug-drug binding. Improvements in imaging techniques, including super-resolution microscopy and cryo-electron tomography, will allow researchers to quantify drug-binding and cellular response to a greater extent. Such capacity will further improve understanding of drug mechanisms and help design effective drugs [52–56].

Personalized Drug Formulations

Criticality plays a most significant role in drug development, namely, developing drugs in a fashion of individualizing medications for each patient with regard to his/her specific genetic, metabolic, and physiological profiles. Personalization of medicine will drive the creation of personalized drug formulations that maximize efficacy and reduce side effects across individual patients [57–62].

Ethical AI Governance

It will become an item of concern as AI has a growing influence in drug design. By setting out the ethical boundaries and guidelines for the responsible and transparent use of AI, there are significant benefits which can be realized through the adoption of AI. Issues of algorithmic bias, data privacy, and decision-making transparency will be important in order to maintain public trust and enable equitable access to emerging therapies.

Bioprinting Technology

Most of all, it is designed for the production of three-dimensional tissue constructs and organ constructs for drug testing. Scientists are able to use 3D printing technologies to create living tissues and design more realistic and functional models of human organs. These bioprinted tissues will provide better conditions for drug efficacy and safety assays, which will, in turn, lead to better preclinical animal studies.

Environmental Impact Assessments

It will be embedded in drug discovery workflows, with a focus on characterizing and mitigating the burden of pharmaceutical production ecologies. Researchers will include environmental factors in the drug development process, e.g., assessing the biodegradability of drugs and the environmental impact of production processes.

Blockchain for Data Integrity

Will enhance drug discovery by providing data security and data trail. Blockchain technology provides an unassailable record of experimental data, enhances transparency in clinical trials, and prevents data manipulation. This technique will allow the reproducibility of published research findings, in turn allowing improved robustness of drug discovery processes. These emerging directions in drug discovery hold the promise of transforming the field, offering new tools and approaches that will accelerate the development of innovative and effective therapies.

Conclusion

Over the past 20 years, drug discovery arguably has taken an enormous step, from classic trial and error settings based more on expertise and luck to increasingly sophisticated setups using ever newer technology never before or soon to be tried again. This progress to understand diseases at the deeper molecular level and develop target therapeutics has been fueled by breakthroughs in molecular biology, genetics, computational tools and chemistry. Drug discovery, however, is known to be one of the most difficult, time-consuming, and expensive processes in biomedical research. It usually requires more than a decade—and billions of dollars—for a new drug to make it through the regulatory process in order to market a product for tens of millions of dollars a year. Nevertheless, it is quite attractive, but the current drug development model is unsustainable for sustaining high attrition rates, a major bottleneck itself. Chronic and multifactorial diseases such as cancer, Alzheimer's disease and diabetes are perhaps the most complex human diseases to study and to formulate therapeutic input on, and represent one of the most harrowing challenges in drug discovery. Moreover, many of these diseases are, to some degree, determined by several genetic and environmental factors such that a single molecular target for intervention cannot be identified. Integrating AI and ML into drug discovery looks like a very promising area. Early stages of drug discovery are being driven faster and better, as hit identification and lead optimization take place in far less time with these technologies. People are also using AI to more quickly design molecules with the specified properties that might speed up the drug development time frame overall, as well as simulate complex biological systems and predict what two different drugs might do.

Among these is also nanotechnology, such as in drug delivery systems being applied to drug discovery. By, for example, tailoring nanoparticles so that they can deliver drugs to diseased cells specifically, and with more precision and in fewer side effects than the rest of the body, drugs and treatments can be increasingly more precise and effective. The advantage in cancer therapy of targeting drug delivery to tumor tissue is especially attractive because it can potentially enhance the therapeutic index of chemotherapeutic agents. Finally, drug discovery in the future has much hope to bring. Personalized medicine, AI, nanotech and sector collaboration are becoming more efficient, targeted, and patient-focused. But as we learn more about disease mechanisms and new technologies continue to become available, one day we will live in a future in which these now untreatable diseases become treatable and patients will be treated with therapies that are safer, more effective and more accessible. However, realization in the future will depend on sustained investment in fundamental science, continued and new interdisciplinary cooperation, and our acceptance of the ethical, economic, and regulatory issues posed by scientific advances.

References

1. Marshall WS, Boymel JL. Oligonucleotide synthesis as a tool in drug discovery research. Drug Discov Today. 1998;3:34–42. doi:10.1016/S1359-6446(97)01116-1.
2. Naksuriya O, Okonogi S, Schiffelers RM, Hennink WE. Curcumin nanoformulations: A review of pharmaceutical properties and preclinical studies and clinical data related to cancer treatment. Biomaterials. 2014;35:3365–3383.
3. Neale C, Camfield D, Reay J, Stough C, Scholey A. Cognitive effects of two nutraceuticals Ginseng and bacopa benchmarked against modafinil: A review and comparison of effect sizes. Br J Clin Pharmacol. 2013;75(3):728–737.
4. Marsden PD. The discovery of urea stibamine. Rev Soc Bras Med Trop. 1986;19(2):115.
5. Taneja B, Yadav J, Chakraborty TK, Brahmachari SK. An Indian effort towards affordable drugs: generic to designer drugs. Biotechnol J. 2009;4(3):348–360.
6. Differding E. Drug discovery alliances in India: Indications, targets, and new chemical entities. ChemMedChem. 2014;9(1):43–60.
7. Misra M. Biosimilars: Current perspectives and future implications. Indian J Pharmacol. 2012;44(1):12–14.
8. Singh M. Centchroman, a selective estrogen receptor modulator, as a contraceptive and for the management of hormone-related clinical disorders. Med Res Rev. 2001;21(4):302–347.
9. Randhawa GK, Kullar JS, Kumar R. Bioenhancers from mother nature and their applicability in modern medicine. Int J Appl Basic Med Res. 2011;1(1):5.
10. Sengupta G, Hazra A, Kundu A, Ghosh A. Comparison of *murraya koenigii* and *tribulus terrestris*-based oral formulation versus tamsulosin in the treatment of benign prostatic hyperplasia in men aged >50 years: A double-blind, double-dummy, randomized controlled trial. Clin Ther. 2011;33(12):1943–1952.
11. Singla D, Dhanda SK, Chauhan JS, Bhardwaj A, Brahmachari SK, Raghava GP. Open source software and web services for designing therapeutic molecules. Curr Top Med Chem. 2013;13(10):1172–1191.
12. Hakim A, Liliasari, Kadarohman A, Syah YM. Making a natural product chemistry course meaningful with a mini project laboratory. J Chem Educ. 2016;93(1):193–196.
13. Adhikari D, Rangra NK. Antimicrobial activities of *Acacia* genus. Asian Pac J Trop Biomed. 2023;13(2):45–59.

14. Kshirsagar N, Pahuja M, Chatterjee NS, Kamboj VP. Gaps in translating basic science research from bench to bedside. Indian J Med Res. 2023;158(3):228.
15. Siagian RC, Bachtiar N, Soewondo P. Strategies of emerging countries to expand the operations to the global market of biopharmaceuticals. Indian Drugs. 2021;58(6):7–18.
16. Devi JR, Devi GN, Bavanilatha M, et al. Pharmacophore-based QSAR modeling of natural leads in antimicrobial drug design. Curr Chin Chem. 2021;1(1):80–84.
17. Madjid AO, Sanni A, Lagnika L. Chemical diversity and pharmacological properties of *Acacia* genus. Asian J Appl Sci. 2020;13(2):40–49.
18. Thakur-Wernz P, Samant S. Relationship between international experience and innovation performance: The importance of organizational learning for EMNEs. *glob.* Strateg J. 2019;9(3):378–404.
19. Differding E. The drug discovery and development industry in India—Two decades of proprietary small-molecule R&D. ChemMedChem. 2017;12(11):786–818.
20. Yaremenko IA, Syroeshkin MA, Levitsky DO, Fleury F, Terent'ev AO. Cyclic peroxides as promising anticancer agents: In vitro cytotoxicity study of synthetic ozonides and tetraoxanes on human prostate cancer cell lines. Med Chem Res. 2017;26(1):170–179.
21. Deore AB, Dhumane JR, Wagh R, Sonawane R. The stages of drug discovery and development process. Asian J Pharm Res Dev. 2019;7:62–67.
22. Svennebring AM, Wikberg JES. Net present value approaches for drug discovery. Springerplus. 2013;2:1–7.
23. Nicolaou KC. Advancing the drug discovery and development process. Angew Chemie. 2014;126:9280–9292.
24. Mohs RC, Greig NH. Drug discovery and development: Role of basic biological research. Alzheimers Dement Transl Res Clin Interv. 2017;3:651–657.
25. Zhong X, Moseley GB. Mission possible: Managing innovation in drug discovery. Nat Biotechnol. 2007;25:945–946.
26. Berdigaliyev N, Aljofan M. An overview of drug discovery and development. Future Med Chem. 2020;12:939–947.
27. Jackson M, Marks L, May GHW, Wilson JB. The genetic basis of disease. Essays Biochem. 2018;62:643–723.
28. Ban TA. The role of serendipity in drug discovery. Dialogues Clin Neurosci. 2006;8:335–344.
29. Weiser J, Weiser AA, Shenkin PS, Still WC. Neighbor-list reduction: Optimization for computation of molecular van der waals and solvent-accessible surface areas. J Comput Chem. 1998;19:797–808.
30. Lombardino JG, Lowe JA. The role of the medicinal chemist in drug discovery—Then and now. Nat Rev Drug Discov. 2004;3:853–862.
31. Holford N, Ma SC, Ploeger BA. Clinical trial simulation: A review. Clin Pharmacol Ther. 2010;88:166–182.
32. McKee AE, Farrell AT, Pazdur R, Woodcock J. The role of the U.S. FDA review process: Clinical trial endpoints in oncology. Oncologist. 2010;15:13–18.
33. Clayden J, Moran WJ, Edwards PJ, Laplante SR. The challenge of atropisomerism in drug discovery. Angew Chem Int Ed. 2009;48:6398–6401.
34. Zisowsky J, Krause A, Dingemanse J. Drug development for pediatric populations: Regulatory aspects. Pharmaceutics. 2010;2:364–388.
35. Hoffer L, Muller C, Roche P, Morelli X. Chemistry-driven hit-to-lead optimization guided by structure-based approaches. Mol Inform. 2018;37.
36. Pickett SD, McLay IM, Clark DE. Enhancing the hit-to-lead properties of lead optimization libraries. J Chem Inf Comput Sci. 2000;40:263–272.
37. Bleicher KH, Böhm HJ, Müller K, Alanine AI. Hit and lead generation: Beyond high-throughput screening. Nat Rev Drug Discov. 2003;2:369–378.
38. Todd S, Stallard N. A new clinical trial design combining phases 2 and 3. Drug Inf J. 2005;39:109–118.

39. Shapiro SZ. The HIV/AIDS vaccine researchers' orientation to the FDA application process. Vaccine. 2002;20:1261–1280.
40. Mahan VL. Clinical trial phases. Int J Clin Med. 2014;5:1374–1383.
41. Zhu T. Hit identification and optimization in virtual screening: Practical recommendations based on a critical literature analysis. J Med Chem. 2013;56:6560–6572.
42. Lee RE. Combinatorial lead optimization of [1,2]-diamines based on ethambutol as potential antituberculosis preclinical candidates. J Comb Chem. 2003;5:172–187.
43. Showell GA, Mills JS. Chemistry challenges in lead optimization: Silicon isosteres in drug discovery. Drug Discov Today. 2003;8:551–556.
44. Cook N, Jodrell DI, Tuveson DA. Predictive in vivo animal models and translation to clinical trials. Drug Discov Today. 2012;17:253–260.
45. Zhang D, Luo G, Ding X, Lu C. Preclinical experimental models of drug metabolism and disposition in drug discovery and development. Acta Pharm Sin B. 2012;2:549–561.
46. Cushman D. Comparisons in vitro, ex vivo, and in vivo of the actions of seven structurally diverse inhibitors of angiotensin converting enzyme (ACE). Br J Clin Pharmacol. 1989;28:115S–131.
47. Holford NHG, Kimko HC, Monteleone JPR, Peck CC. Simulation of clinical trials. Annu Rev Pharmacol Toxicol. 2000;40:209–234.
48. Herbert RD. Randomisation in clinical trials. Aust J Physiother. 2005;51:58–60.
49. Shapiro SZ. The HIV/AIDS vaccine researchers' orientation to the process of preparing a US FDA application for an investigational new drug (IND): What it is all about and how you start by preparing for your pre-IND meeting. Vaccine. 2002;20:1261–1280.
50. Yip D. A phase 0 trial of riluzole in patients with resectable stage III and IV melanoma. Clin Cancer Res. 2009;15:3896–3902.
51. Ivy SP, Siu LL, Garrett-Mayer E, Rubinstein L. Approaches to phase 1 clinical trial design focused on safety, efficiency, and selected patient populations: A report from the clinical trial design task force of the national cancer institute investigational drug steering committee. Clin Cancer Res. 2010;16:1726–1736.
52. Seymour NE. Virtual reality training improves operating room performance results of a randomized, double-blinded study. Ann Surg. 2002;236:458–464.
53. Atmakuri LR, Peeriga R, Begum S, Vallamkonda B, Baratam A. Novel bioanalytical LC-MS/MS method for determination of metoprolol in human plasma. J Appl Pharm Sci. 2024;14(12):131–138.
54. Peeriga R, Venkata Bangaru GK. Implementation of the POCSO act in schools. In: Child Sexual Abuse: A Public Health Problem in India. Springer Publications, Singapore. 2024. p. 391–413.
55. Peeriga R, Yarlagadda LC, Alla NR. Protection of children from sexual exploitation. In: Child Sexual Abuse: A Public Health Problem in India. Springer Publications, Singapore. 2024. p. 191–201.
56. Peeriga R, Shiek Arabath SAM, Manubolu K, Thelappilly BB, Yarlagadda LC. Insilico assessment of phytoconstituents in *myxopyrum smilacifolium* Blume against arthritis. Biomed Pharmacol J. 2024;17(1):235–241.
57. Manubolu K, Balagani PK, Gope ER, Peeriga R, Sridevi AR. Unlocking the potential of aquasomes: A comprehensive review on innovative nanocarriers in drug delivery and beyond. Int J Chem Biochem Sci. 2023;24(6):405–410.
58. Manubolu K, Peeriga R, Bonthu MG, Gope ER, Kadirvel D. Evaluation of anti-inflammatory activity of *Millingtonia hortensis* leaf extract. Int J Chem Biochem Sci. 2023;24(6):380–385.
59. Peeriga R, Chandrasekhar KB. Comparative study of anti-inflammatory activity of petroleum ether extract of *myxopyrum smilacifolium* Blume and ethanolic leaf extract of *pamburus missionis* swingle. J Pharm Sci Res. 2017;9(6):955–957.
60. Peeriga R, Manubolu K. (2025). Design strategies for waste reduction and enhanced recyclability in pharmaceutical packaging. In: Yingngam, B., Aslam, M.S., Haghi, A.K.

(eds) Sustainable Pharmaceutical Product Development and Optimization Processes. Springer, Singapore.

61. Manubolu K, Peeriga R, Chandrasekhar KB. A Short Guide to Clinical Pharmacokinetics. 1st ed. 2024. Springer. Singapore.
62. Manubolu K, Peeriga R. (2025). Ecodesign principles. In: Yingngam, B., Aslam, M.S., Haghi, A.K. (eds) Sustainable Pharmaceutical Product Development and Optimization Processes. Springer, Singapore.

Index

Note:- Page numbers in *italics* and **bold** refer to figures and tables

FSC
www.fsc.org
MIX
Papier | Fördert gute Waldnutzung
FSC® C083411

Kolibri 360 GmbH
Ferdinand-Jühlke-Straße 7
99095 Erfurt, Deutschland
produktsicherheit@kolibri360.de